CHEST
RADIOLOGY

PLAIN FILM PATTERNS
AND DIFFERENTIAL
DIAGNOSES

FOURTH
EDITION

CHEST
RADIOLOGY

PLAIN FILM PATTERNS
AND DIFFERENTIAL
DIAGNOSES

FOURTH EDITION

James C. Reed, M.D.
Professor and Chairman
Diagnostic Radiology
University of Kentucky College of Medicine
Lexington, Kentucky

with 397 illustrations

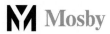 Mosby

St. Louis   Baltimore   Boston   Carlsbad   Chicago   Naples   New York   Philadelphia   Portland
London   Madrid   Mexico City   Singapore   Sydney   Tokyo   Toronto   Wiesbaden

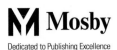

Mosby

Dedicated to Publishing Excellence

A Times Mirror Company

Vice President and Publisher: Anne S. Patterson
Executive Editor: Robert A. Hurley
Managing Editor: Elizabeth Corra
Associate Developmental Editor: Mia Cariño
Project Manager: Linda Clarke
Production Editor: Jennifer Harper
Production: Graphic World Publishing Services
Designer: Carolyn O'Brien
Manufacturing Manager: William A. Winneberger, Jr.

Fourth Edition
Copyright © 1997 by Mosby–Year Book, Inc.

Previous editions copyrighted 1981, 1987, 1991

All rights reserved. No part of this publication may be reproduced, stored in a retrieval system, or transmitted, in any form or by any means, electronic, mechanical, photocopying, recording, or otherwise, without written permission of the publisher.

Permission to photocopy or reproduce solely for internal or personal use is permitted for libraries or other users registered with the Copyright Clearance Center, provided that the base fee of $4.00 per chapter plus $.10 per page is paid directly to the Copyright Clearance Center, 27 Congress Street, Salem, MA 01970. This consent does not extend to other kinds of copying, such as copying for general distribution, for advertising or promotional purposes, for creating new collected works, or for resale.

Printed in the United States of America
Composition by Graphic World, Inc.
Printing/binding by Maple-Vail Book Manufacturing Group

Mosby–Year Book, Inc.
11830 Westline Industrial Drive
St. Louis, Missouri 63146

Library of Congress Cataloging-in-Publication Data

Reed, James Croft, 1942–
    Chest radiology : plain film patterns and differential diagnoses /
James C. Reed. — 4th ed.
        p.   cm.
    Includes bibliographical references and index.
    ISBN 0–8151–7122–6
    1. Chest—Radiography.   2. Diagnosis, Radioscopic.   I. Title.
    [DNLM: 1. Thoracic Radiography.   2. Diagnosis, Differential.   WF
975R324c   1996]
RC941.R4   1996
617.5'40757—dc20
DNLM/DLC
for Library of Congress   96–29141
                                                                           CIP

97 98 99 00 01 / 9 8 7 6 5 4 3 2 1

To my wife, Sharon, and our children
James, Peter, Brent, and Cameron

Preface to the Fourth Edition

Progress in the diagnosis and treatment of chest diseases continues to expand the scope of chest radiology. In an effort to avoid confusing terminology I have reconsidered an old semantic concern for description of basic observations. The term *density* is correctly used to describe the mass of a substance per unit volume. The radiologist recognizes that an increase in tissue may cast a shadow or opacity that appears white on the film. Such a shadow is frequently described as a density, but density has an opposite meaning when it is used to describe film blackening or optical density. The term *density* has therefore been a recurring source of confusion. While *density* is still often used to describe a white abnormality on exams such as mammograms, the glossary of terms published by the Fleischner Society has shown a strong preference for the term *opacity*. New advances in our understanding of diffuse pulmonary diseases have also led to some updates in pathologic and radiologic descriptive terminology.

Our advancing knowledge of diseases such as AIDS continues to expand our understanding of the diversity of patterns of chest disease. Many common diseases including lung cancer, tuberculosis, and AIDS-related diseases produce a variety of plain film patterns. AIDS-related diseases are considered causes of mediastinal adenopathy, diffuse air-space disease, multifocal opacities, and hyperlucent abnormalities. The major technical advances to affect chest disease are in CT. High-resolution thin section CT has replaced bronchography for the diagnosis of bronchiectasis and has advanced our understanding of the patterns and distributions of diffuse pulmonary diseases. Single-breath hold spiral CT has reduced artifacts and provides a new area for further research. The plain film, however, continues to be the most frequently performed of all radiologic procedures, and while it appears to be simple to perform, it is often the most challenging of radiologic exams to interpret.

James C. Reed, M.D.

Preface to the Third Edition

In the last decade we have seen the emergence of exciting new techniques and the appearance of new diseases. AIDS has profoundly affected many aspects of our society and the practice of medicine, including interpretation of the plain chest film. Computer technologies are changing the way we examine patients, and offer a host of new imaging options. Computed radiography is addressing some old technical problems and should provide better quality bedside plain films. High-resolution CT is very sensitive for confirming abnormalities that are only suspected from plain film or the clinical information, particularly fine reticular or nodular interstitial diseases and early emphysema. To optimize our use of these new technologies, we still need a thorough understanding of the diseases and their plain film patterns. This edition continues to emphasize plain film interpretation and uses radionuclide scans, ultrasound, CT, MR, and angiography to provide clarification of the patterns and to confirm specific diagnoses.

James C. Reed, M.D.

Preface to the Second Edition

This book utilizes a unique format in order to walk the reader through the differential diagnoses of 23 common plain film patterns of chest disease.

Each chapter opens with one or more unidentified radiographs. A series of questions follow, all designed to help identify the pattern of disease presented on the film. For those desiring immediate answers, the legends for the introductory radiographs are at the end of each chapter. So, too, are the answers to the multiple choice, yes-no, and true-false questions.

Sandwiched between the presentation of the case at each chapter's beginning and the answers at the end are a tabular listing of differential considerations and a discussion of the problem case. The discussion follows a step-by-step approach to eliminating inappropriate diagnoses and arriving at the correct one or by suggesting that other radiologic procedures and laboratory tests be performed, concluding with a summary. This section makes reference to several additional radiographs, all of which are fully identified and grouped after the discussion and summary.

It has been my intention to simulate within the confines of a book the radiologist's decision-making process of going from film to diagnosis. Although limitations of the format make it impossible to realistically reenact the process, it is hoped that your trip through these pages is both instructive and enjoyable.

The second edition of this book has expanded some of the differentials, and emphasized the impact of the newer modalities, particularly CT scanning, on the diagnosis of chest disease. While the role of MR appears to be limited mainly to the evaluation of the mediastinum,[208,214,527] CT has impacted almost all of the patterns in chest radiology. While a number of cases have been added to demonstrate the use of CT, the emphasis of this text continues to be the plain film patterns and their differential diagnoses.

The reference list is also substantially expanded because of the continued rapid growth of the medical literature related to chest radiology. Since this is intended to be an introductory text, a large number of topics are considered in a simplistic manner. The reference list is intended to be used as a suggested reading list. This will provide the reader with a more comprehensive work on a particular entity.

James C. Reed, M.D.

Preface to the First Edition

This manual is designed to provide a comprehensive differential diagnosis for 23 of the most common radiologic patterns of chest disease. Each chapter is introduced with problem cases and a set of questions, followed by a tabular listing of the appropriate differential considerations. The discussion centers on the problem case and demonstrates how the radiologist can use additional radiologic procedures along with correlative clinical and laboratory data to narrow the differential diagnosis or to suggest a specific diagnosis.

The book aims to provide a thorough background in the differential diagnosis of chest disease for residents in radiology, internal medicine, pulmonary medicine, family medicine, and emergency medicine. It also offers the practicing radiologist an updated review of the radiologic patterns of chest disease and a concise reference on differential diagnosis.

ACKNOWLEDGMENTS

It is impossible to acknowledge adequately all of the sources of inspiration, background, and support for this text. It began when Captain Q. E. Crews, Jr., M.C., U.S.N., and Dr. Elias G. Theros appointed me to the faculty at the Armed Forces Institute of Pathology. Dr. Theros created a stimulating environment and inspired early interest in chest radiology. Many of the ideas in this text were developed in the rich and dynamic atmosphere of the AFIP. My interaction with Drs. Theros, Madewell, Allman, Olmsted, and Korsower in radiology and Drs. Johnson, Hockholzer, Sobonya, Kagan-Hallet, and Daroca in pathology provided the framework on which this text has been built.

Preparation of the text and illustrations were accomplished during my tenure on the radiology faculty at Duke University. Special mention must be given to Dr. Charles E. Putman, who arranged for photographic support, David Page, who prepared the illustrations, Brenda Peele and Susan Morrison, who typed the text, and Dr. Lawrence Hedlund, whose editorial suggestions and proofreading were invaluable.

The list of friends providing support for a text cannot be complete, nor would enumeration express my gratitude adequately.

Finally, the completion of the text is due in no small measure to the untiring support and encouragement of my wife, Sharon.

James C. Reed, M.D.

Acknowledgments

The preparation of the manuscript and illustrations of the fourth edition would not have been possible without assistance in word processing from Willie Riddle and photographic production by Phyllis Gillespie.

James C. Reed, M.D.

Contents

PART II
PULMONARY OPACITIES

PART I

CHEST WALL, MEDIASTINUM, AND PLEURA

CHAPTER 1

Introduction

Many of the pioneers in radiology have struggled with the problems of differential diagnosis of chest disease. Despite the fact that chest roentgenography was one of the first radiologic procedures available to the physician, the problems of interpreting chest roentgenograms continue to be perplexing as well as challenging. The volume of literature on the subject indicates the magnitude of the problem and documents the many advances that have been made in this subspecialty of radiology. A casual review of the literature quickly reveals the frustrations a radiologist encounters in evaluating the several patterns of chest disease. There are as many efforts to define the patterns of chest radiographs as there are critics of the pattern approach. Since radiologists basically view the shadows of gross pathology, it is not surprising that the patterns are frequently nonspecific, and that those who expect to find a one-to-one histologic correlation of the roentgenogram with the microscopic diagnosis will be frustrated. It is much more important to develop an understanding of gross pathology to predict which patterns are likely in a given pulmonary disease. With this type of understanding of pulmonary diseases, we are better qualified to use nonspecific patterns in developing a differential diagnosis.

Colonel William LeRoy Thompson of the Armed Forces Institute of Pathology first adumbrated the concept of radiologic differential diagnosis. Later, Reeder and Felson amplified and popularized the approach in their book *Gamuts in Radiology* by providing an extensive list of the various patterns and their differential diagnoses.

This manual illustrates the common patterns of chest disease in order to facilitate their recognition. After recognition, the second step in the evaluation of a pattern is to develop an appropriate differential diagnosis. The differential diagnosis must include all of the major categories of disease (Chart 1–1) that might lead to the identified pattern. Next, the differential must be significantly narrowed by (1) careful analysis of the film for additional radiologic findings, (2) consideration of the evolving patterns of the disease by examination of serial roentgenograms, and (3) correlation of patterns with clinical and laboratory data (Chart 1–2). With this narrowed differential, we will be able to function as con-

CHART 1–1.
Categories of Diseases

   I. Inflammatory
  II. Vascular
     A. Thromboembolic
     B. Cardiovascular
     C. Collagen-vascular
 III. Neoplastic
 IV. Traumatic
  V. Developmental
 VI. Idiopathic

CHART 1–2.
Algorithmic Application of Chest Patterns

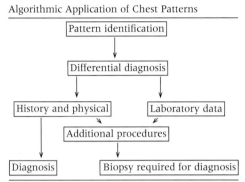

sultants, suggesting further procedures that may lead to a precise diagnosis. These procedures vary from simple roentgenographic examinations such as oblique films to percutaneous or transbronchial biopsy under fluoroscopic control.

A radiologist does not need to be reminded of the various procedures available for investigating diseases of the chest, but should have a thorough understanding of the radiologic differential diagnosis in order to determine which procedures may solve a specific problem. It should be obvious that the first step in evaluating many abnormalities identified on the standard posteroanterior (PA) and lateral chest x-ray film is to confirm that the abnormality is real. A newcomer to radiology frequently forgets the value of simple techniques such as oblique views, repeated PA chest films with nipple markers, fluoroscopy, full chest lordotic views, the overpenetrated Bucky chest technique, and, most important, the examination of old films. These simple procedures should be done to confirm the presence of an abnormality before considering more complicated procedures such as radionuclide scanning, arteriography, computed tomographic (CT) scanning, magnetic resonance imaging (MRI), or biopsy. In fact, the later procedures are special procedures that should be undertaken to answer specific questions.

One of the most important radiologic decisions to be made, after deciding that a shadow is a true abnormality, is to localize the abnormality. Localization to soft tissues, the chest wall, pleura, diaphragm, mediastinum, hilum, peripheral vessels, or the lung parenchyma is absolutely necessary before a logical differential diagnosis can be developed. Once the abnormal shadow is localized to a specific anatomic site, it is necessary to classify or describe the pattern. Some of the patterns of parenchymal lung disease considered in this text are nodules, masses, infiltrates, cavities, calcifications, and atelectasis. If the pattern is nonspecific, a moderately long differential must be offered. As mentioned earlier, one of the objectives of this manual is to further refine pattern analysis and develop methods of improving diagnostic specificity. For example, in the analysis of parenchymal lung disease, assessment of the distribution—deciding whether the process is localized or diffuse, peripheral or central, in the upper vs. lower lobes, or alveolar vs. interstitial—is extremely helpful. In correlating these features we are able to eliminate a number of possible diagnoses from initial consideration. Once the differential has been narrowed on the basis of identification of the disease pattern and distribution, examination of old films is valuable. Unfortunately, a common mistake is oversight of the very dynamic changes in the patterns of chest disease. A typical case history may be as follows: This is the first admission for this patient, and therefore the first chest x-ray. The knowledge that a solitary nodule was present on a film taken 2 years earlier at another hospital, or even 5 or 10 years earlier at still other hospitals, could completely resolve the problem of how to manage the patient. It is not always necessary to make a precise diagnosis, particularly in a case such as the one just described. The diagnosis of old granuloma, whether secondary to tuberculosis or histoplasmosis, is almost always adequate for the clinical management of the patient. Without old films the solitary nodule is a frustrating problem because the differential is long and, more important, cancer cannot be ruled out, whereas with the old film the diagnosis is obvious.[213,493]

Careful clinical correlation is also important in understanding the evolution of a pulmonary disease. For example, in evaluating a patient with a solitary pleural-based nodule on admission, a history of pleuritic chest pains 6 weeks earlier drastically changes the probable diagnosis. An additional history of thrombophlebitis and multiple episodes of pleuritic chest pain makes the diagnosis of pulmonary embolism with a resolving infarct almost certain.[649]

It is hoped that the 23 problems in differential diagnosis that follow this introductory chapter will be instructive as to how the radiologist can interpret the pattern on a single chest x-ray film, develop a moderately long differential diagnosis, narrow the differential diagnosis to a reasonable number of possibilities, and make recommendations for further procedures, leading to a single diagnosis.

CHAPTER 2

Chest Wall Lesions

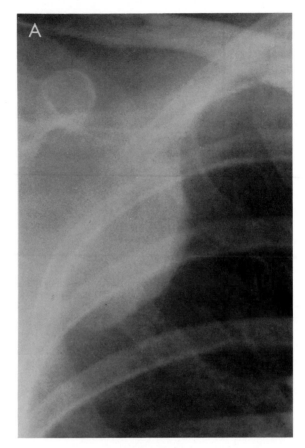

FIG 2–1, A

QUESTIONS

1. The most likely diagnosis in the afebrile patient in Figure 2–1, *A* is:
   a. Neurofibroma.
   b. Lipoma.
   c. Multiple myeloma.
   d. Actinomycosis.
   e. Chondrosarcoma.

Mark the following questions *True* or *False.*

2. _____ Chest wall lesions may sometimes be distinguished from pulmonary nodules by identification of an incomplete border.
3. _____ Lipoma is a common chest wall lesion.
4. _____ Neurofibroma of an intercostal nerve will probably cause rib destruction.

5. _____ Rib detail films are rarely needed to identify the rib destruction of a primary bone tumor in the chest wall.

6. _____ Multiple myeloma and metastases are among the most common causes of a chest wall mass with associated rib destruction in an adult.

7. _____ Ewing's tumor and neuroblastoma should be considered when a chest wall mass is observed in a child.

CHART 2–1.
Pattern: Chest Wall Lesions

- I. Nipples,[409] supernumerary nipples[230]
- II. Artifact
- III. Skin lesions (e.g., moles, neurofibromas, extrathoracic musculature)[97]
- IV. Mesenchymal tumors (muscle tumors, fibromas, lipomas,[147] desmoid tumor[116])
- V. Neural tumors (schwannoma,[468] neurofibroma, neuroblastoma)
- VI. Hodgkin's and non-Hodgkin's lymphoma[463]
- VII. Vascular tumors (hemangioma, hemangiopericytoma)
- VIII. Bone tumor (metastasis,[344] multiple myeloma, Ewing's sarcoma, fibrous dysplasia, chondrosarcoma, osteosarcoma [rare], fibrosarcoma, solitary plasmacytoma)
- IX. Hematoma
- X. Rib fractures
- XI. Infection (actinomycosis,[633] aspergillosis,[10] nocardiosis, blastomycosis, tuberculosis, osteomyelitis [rare])[236]
- XII. Thoracopulmonary small cell ("Askin") tumor[168]
- XIII. Invasion by contiguous mass (lung cancer)[181,327]

DISCUSSION

Chest wall opacities may be observed as a result of shadows that arise from both extrathoracic and intrathoracic normal and abnormal structures. Common extrathoracic causes of radiographically visible opacities include nipples, moles, and various cutaneous lesions (e.g., neurofibromas of von Recklinghausen's disease). The extrathoracic causes of chest wall opacities are seen as soft tissue opacities with an incomplete sharp border. The border is produced by the interface of the mass with air and is lost where the mass is continuous with the soft tissues of the chest wall. Cutaneous lesions should not have the tapered borders that are seen in Figure 2–1, *A*. The tapered border indicates displacement of the pleura inward by the mass. Physical examination is also essential in the evaluation of cutaneous lesions. Nipple shadows may be easily identified when they are symmetric and when their borders are incomplete, but caution is warranted.[409] Repeat examination with small lead nipple markers, and oblique views should be performed if there is any possibility of confusing a nipple shadow with a pulmonary nodule.

Intrathoracic lesions are radiologically visible because of their interface with aerated lung. Like the cutaneous lesion, their borders are incomplete where they are contiguous with the chest wall (Fig 2–2, *A*).[141] Thus, the incomplete border is helpful in distinguishing chest wall lesions from pulmonary lesions (answer to question 2 is True), but not in distinguishing cutaneous from intrathoracic chest wall lesions. The tapered superior and inferior borders, however, are valuable signs for confirming an intrathoracic extrapulmonary location. Unfortunately, the tapered border may not be observed if the lesion is seen en face; in fact, the lesion may not be visible at all. Lateral and oblique coned-down views are frequently helpful in eliciting this sign (Fig 2–2, *B* and *C*).

Lipomas are common chest wall lesions and may be seen as either subcutaneous or intrathoracic masses (Fig 2–3, *A*). (Answer to question 3 is *True*.) They may even grow between the ribs, presenting as both intrathoracic and subcutaneous masses. Physical examination reveals a soft, movable mass when there is a significant subcutaneous component. Computed tomography (CT) should show the extent of the mass and, more important, confirm that the lesion is of fat density[147] (Fig 2–3, *B*).

A key observation in Figure 2–1, *B* is rib destruction.[164,167] This finding excludes lipoma and other benign tumors, such as neurofibroma, from the diagnosis. Benign neural tumors such as schwannoma and neurofibroma may erode ribs inferiorly and even produce a sclerotic reaction (Fig 2–4), but should not destroy the rib, as shown in Figure 2–1, *B*. (Answer to question 4 is *False*.) Rib destruction is not always obvious on a straight PA film and may be better visualized with coned-oblique or rib detail film. (Answer to question 5 is *False*.)

The rib destruction seen in Figure 2–1, *A* and *B* is suggestive of either an aggressive tumor or an inflammatory process. Metastases and small round cell tumors are the most common tumors to produce the pattern of chest wall destruction seen in this case. The most common primary tumors to metastasize to the chest wall are lung, breast, and renal cell, but knowledge of a primary tumor is essential since any tumor that spreads by hematogenous dissemination may produce a chest wall lesion (Fig 2–5, *A* and *B*). Multiple myeloma, plasmacytoma, and Ewing's tumors are primary round cell tumors that may arise in the bones of the chest wall. The differential diagnosis in the adult patient with a chest wall mass and bone destruction is most often metastasis vs. multiple myeloma. (Answer to question 6 is *True*.) In a child, however, the pattern is more suggestive of metastatic neuroblastoma or Ewing's tumor. (Answer to question 7 is *True*.) Figure 2–1 shows a typical example of multiple myeloma. (Answer to question 1 is *c*), but there are a number of common variations. Myeloma may occur with complete loss of a rib, large expanded ribs, or only a small ill-defined area of bone destruction. The patient may even present with a pathologic fracture of the involved rib. Occasionally the soft tissue mass may be rather large and the bone lesion minimal. Lymphoma is another tumor that may infrequently produce a peripheral soft tissue mass with incomplete or tapered borders and extend through the chest wall.[463] This would indicate an advanced stage of lymphoma and is not an expected abnormality at the time of presentation. The chest wall extension may not be seen on the plain film, but it can be confirmed with a CT scan (Fig 2–6, *A* and *B*).

Benign and malignant bone tumors may arise in the scapula, sternum, vertebra, and ribs. Some of the common benign rib lesions—such as benign cortical defect and fibrous dysplasia—do not produce soft tissue masses, but he-mangiomas and osteochondromas do produce soft tissue opacies that project inward and should be considered in the differential diagnosis of intrathoracic chest wall masses. Hemangiomas may produce a significant extraosseous mass and resemble other chest wall masses, but they can best be identified by their typically reticular, or "basket weave," pattern of bone destruction. Osteo-chondromas may elevate the pleura and present as an intrathoracic chest wall mass. The typical pattern of the calcified matrix should confirm the diagnosis of osteochondroma (Fig 2–7). Hereditary multiple exostoses are the result of an autosomal dominant disorder that frequently involves multiple flat bones. These patients may have deformity of the ribs and multiple osteochondromas. They are also at increased risk for the development of chondrosarcoma. Ma-lignant transformation of osteochondromas in this group of patients has been reported to vary from 3% to 25%. Signs of malignancy include pain, swelling, soft tissue mass, and growth (Fig 2–8). Both osteosarcoma and chondrosar-coma may arise from the bones of the chest wall in patients without any known risk factors. Chondrosarcoma is the most common primary bone tu-mor of the scapula, sternum, and ribs. Eight percent of all chondrosarcomas are reported to arise from the ribs.

Inflammatory lesions of the chest wall may arise from puncture wounds, hematogenous seeding, or direct extension from intrathoracic infections. Sep-ticemia by bacterial infections and even miliary spread of tuberculosis may cause osteomyelitis of the spine or ribs with chest wall involvement, but infectious chest wall masses most often arise from empyemas or pneumonias with empyemas. Actinomycosis is one of the more aggressive granulomatous infections and may produce a parenchymal infiltrate, pleural effusion, chest wall mass, rib destruc-tion, and even cutaneous fistulas.[178,633] Occasionally air-fluid levels are seen in the soft tissues. Other granulomatous infections that produce a similar appearance in-clude aspergillosis,[10] nocardiosis, blastomycosis, and, rarely, tuberculosis. Patients with these infections usually have a febrile course, although it may be somewhat indolent.

Hematoma is usually suggested by a history of trauma and is frequently asso-ciated with rib fractures. Care must be taken not to overlook an underlying lytic lesion that would indicate that the fracture is pathologic. Occasionally, old rib fractures may be mistaken for nodules because of their callus. These are best eval-uated with coned-down views of the ribs. Rarely chest wall desmoid tumor oc-curs as a late complication of trauma.[318] Desmoid tumors are locally invasive but histologically benign chest wall masses.[116]

Primary lung abnormalities sometimes invade the pleura and chest wall with rib destruction and resemble primary chest wall abnormalities. This is observed with both infections and primary lung tumors. The apical lung cancer (Pancoast's tumor) is best known for this presentation. When a lung cancer invades the pleura, it may spread along the pleura in a manner that produces a tapered border. However, close observation often reveals irregular or even spiculated bor-ders, which should strongly suggest the pulmonary origin of the tumor (Fig 2–9). CT is sometimes required to visualize the irregular interface with the lung and confirm the pulmonary origin of the tumor.

SUMMARY

1. The incomplete border sign is suggestive of an extrapulmonary process.

2. Chest wall masses have smooth, tapered borders that are helpful in distinguishing them from pulmonary lesions. These are best seen with tangential views.

3. Benign chest wall tumors such as lipoma, schwannoma, and neurofibroma should not destroy ribs but may erode the inferior surface of a rib.

4. Chest wall tumors that destroy ribs are most commonly metastases or multiple myelomas in adults and Ewing's tumor or neuroblastoma in children.

5. Rib destruction may be subtle, requiring coned-down views, CTs, and even radionuclide bone scans for visualization.

6. Actinomycosis, aspergillosis, nocardiosis, tuberculosis, and blastomycosis may all produce chest wall lesions with rib destruction. The history and physical findings should alert the radiologist to these possibilities.

7. A CT scan is often required to confirm chest wall involvement by metastases, myeloma, lymphoma, and even benign masses.

8. Lung, breast, and renal cell tumors are the most common primary tumors to metastasize to the chest wall.

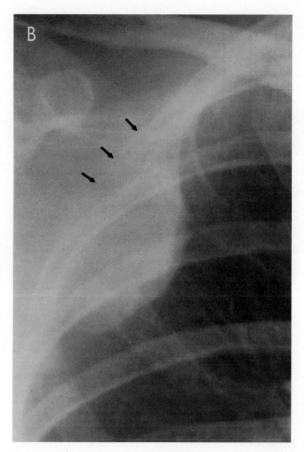

FIG 2–1
B, Same film seen in Fig 2–1, *A* shows rib destruction *(arrows)* and confirms chest wall involvement. These observations narrow the differential to metastasis vs. multiple myeloma. Myeloma is the diagnosis.

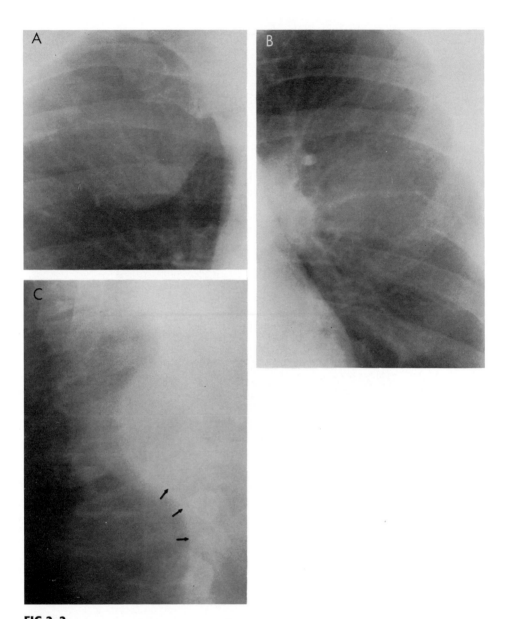

FIG 2–2
A, This myeloma illustrates the incomplete border sign, which is useful in distinguishing pulmonary from extrapulmonary masses. Note the sharp inferior border and absence of a superior border. **B,** Entire border of a chest wall mass may appear incomplete owing to tapering. Note bone destruction. This is another example of myeloma. **C,** Coned-down lateral view of case illustrated in **B** reveals tapered borders *(arrows)*, which result from displacement of both layers of the pleura, a valuable sign for distinguishing pulmonary from extrapulmonary masses.

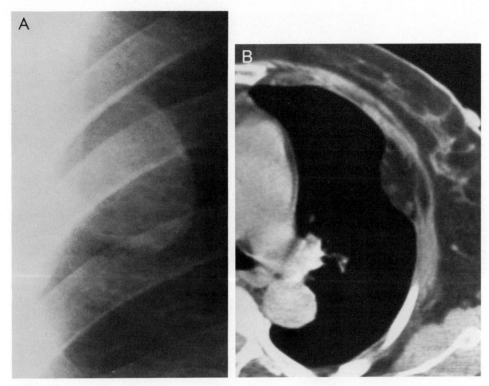

FIG 2–3
A, Chest wall lipoma appears to be of tissue opacity, in contrast to aerated lung. Location of lipoma against the lateral chest wall and its incomplete border (sharp medial but absent lateral border) suggest that it is nonpulmonary. There is no rib destruction to confirm chest wall origin. Both chest wall and pleural masses should be considered in differential. **B,** CT scan of another patient with a chest wall lipoma shows a mass that is of greater opacity than the aerated lung but less opaque than the musculature of the chest wall. This intermediate fat density mass is shown to extend through chest wall muscles. (Case courtesy of Thomas L. Pope, Jr., M.D.)

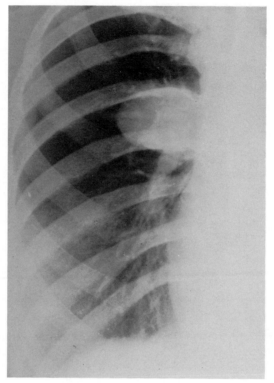

FIG 2–4
Benign schwannoma has not destroyed the rib but has eroded its inferior cortex. Note sclerotic border, which virtually ensures the benign nature of the lesion.

FIG 2–5
A, PA film shows a large soft tissue opacity projected over the left upper chest. The inferior border is sharply defined, appearing to follow the inferior cortex of the fifth left rib, and the fourth rib is missing. The mass has no superior, medial, or lateral borders; therefore, this is another variation of the incomplete border sign. **B,** CT confirms a posterior soft tissue mass with rib destruction. This is a common appearance for a chest wall metastasis, but in this case the primary is a rare cutaneous Merkel's cell tumor. **C,** Lower CT image with lung windows shows how the mass appears to change shape as it extends around the chest wall following the rib. The only border of the mass that is visible on the plain film is produced by the interface of the mass with the lung.

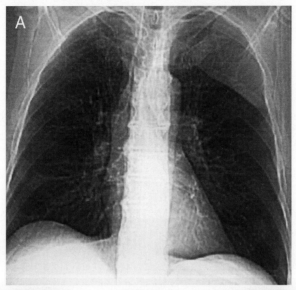

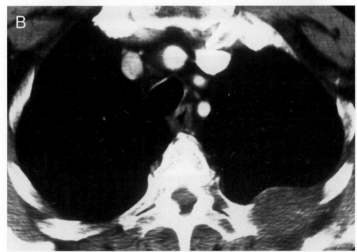

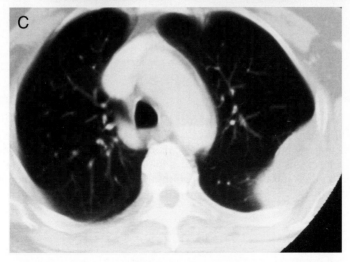

See legend on page 14

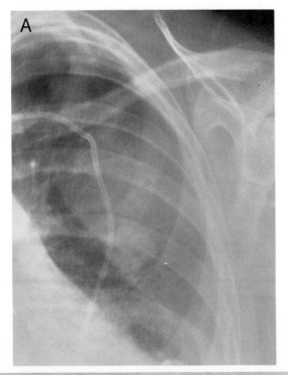

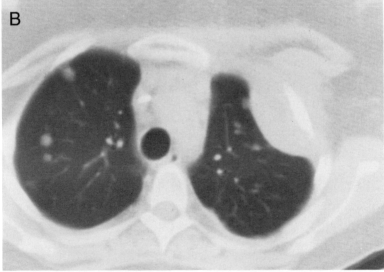

FIG 2–6
A, Advanced Hodgkin's lymphoma has caused this large soft tissue mass. The incomplete borders indicate an extrapulmonary location, but the plain film reveals no evidence of the chest wall extension. **B,** CT scan shows the large, peripheral soft tissue opacity to have tapered borders and to extend through the chest wall. Multiple pulmonary nodules were also confirmed.

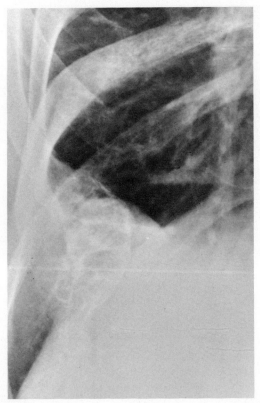

FIG 2–7
This mass has protruded into the thorax, elevating the pleura, as evidenced by the tapered borders. The calcified matrix has a speckled, reticulated appearance that is typical of a cartilage matrix. In addition, there is a well-defined calcified cortex. These features are diagnostic of an osteochondroma.

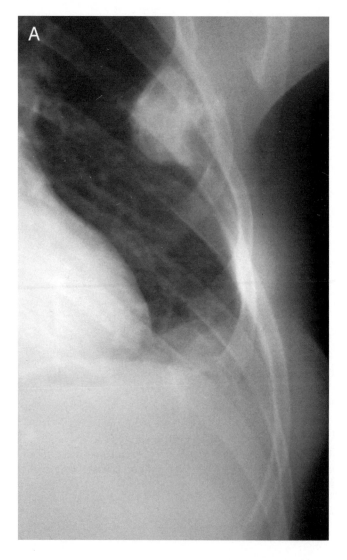

FIG 2-8
A, Multiple osteochondromas produce calcified soft tissue masses. These masses may cause considerable chest wall deformity with spreading of ribs. They may also cause intrathoracic and extrathoracic soft tissue masses. This patient with hereditary multiple exostoses has two large masses. The smaller superior mass is an osteochondroma. The large inferior mass obliterates the costophrenic angle and extends into the extrathoracic soft tissues. Because of recent growth, a biopsy was performed confirming the diagnosis of chondrosarcoma. **B,** CT of the smaller superior osteochondroma shows a typical pattern of calcification. **C,** CT of the larger inferior chondrosarcoma shows a large soft tissue mass with irregular bands of calcified matrix.

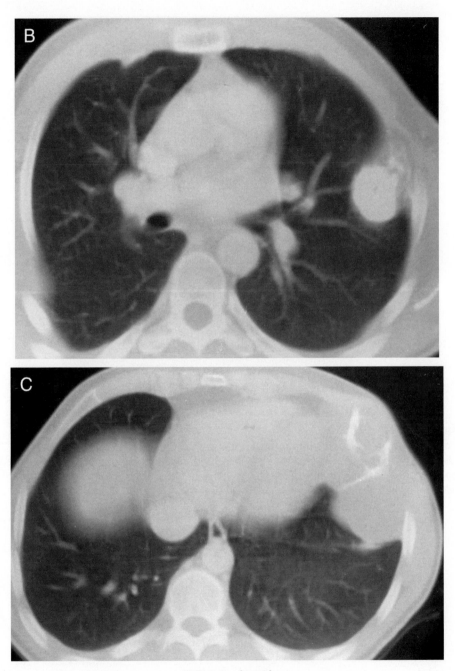

FIG. 2-8   (cont.)

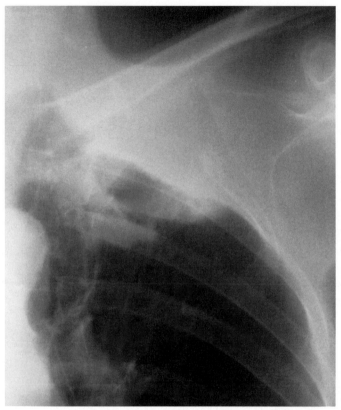

FIG 2–9
Coned view of a Pancoast's tumor reveals rib destruction and tapered borders resembling the myeloma seen in Figure 2–1, but the additional finding of a poorly marginated opacity extending into the lung indicates that this is most likely a lung mass that has invaded the chest wall rather than a true chest wall mass.

ANSWER GUIDE

LEGEND FOR INTRODUCTORY FIGURE

FIG 2-1, A
Mass is typical of chest wall mass because of the smooth, tapered medial border. The tapered border indicates an intrathoracic location. See Figure 2-1, B.

ANSWERS

1, c; 2, T; 3, T; 4, F; 5, F; 6, T; 7, T.

CHAPTER 3

Pleural and Subpleural Masses

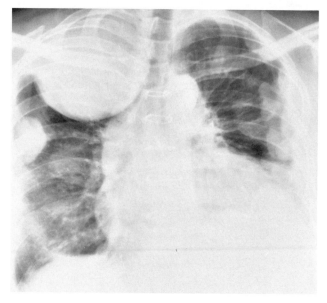

FIG 3–1

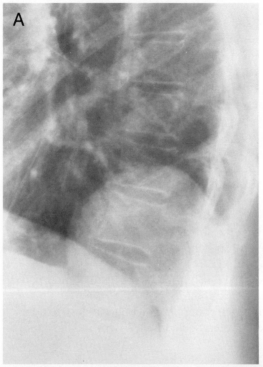

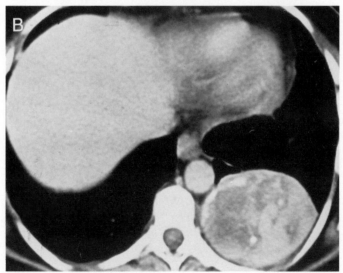

FIG 3–2

QUESTIONS

1. Referring to Figure 3–1, which of the following is the least likely diagnosis?
   a. Metastatic melanoma.
   b. Metastatic breast carcinoma.
   c. Malignant thymoma.
   d. Malignant mesothelioma.
   e. Metastatic ovarian carcinoma.
2. Referring to Figure 3–2, *A* and *B,* the most likely diagnosis for this case is:
   a. Rounded atelectasis.
   b. Localized fibrous tumor of the pleura.
   c. Multiple myeloma.
   d. Infarct.
   e. Mesothelial cyst.
   Mark the following questions *True* or *False*.
3. _____Malignant mesothelioma may present with either solitary or multiple pleural nodules.
4. _____A shaggy, irregular border favors a subpleural parenchymal lung lesion over a pleural lesion.
5. _____Mesothelioma frequently causes bone destruction.
6. _____Pleural lesions may be confused with mediastinal masses.

CHART 3–1.
Solitary Pleural Opacity

   I. Loculated pleural effusion
  II. Metastasis[140]
 III. Mesothelioma[53,57] (benign or malignant)
  IV. Lipoma[166,172,209,490]
   V. Organized empyema[537,621,640]
  VI. Hematoma
 VII. Mesothelial cyst
VIII. Neural tumor (schwannoma and neurofibroma)[483]
  IX. Localized fibrous tumor of the pleura

CHART 3–2.
Multiple Pleural Opacities (Each >2 cm)

   I. Loculated pleural effusion
  II. Metastases (particularly from adenocarcinomas)
 III. Malignant thymoma (rare)
  IV. Mesothelioma (malignant)[287,520]
   V. Pleural plaques (asbestos-related)
  VI. Splenosis[298]

CHART 3–3.
Subpleural Parenchymal Lung Opacities

    I. Infarct[244]
   II. Granuloma (tuberculosis, fungus)
  III. Inflammatory pseudotumor
  IV. Metastasis
   V. Rheumatoid nodule
  VI. Primary carcinoma of the lung including
       Pancoast's tumor[206]
 VII. Lymphoma[59, 588]
VIII. Round atelectasis[394]

DISCUSSION
Solitary Pleural Opacity

The radiologic evaluation of a solitary pleural mass (Chart 3–1) is compli-cated by the paucity of reliable signs for accurate localization.[537, 606] The mass should be in a peripheral location, which may be confirmed by identifying the incomplete border sign (see Fig 2–2, *A–C*). The peripheral position is easily recognized when the mass is against the lateral chest wall, but the correct location may be more difficult to identify when the mass is either anterior or posterior (Fig 3–3, *A*). The lateral view (see Fig 3–2, *A*) or even a CT scan[133, 321] (Fig 3–3, *B*) may be needed to confirm the peripheral location. A peripheral mass requires consideration of three locations: (1) the chest wall, (2) the pleura, and (3) the subpleural area of the lung. Smooth, incomplete tapered borders with obtuse pleural angles localize a mass to either the chest wall or pleura, while shaggy borders and acute pleural angles confirm the diagnosis of a subpleural pe-ripheral lung mass (Figs 3–4, *A* and *B*, and Fig 3–5). One pitfall is that a peripheral lung mass such as a metastasis may have smooth borders. Some metastatic tumors and even lymphoma can also disseminate to both lung and pleura. The foregoing signs for localizing peripheral masses are somtimes indeterminate on the plain film, but they are also applicable in CT interpretation. In fact, CT is often required for the precise localization of abnormalities that are seen on the plain film.

Some pleural tumors lack the broad-based pleural signs described above be-cause they have a small area of attachment to either pleural surface and appear more round. The case shown in Figure 3–2, *A* and *B*, was described at surgery as a pedunculated pleural mass. Berne and Heitzman[48] reported that pedunculated pleural tumors may be fluoroscopically observed to change shape or move with respiration. This motion may also be recorded on inspiration and expiration films. Documentation of free movement in the pleural space would distinguish chest wall from pleural masses.

Probably the most confusing pleural tumor is the one that presents in a medial location. This position is more suggestive of a mediastinal mass. Since both pleural masses and mediastinal masses are seen because of their interface with the lung, both will have a sharp, incomplete border, frequently tapered. There-fore, diagnosis of a medially located mesothelioma can be made only by biopsy. Similarly, mesothelioma arising from an interlobar fissure is difficult to correctly identify as a pleural mass. This is best accomplished by identification of the fissures on the lateral film, or even with a CT scan.

The distinction of loculated pleural fluid from a solid pleural tumor may also be difficult.[621] The most practical approach to this problem is to review serial films. Because localized collections of pleural fluid may change rapidly, they are frequently referrred to as "vanishing tumors." These collections may occur in either the lateral pleural space or the interlobar fissures. Both PA and lateral films are required for their localization, since a localized effusion in the fissure may mimic an intrapulmonary lesion. Ultrasound may be useful for determining that a lesion is fluid filled rather than solid, but successful ultrasound examination requires that the mass be contiguous with the chest wall (Fig 3–6, *A–C*). Computed tomographic scans have also been useful in separating pulmonary from pleural opacities and correctly identifying pleural fluid collections (Fig 3–7). The laterally located collections are easily accessible to direct needle puncture, which not only rules out a mass lesion but also provides fluid for culture when an empyema is suspected. Correlation with the clinical history is also important. A history of recent pneumonia is evidence in favor of a loculated empyema.[246, 537]

Pleural tumors, cysts, and loculated effusions all appear homogeneous on plain films, but should be distinguished with ultrasound, CT, or magnetic resonance (MR) scans. Pleural tumors may be regarded as solid, but they are not always entirely homogeneous. The large mass shown in Figure 3–2, *A* and *B* is shown by CT to be heterogeneous, with soft tissue opacity, a calcification, and areas of low attenuation caused by necrosis. It does not have uniform low attenuation that would be expected with a mesothelial cyst.

Localized fibrous tumor of the pleura (previously called solitary mesothelioma) probably arises from submesothelial mesenchymal cells rather than mesothelial lining cells and is usually benign, although 37% of such tumors have been reported to be malignant.[133]

Localized fibrous tumor of the pleura should present as a well-circumscribed peripheral mass and should never invade the chest wall or lung. The case shown in Figure 3–2 is a benign localized fibrous tumor of the pleura. (Answer to question 2 is *b.*) The plain films in this case are not adequate for exclusion of a chest wall mass, but the CT shows the mass to be separate from the chest wall and thus makes multiple myeloma an unlikely choice. The CT appearance of this heterogeneous mass further excludes mesothelial cyst. Both pulmonary infarcts and rounded atelectasis are pulmonary processes that typically have a subpleural location. They usually have poorly marginated borders, and the CT scan should confirm their pulmonary origin.[394]

Malignant solitary mesothelioma may be radiographically similar but is probably not related to the localized fibrous tumor of the pleura. When it occurs in combination with a history of asbestos exposure, it probably should be considered an early stage of the malignant mesothelioma. At this early localized stage, a malignant solitary mesothelioma would not be expected to extend into either chest wall or lung.

A solitary pleural metastasis would be impossible to differentiate on the basis of its radiologic features from the mass seen in this case. The similarity of a solitary metastasis is illustrated in Figure 3–3, *A* and *B*. Metastatic disease is the most common cause of a pleural mass, with lung and breast cancer accounting for 60% of cases.

Multiple Pleural Opacities

Multiple pleural opacities (Chart 3–2) are usually the result of loculated effusion, pleural masses, or a combination of the two. The radiologic appearance is that of multiple, separate, sharply circumscribed, smooth tapered opacities (see Fig 3–1) or of diffuse pleural thickening with lobulated inner borders. Loculated pleural effusion is probably the most common cause of this appearance. The causes of loculated effusion include empyema, hemorrhage, and neoplasms. Lateral decubitus films are of little value in recognizing the condition, since some free fluid may coexist with either loculated collections of fluid or solid masses. Sequential films showing a change over a short period of time should confirm the presence of loculated fluid collections (Fig 3–8). Ultrasound and CT scans may be useful for confirming the presence of loculated fluid collections and for thoracentesis or drainage procedures. As with a solitary pleural opacity, a history of previous pneumonia or a distant primary tumor may suggest the correct cause of the pleural thickening.

Metastasis is the most common cause of multiple pleural nodules. Adenocarcinomas are particularly known for their tendency to produce pleural metastases. Knowledge of either a primary lung tumor or an extrathoracic primary tumor such as breast cancer or melanoma should strongly suggest the diagnosis. The radiologic combination of bilateral lobulated pleural thickening and a previous mastectomy would virtually assure the diagnosis of metastatic breast carcinoma; however, metastatic breast cancer is often unilateral (Fig 3–9).

Malignant thymoma typically spreads contiguously, invades the pleura, and spreads around the lung with the radiologic appearance of multiple pleural masses (see Fig 3–1).

In the terminal stages of lymphoma, spread to the pleura is not uncommon.[59, 606] This is most often in the form of pleural effusion,[588] but nodular masses may also be observed.

Multiple myeloma often presents with multiple extrapulmonary masses (see Chapter 2) and may mimic multiple pleural masses. It is not likely to result in the appearance of diffuse nodular pleural thickening as seen in either pleural metastases or mesothelioma (see Figs 3–1 and 3–10). Bone destruction is a reliable feature of multiple myeloma (see Fig 2–1).

Diffuse malignant mesothelioma is another important cause of lobulated or nodular pleural thickening (Fig 3–10).[133, 140, 264, 444] In contrast to the condition illustrated in Figure 3–1, diffuse malignant mesothelioma is virtually always unilateral. (Answer to question 1 is *d*). However, radiologic distinction of mesothelioma from diffuse pleural metastases and, rarely, local spread of a bronchioloalveolar carcinoma[133, 268] is often impossible. Either may have an associated bloody pleural effusion. Even the histologic distinction of these two lesions may be difficult, requiring special stains. Recent CT studies have shown these tumors to be more extensive than suspected from plain films, with extension into the lung, chest wall, and mediastinum[9] (Fig 3–11, *A* and *B*).

The association of asbestos exposure with both primary carcinoma of the lung and malignant mesothelioma is well known.[53, 264, 395, 536] Since the incidence of both primary lung and pleural tumors is increased by asbestos exposure, a history of exposure is of no value in making the distinction of metastasis vs. mesothelioma. Another curious feature of the relationship between asbestos exposure and these tumors is that patients who develop the neoplasms usually do not have the typical pulmonary findings of asbestosis (see Chapters 18–19).

Asbestos-related pleural plaques may be flat or nodular. They are easily over-looked or mistaken for artifacts in the early stages of the disease.[203] These plaques most commonly cause areas of flat pleural thickening, but occasionally they pro-duce a nodular appearance. They do not spread around the lung and are not seen in the apex. While they may be confused with the early stages of mesothelioma, they should not be confused with advanced cases such as that illustrated in Figure 3–10.

Splenosis[300, 513] occurs after the autotransplantation of splenic tissue into the pleural space following combined splenic and diaphragmatic injuries. The pres-ence of multiple masses in the left pleural space requires questioning of the pa-tient for a history of prior severe upper abdominal or lower thoracic trauma. This is particularly important when the patient has undergone splenectomy and repair of a ruptured diaphragm.

Subpleural Parenchymal Lung Nodules

Another group of lesions to be considered in the evaluation of a pleural lesion is the subpleural lung lesion (Chart 3–3). Sometimes these lesions are so sharply defined that they completely mimic a true pleural mass. Additional signs that sug-gest the true nature of the lesion are (1) ill-defined or shaggy borders, (2) associ-ated linear opacities, (3) a heterogeneous texture, such as small areas of lucency or air-bronchograms, and (4) acute pleural angles. These clues to a pulmonary origin of the nodule may be enhanced by CT scan. Computed tomography en-hances the texture of the mass and its interface with the surrounding lung.[206] This provides a sensitive means for detecting local invasion of lung parenchyma and even confirming a pulmonary origin of the nodule (see Fig 3–5, A–C). Computed tomography has the added advantage of being more sensitive for the detection of very small lesions. The latter fact is most important in evaluating patients with a known primary neoplasm.

Neoplasms, including metastases and primary lung cancer, often develop in a peripheral subpleural location. The frequency with which metastases occur in this setting was not appreciated prior to the use of CT scanning for staging metastatic disease. Metastatic nodules are typically well-circumscribed opacities. Some have acute pleural angles and can be labeled intrapulmonary, while others have more obtuse angles indicating pleural involvement (see Fig 3–3, B). Because they are incompletely surrounded by air and are often small, the plain film is not sensitive to subpleural metastases.

Apical primary carcinoma of the lung (Pancoast's or superior sulcus tumor)[442] represents a common presentation of a peripheral subpleural primary lung can-cer. These masses grow by contiguous invasion and are distinguished radiologi-cally from pleural masses by their irregular, poorly marginated, or even spiculated borders (see Fig 3–4, A–C). Since they are locally very invasive, they often spread through the pleura into the chest wall. The plain film finding of bone destruction indicates advanced disease (Fig 3–12). In the absence of bone involvement on the plain film, CT and MR scans are used for detecting extension into the soft tissues of the chest wall, particularly in seeking brachial plexus invasion. The superiority of CT over plain film for staging these tumors is well documented, but the axial display of CT does not optimally show the pleural fat planes. Coronal MR scans may provide the optimal means for detecting penetration of the mass through the apical pleura.

The cell types of apical lung cancer include adenocarcinoma, bronchioloalveolar cell carcinomas, and squamous cell carcinomas. These tumors are accessible to needle-aspiration biopsy, which yields a diagnosis in a high percentage of cases. Scar carcinoma is another variant of lung cancer that often occurs in the apices. This variant includes all lung cancers that arise around a preexistent scar. Scar carcinoma may be suggested by serial films that reveal an old calcified scar from previous granulomatous infection and an associated growing soft tissue opacity. Lymphoma may also cause an irregular apical mass that resembles a superior sulcus or Pancoast's tumor. It is usually associated either with evidence of lymphadenopathy or with a history of previously treated nodal disease.

Organizing pulmonary processes, including organizing pneumonia, inflammatory pseudotumor, granulomas, infarcts, and rounded atelectasis, must also be considered in the differential diagnosis of subpleural pulmonary opacities. Granulomas are often peripheral, and may resemble either metastases or primary lung tumors. Likewise, infarcts may organize into well-circumscribed subpleural opacities that are radiologically indistinguishable from granulomas, metastases, or lung cancers, but they more typically form pleural-based triangular opacities. This characteristic triangular or wedge-shaped opacity may be more confidently identified by CT. A history of prior pleuritic chest plain or thrombophlebitis should provide further confirmatory evidence of an infarct.

Rounded atelectasis or folded lung is another benign cause of peripheral lung opacities that resemble lung cancer.[73] These opacities are associated with pleural thickening and may be caused by retracting pleural fibrosis. They are usually spherical with irregular borders, typically extend to the pleura with an acute angle, and are most often posterior. Air bronchograms may be observed at the periphery. This phenomenon is usually seen in patients with a history of asbestos exposure and must be distinguished from mesothelioma and lung cancer. Computed tomography may be diagnostic in revealing the associated pleural thickening and characteristic retraction of pulmonary vessels and bronchi into a curved shape following the contour of the mass of scarred, collapsed lung[79,394] (Fig 3–13). Confirmation of stability with old film is essential, since lung cancer may appear to be nearly identical, sometimes requiring biopsy.

SUMMARY

1. Pleural opacities may be confused with either chest wall lesions or subpleural parenchymal lung lesions.

2. Identification of bone destruction or extension of the mass through the ribs is the most reliable plain film method of localizing a chest wall lesion.

3. A solitary pleural opacity may be caused by a loculated fluid collection or a solid mass such as a metastasis, mesothelioma, or lipoma.

4. Localized fibrous tumor of the pleura (solitary benign mesothelioma) has no association with asbestos exposure. Malignant solitary mesothelioma represents the early phase of diffuse mesothelioma, is related to asbestos exposure, and requires histologic diagnosis.[142]

5. Multiple pleural opacities result from loculated effusion, malignant mesothelioma, and metastases from adenocarcinomas (particularly lung or breast primaries) or melanoma, or spread from a malignant thymoma.

6. Splenosis is a rare cause of multiple pleural masses that should be suspected on the basis of a history or prior splenic injury and thoracoabdominal surgery.

7. Ill-defined or shaggy borders, associated linear opacities, and a heterogeneous appearance with air bronchograms should be reliable findings for the identification of a subpleural parenchymal lung process that may have secondarily involved the pleura. These findings should suggest tuberculosis, fungal infection, an organizing infarct, or even a primary lung tumor.

8. Rounded atelectasis is associated with pleural scarring, occurs in patients with a history of asbestos exposure, and must be distinguished from primary lung cancer or mesothelioma.

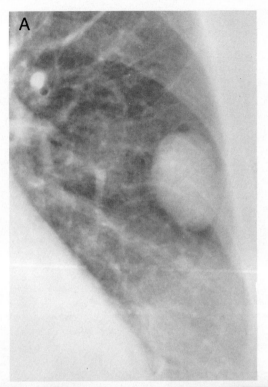

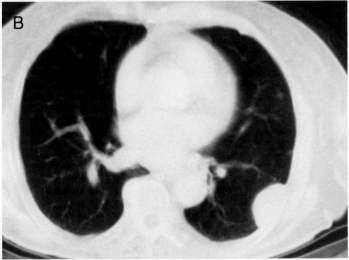

FIG 3-3
A, This solitary metastasis from a malignant fibrous histiocytoma presents as a sharply circumscribed peripheral mass. Its pleural location may be suspected because of the less definite lateral borders, but this cannot be confirmed on the PA film. **B,** CT scan shows the mass to have a broad pleural attachment with obtuse pleural angles, confirming its pleural origin.

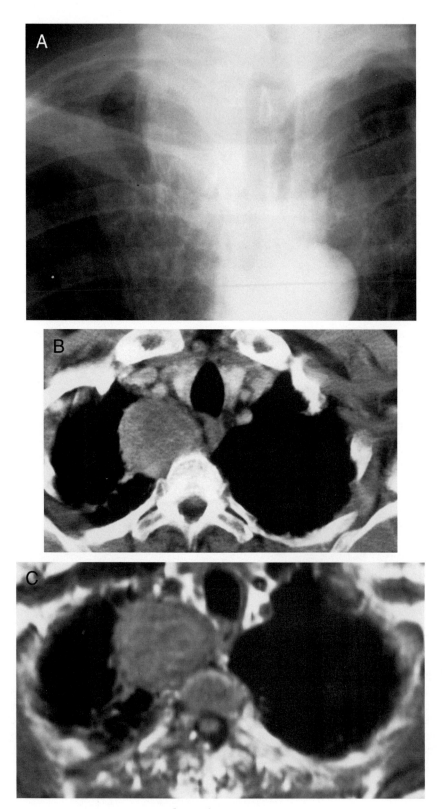

See legend on page 33

FIG 3–4

A, This right apical opacity extends to the medial and apical pleura. It could arise from the mediastinum, pleura, or lung. The streaky linear opacities along its lateral border could represent either atelectatic lung caused by compression or extension of the mass into surrounding lung tissue. **B,** CT demonstrates the relationship of the mass to mediastinal structures and shows an irregular linear opacity extending through the lung to the lateral pleura. This is most suggestive of a lung mass that has extended through the pleura into the mediastinum. **C,** T-1–weighted axial MR shows similar extension across the mediastinum with displacement of the esophagus. Biopsy confirmed primary lung cancer. This case illustrates the difficulty of precise localization of some masses even with CT and MR.

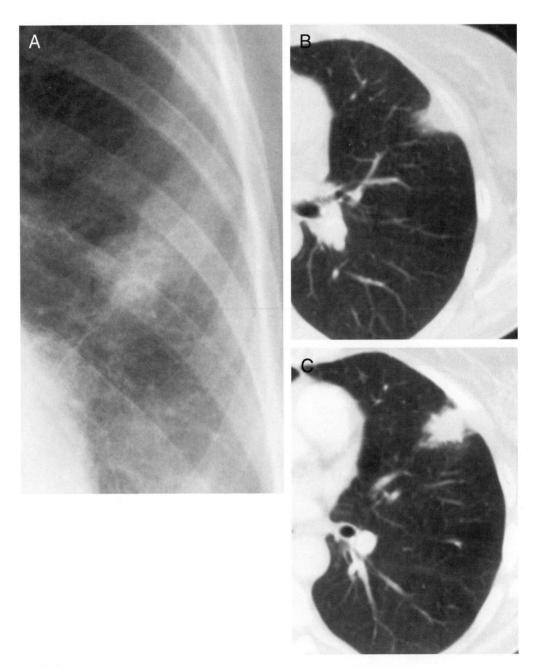

FIG 3–5
A, PA chest shows a poorly defined opacity in the periphery of the left upper lobe. **B,** CT section of the upper portion of the opacity shows a tapered border suggesting either a pleural mass or pleural extension of a lung mass. **C,** A lower CT section shows irregular margins confirming a subpleural origin of a pulmonary mass. Biopsy confirmed primary lung cancer.

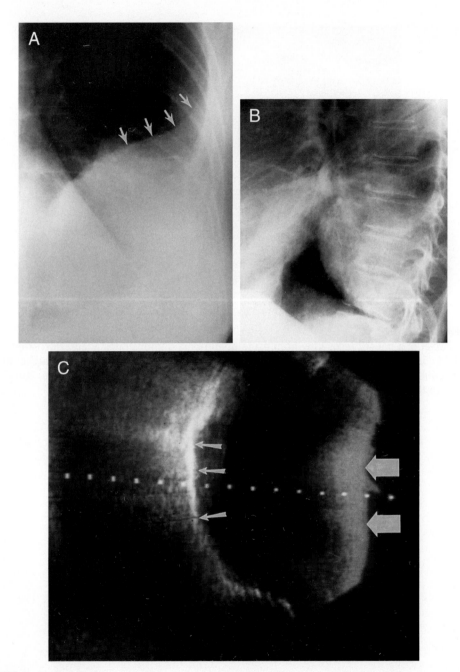

FIG 3–6
A, This large masslike opacity fills the left lower chest, obscuring the costophrenic angle. The smooth tapered superior lateral border (arrows) suggests a pleural opacity. **B,** The lateral film further confirms a well-circumscribed opacity suggestive of a pleural mass, but the history of a recent left lower lobe pneumonia favors the diagnosis of a loculated effusion. **C,** Ultrasound demonstrates a large sonolucency between the posterior chest wall (thick arrows) and the lung (thin arrows). This confirms the presence of a loculated effusion consistent with an empyema.

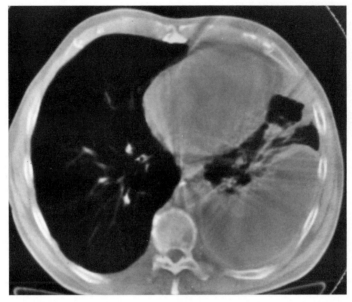

FIG 3–7
CT scan of a patient recovering from acute pneumonia demonstrates a large, loculated fluid collection. Note the low attenuation of the fluid, surrounded by a band of higher attenuation lung. There are also residual pulmonary opacities from the pneumonia, anterior to the pleural fluid.

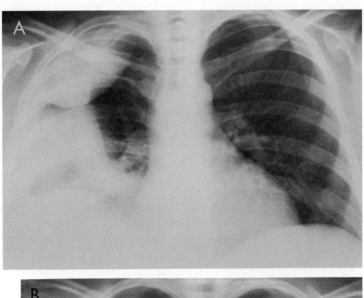

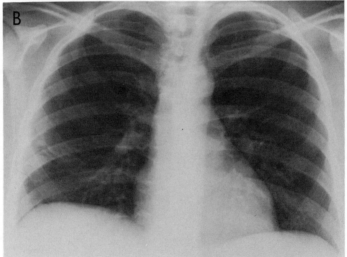

FIG 3–8
A, This diffuse, masslike pleural thickening was the result of hemothorax in a hemophiliac. **B,** Follow-up PA chest film after 2 weeks from the case illustrated in **A** reveals complete resolution of the pleural thickening, confirming a suspected diagnosis of pleural effusion.

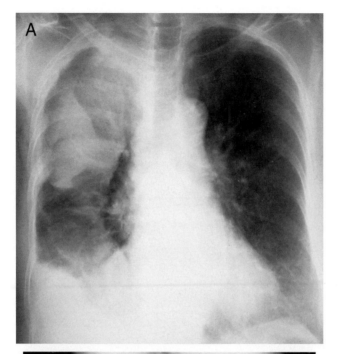

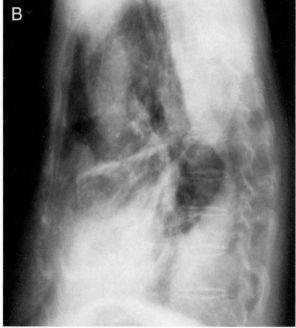

FIG 3–9
A, Patient with prior right mastectomy for breast cancer has developed extensive opacification of the right hemithorax with nodular thickening of the lateral pleura. **B,** Lateral
view shows the largest portion of the opacity to represent posterior pleural thickening.
There is also thickening of the minor fissure. This metastatic breast cancer has spread
around the pleura, resembling the appearance expected with diffuse malignant
mesothelioma (compare with Fig 3–10).

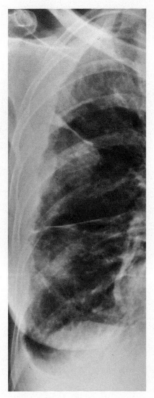

FIG 3–10
Diffuse nodular pleural thickening with thickening of interlobar fissures was unilateral in this case of diffuse malignant mesothelioma. Solitary mesothelioma may be either benign or malignant, but diffuse mesothelioma is always malignant.

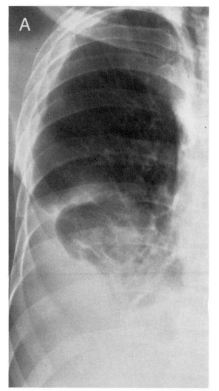

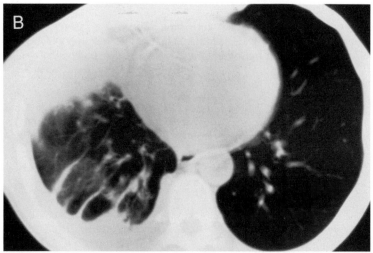

FIG 3–11
A, This diffuse mesothelioma appears less nodular than that seen in Figure 3–9, possibly because of the associated pleural effusion. The linear opacities in the right lung could be the result of compressive atelectasis or extension of the tumor. **B,** CT scan confirms the presence of peripheral linear pulmonary opacities that are continuous with the pleural tumor. These occur when mesothelioma follows the interlobar fissures and invades the interlobular septae.

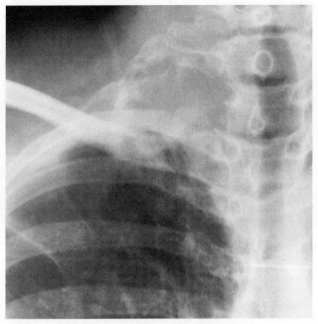

FIG 3–12
Superior sulcus, or Pancoast's tumors are primary lung cancers that often invade the pleura and chest wall. Notice the poorly marginated inferior border of the mass, which distinguishes it from a chest wall or pleural mass. The tumor has destroyed multiple ribs and vertebrae.

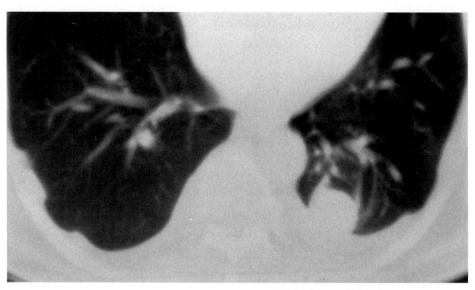

FIG 3-13
Rounded atelectasis causes a peripheral, masslike opacity with associated pleural thickening. The volume loss leads to retraction of surrounding pulmonary vessels with a characteristic CT appearance. Also note the plaques of pleural thickening, which are the result of asbestos exposure.

ANSWER GUIDE

LEGENDS FOR INTRODUCTORY FIGURES

FIG 3–1
Multiple bilateral pleural masses are the result of contiguous spread of malignant thymoma. Observe the sharply defined interface with the lung and the incomplete borders. The large right apical mass has obtuse pleural angles. These features confirm an extrapulmonary origin. The prior sternotomy was for resection of the primary mediastinal tumor.

FIG 3–2
A, This localized fibrous tumor of the pleura is seen as a sharply circumscribed mass in the left posterior pleural space. Other differential considerations include loculated pleural fluid and a solitary metastasis. **B,** CT scan from the same case confirms that the opacity is a heterogeneous mass with soft tissue, a calcification, and low-attenuation areas of necrosis. The mass is bounded posteriorly by the pleural fat and does not involve the chest wall. The CT findings rule out the options of a mesothelial cyst, myeloma, infarct, and rounded atelectasis. The correct answer to question 2 is *b*.

ANSWERS

1, d; 2, b; 3, T; 4, T; 5, F; 6, T.

C H A P T E R 4

Pleural Effusions

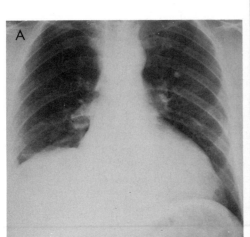

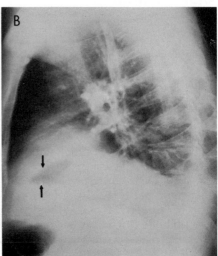

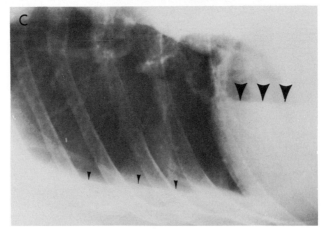

FIG 4–1

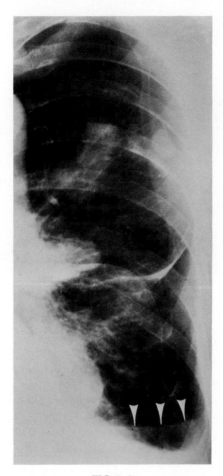

FIG 4–2

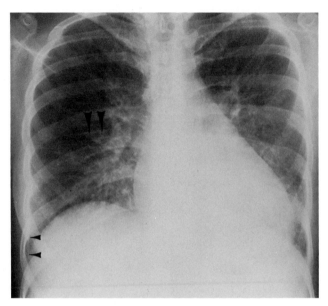

FIG 4–3

QUESTIONS

1. The most likely diagnosis in the case illustrated in Figure 4–1 is:
   a. Right lower lobe pneumonia.
   b. Pulmonary embolism.
   c. Subphrenic abscess.
   d. Lymphoma.
   e. Diaphragmatic hernia.
2. Which of the following examinations would be least useful in further evaluation of the case illustrated in Figure 4–1?
   a. Abdominal ultrasound.
   b. Cross-table lateral.
   c. Right lateral decubitus film.
   d. Expiratory film.
   e. CT scan.
3. Which of the following is most likely to result in the radiologic combination of pleural effusion and subsegmental atelectasis?
   a. Bacterial pneumonia with empyema.
   b. Pulmonary embolism.
   c. Congestive heart failure.
   d. Tuberculosis.
4. The most likely diagnosis in the case illustrated in Figure 4–2 is:
   a. Multiple myeloma.
   b. Actinomycosis.
   c. Metastases.
   d. Mesothelioma.

5. The least likely diagnosis in the case illustrated in Figure 4–3 is:
   a. Pulmonary embolism.
   b. Systemic lupus erythematosus.
   c. Congestive heart failure.
   d. Pancreatitis.

CHART 4–1.
Pleural Effusion

   I. Congestive heart failure[4, 414]
   II. Thromboembolic disease[668]
   III. Infection
      A. Bacteria (*Klebsiella pneumoniae, Staphylococcus aureus, Streptococcus pyogenes, Nocardia aster-oides,*[26] *Streptococcus pneumoniae [Diplococcus],*[598] anaerobic,[340] and other necrotizing bacterial infections)
      B. Tuberculosis[284]
      C. Viral (uncommon)
      D. Mycoplasma (uncommon)
      E. Fungus (blastomycosis, actinomycosis,[178] coccidioidomycosis,[457] histoplasmosis, cryptococco-sis[524] [effusion secondary to fungal infection is rare], malaria)
      F. Parasites (*Entamoeba histolytica,*[651] *Echinococcus, Paragonimus,*[289, 291] malaria)
      G. Infectious mononucleosis[341]
   IV. Neoplasms
      A. Metastases
         1. Bronchogenic
         2. Distant (e.g., breast, gastrointestinal, pancreatic)
      B. Multiple myeloma
      C. Mesothelioma
      D. Chest wall: primary bone (Ewing's sarcoma, chondrosarcoma, osteosarcoma, fibrosarcoma)
      E. Lymphoma[635]
      F. Waldenström's macroglobulinemia
   V. Collagen-vascular disease (autoimmune)
      A. Systemic lupus erythematosus[644]
      B. Rheumatoid arthritis[77, 553]
      C. Wegener's granulomatosis[377]
      D. Systemic sclerosis
   VI. Trauma
      A. Chest wall trauma[418]
      B. Rupture of the esophagus
      C. Rupture of the thoracic duct
      D. Laceration of great vessels (e.g., aorta, vena cava, pulmonary veins)
   VII. Abdominal diseases
      A. Pancreatitis
      B. Pancreatic neoplasms
      C. Pancreatic pseudocyst
      D. Pancreatic abscess
      E. Subphrenic abscess
      F. Abdominal or retroperitoneal surgery (e.g., renal surgery, splenectomy)
      G. Urinary tract obstruction with extension of retroperitoneal urine[29]
      H. Ovarian tumors (e.g., Meigs' syndrome)
      I. Cirrhosis of the liver
      J. Peritoneal dialysis
      K. Renal disease
         1. Renal failure
         2. Acute glomerulonephritis
         3. Nephrotic syndrome
      L. Whipple's disease

(Continued.)

Chart 4–1. (cont.).

VIII. Diffuse pulmonary diseases
    A. Lymphangiomyomatosis[410, 563]
    B. Asbestosis (rare)
    C. Usual interstitial pneumonitis (rare)
    D. Sarcoidosis (reported to be 4% of cases)[647]
IX. Drug reactions
    A. Nitrofurantoin
    B. Methysergide
    C. Busulfan
    D. Procainamide
    E. Hydralazine
    F. INH (isoniazid)   } Lupus reactions[511]
    G. Dilantin
    H. Propylthiouracil
    I. Procarbazine[134]
X. Other
    A. Postmyocardial infarction syndrome (Dressler's) and postpericardiotomy syndrome
    B. Coagulation defect
    C. Radiation therapy (very rare)[19, 643]
    D. Idiopathic
    E. Pleural fistulas (bronchial, gastric, esophageal, subarachnoid)[246, 401, 650]
    F. Empyema from retropharyngeal and neck abscess[477]
    G. Empyema in postpneumonectomy space[253]

CHART 4–2.
Pleural Effusion With Large Cardiac Silhouette

  I. Congestive heart failure
 II. Pulmonary embolism with right-sided heart enlargement
III. Myocarditis or pericarditis with pleuritis
    A. Viral infection
    B. Tuberculosis
    C. Rheumatic fever
IV. Tumor: metastasis, mesothelioma
 V. Collagen vascular disease
    A. Systemic lupus erythematosus[644] (pleural and pericardial effusion)
    B. Rheumatoid arthritis[77, 553]
VI. Postpericardiotomy syndrome

CHART 4–3.
Small Pleural Effusion With Subsegmental Atelectasis

  I. Postoperative (thoracotomy, splenectomy, renal surgery)
 II. Pulmonary embolism
III. Abdominal mass
IV. Ascites
 V. Rib fractures

CHART 4–4.
Pleural Effusion With Lobar Opacities

  I. Pneumonia with empyema[598]
 II. Pulmonary embolism
III. Neoplasm
    A. Bronchogenic carcinoma (common)
    B. Lymphoma
 IV. Tuberculosis

CHART 4–5.
Pleural Effusion With Hilar Enlargement

  I. Pulmonary embolism
 II. Tumor (bronchogenic carcinoma, lymphoma,
    metastasis)
III. Tuberculosis[284]
 IV. Fungal infections (rare)
  V. Sarcoidosis

DISCUSSION

The differential diagnosis of pleural effusion entails consideration of a long list of entities (Chart 4–1),[489] but the radiologist should not be discouraged.[500] Pleural effusion is frequently associated with additional radiologic findings that may be very specific. The first step in evaluating a pleural effusion is to confirm its presence. The upright chest film may reveal a variety of findings, from complete opacification of the chest to blunting of a costophrenic angle with a sulcus, apparent elevation of the diaphragm (see Fig 4–1, *A*), or opacity in the interlobar fissures (Fig 4–4, *A–C*),[114, 473] We are accustomed to looking at the lateral costophrenic angles for blunting, but the posterior angles should be carefully examined since the posterior angle is much deeper and may be blunted below the level of the lateral angle (see Fig 4–1, *B*). Blunting of the costophrenic angle or thickening of the pleural space may represent free fluid. This can be determined directly if decubitus views show a change in contour (see Fig 4–1, *C*). Previous films that indicate that the blunting is a new finding also provide a good indicator of pleural effusion. Loculated effusions are difficult to confirm with plain film, but ultrasound, CT, and even MR imaging may be used to verify a localized collection of pleural fluid.[273]

Pleural Effusion with Large Cardiac Silhouette

Congestive heart failure is probably the most common cause of pleural effusion, and it usually presents with a specific combination of cardiac and vascular findings. These cardiovascular changes include cardiomegaly, prominence of upper lobe vessels, constriction of lower lobe vessels, and prominent hilar vessels (see Fig 4–3). In addition, there may be signs of interstitial edema, including a fine reticular pattern, Kerley lines (septal), perihilar haze, and peribronchial thickening (see Fig 4–3). There may even be evidence of alveolar edema with confluent, ill-defined opacities with a perihilar distribution and air bronchograms. The combination of cardiomegaly, pulmonary vascular changes, and pleural effusion is almost certainly diagnostic of congestive heart failure. Correlation with the clinical history is very important for confirming or excluding the diagnosis of chronic renal failure with secondary cardiac failure.

The pleural effusions resulting from congestive heart failure may be either bilateral or unilateral. Unilateral effusions are most commonly on the right. Unilateral left pleural effusion in congestive failure has been called a great rarity. It has even been cited as a reason to consider other diagnoses, but it actually occurs in 10% to 15% of patients who develop pleural effusions secondary to congestive heart failure. Recurrent effusions caused by congestive failure tend to duplicate the appearance of the effusion seen in the previous episode of failure.

The combination of enlargement of the cardiac silhouette, pleural effusion in the absence of pulmonary vascular congestion, and signs of pulmonary interstitial or alveolar edema may be consistent with congestive heart failure. However, the presence of pleural effusion and cardiac enlargement alone is less specific and therefore requires more careful review of serial films and correlation with clinical data to narrow the differential diagnosis (see Chart 4–2). Since interstitial and alveolar edema may rapidly resolve in response to diuretics, these signs of congestive failure may disappear, leaving residual pleural effusion and cardiomegaly. Serial roentgenograms frequently confirm this possibility.

The diagnosis of pulmonary embolism is more difficult to confirm.[70] Obviously, right-sided heart enlargement and pleural effusion are suggestive of embolism. However, a patient with congestive heart failure may have right heart enlargement and pleural effusion, and is also at increased risk for developing a pulmonary embolism. If the effusion is atypical (e.g., predominantly left-sided) or if it increases after the pulmonary edema has begun to clear, the possibility of embolism should be considered. Any combination of additional clinical information indicating the development of chest pain, hemoptysis, sudden shortness of breath, pleural friction rub, a decreased arterial Po_2, or thrombophlebitis should be considered strong evidence for pulmonary embolism and thus indicate more definitive evaluation.[423] In the case illustrated in Figure 4–5, *A–C*, the combination of plain film and clinical findings lead to performance of the diagnostic pulmonary arteriogram.

The combination of cardiac silhouette enlargement, due either to pericardial effusion or cardiac enlargement, and pleural effusion may also be seen in patients with inflammatory diseases, in particular viral and tuberculous infections and poststreptococcal infections (rheumatic fever). History of a current or recurrent febrile illness and physical findings of pericarditis or myocarditis are helpful in suggesting these possibilities.

Metastatic tumors and mesothelioma occasionally involve both the pericardium and pleura, resulting in pericardial and pleural effusions. The association of multiple pulmonary masses or a lobulated appearance of the pleura strongly suggests this possibility (see Fig 4–2). The additional history of a distant primary tumor is strong supportive evidence for metastasis, whereas a history of asbestos exposure favors the diagnosis of mesothelioma.

Pleural and pericardial effusions are the most common radiologic manifestations of systemic lupus erythematosus. This diagnosis is rarely suggested by the radiologist. In the absence of other radiologic or clinical features of the common causes of pleural effusion with cardiac enlargement, this diagnosis may be considered. Confirmation of the pericardial effusion with ultrasound is frequently a useful procedure. Correlation with clinical and laboratory data is required to confirm the diagnosis. In answer to question 5, the combination of cardiac enlargement and pleural effusion is compatible with congestive heart failure, pulmonary embolism, and systemic lupus erythematosus, but should not be expected in pancreatitis.

Pleural Effusion with Atelectasis

Pleural effusion in combination with atelectasis suggests a more limited differential. The degree of atelectasis is an important consideration, since the differential for the combination of pleural effusion with subsegmental atelectasis (Chart 4–3) is much more limited than that for effusion and lobar atelectasis (Chart 4–4). The combination of subsegmental atelectasis and pleural effusion requires especially careful correlation with the clinical data, since it may indicate pulmonary embolism. The postoperative patient requires the most careful clinical correlation, since subsegmental atelectasis is frequently secondary to a combination of thoracic splinting and small airway mucous plugging, but the coexistence of pleural effusions requires a separate explanation. Obviously, a thoracotomy will explain effusion, and sympathetic effusion related to abdominal surgery is a well-known entity. In the latter situations the timing of development of the effusion should be considered. Late development or increasing pleural effusion must be considered evidence of a complication such as pulmonary embolism. In answer to question 3, pulmonary embolism is suggested by the combination of pleural effusion and subsegmental atelectasis.

Lobar atelectasis and pleural effusion also require careful clinical correlation. Acute onset of these abnormalities in a patient who is at bed rest and has thrombophlebitis and dyspnea, hemoptysis, or chest pain of acute onset should obviously suggest pulmonary embolism. However, a history of gradually increasing dyspnea and productive cough, possibly with blood-tinged sputum, that has evolved over a period of months must be considered evidence of a central tumor with obstructive atelectasis or even obstructive pneumonia. In these cases, the effusion may be an empyema secondary to the obstructive pneumonias or a malignant effusion. Tuberculosis is another consideration for this combination of lobar atelectasis and pleural effusion. It is certainly not a rare cause of pleural effusion, and may produce bronchial obstruction either by direct granulomatous reaction in and around the bronchus or by nodal compression of a bronchus. The combination of hilar enlargement, especially hilar adenopathy with pleural effusion, may be even more specific, suggesting primary lung cancer, metastases, lymphoma, or granulomatous diseases (Chart 4–5). In these cases with pleural effusion and atelectasis or adenopathy, there are two approaches to the diagnosis: (1) thoracentesis, with cultures of the fluid, or (2) bronchoscopy, with cultures and biopsy of specimens from the occluded bronchus, or enlarged nodes.

Parapneumonic Effusions and Empyema

Parapneumonic effusions and empyema develop in response to pneumonias. Parapneumonic effusions have a low white blood cell count and low protein content, are sterile, and resolve completely in response to antibiotic therapy. In contrast, empyemas have an elevated white blood cell count and high protein content, and organisms may be cultured from the fluid. Thoracentesis specimens should be cultured for bacteria, fungi, and tuberculosis. Empyema is an active pleural infection that often requires pleural drainage to prevent chronic pleural scarring.[482]

The radiologic appearance of parapneumonic effusions and empyemas may be indistinguishable. However, empyemas should be suspected when there is rapid accumulation of a large quantity of pleural fluid (Fig 4–6, A–B). CT is often required for precise localization of loculated empyemas (Fig 4–7, A–B).

Empyemas are most often secondary to pneumonias, but may also be caused by extension of infection from pharyngeal abscess, mediastinitis, or abdominal infection. They are also complications of penetrating chest trauma, pulmonary resections, thoracostomy tube placement, sclerosis of malignant effusions, and esophageal perforation.

Chronic or Recurrent Pleural Effusion

It is well known that the isolated finding of pleural effusion is nonspecific and may be secondary to many of the entities listed in Chart 4–1. Even the infectious diseases may present with absolutely no evidence of underlying pulmonary disease. Tuberculosis is notorious for this presentation and may require multiple cultures for accurate diagnosis. It is also a well-known cause of chronic or recurrent effusion. Rheumatoid disease of the pleura is another very elusive diagnosis unless the patient has obvious joint abnormalities. In the absence of joint abnormalities, the rheumatoid effusion may be diagnosed only after an extensive laboratory evaluation to exclude infectious causes such as tuberculosis, and with positive results of serologic studies.[77] Other collagen-vascular diseases that cause chronic or recurrent effusions include lupus erythematosus, Wegener's granulomatosis, and systemic sclerosis.

Malignant pleural effusions[378] should be suspected in patients with a known primary tumor, but effusion may also be the presenting abnormality in patients with lung cancer, mesothelioma, and even distant primaries such as ovarian carcinoma. The radiologic combination of multiple pulmonary nodules and pleural effusion virtually confirms the diagnosis of metastatic disease. Sometimes, unique combinations indicate a specific primary tumor. The combination of pleural effusion, multiple pulmonary nodules, and spontaneous pneumothorax seen in Figure 4–2 is strongly suggestive of metastatic osteosarcoma. (Answer to question 4 is *c*.) Since patients with malignant effusions are also at risk for opportunistic infections and are often treated with toxic drugs, malignant effusions must be differentiated from empyema and drug reactions.

Abdominal Diseases

Abdominal diseases must be considered in the evaluation of pleural effusion.[50] A minimal radiologic examination of patients with abdominal diseases should include films of the abdomen with the patient in the supine and upright positions, as well as PA and lateral chest films. Figure 4–1 illustrates a case of pleural effusion secondary to abdominal disease. In addition to the apparent elevation of the right hemidiaphragm and blunting of the right costophrenic angle, air is seen over the right upper quadrant of the abdomen. A localized extraluminal collection of air is good evidence of a subphrenic abscess. (Answer to question 1 is *c*.) A cross-table lateral film or a lateral decubitus film (see Fig 4–1, *C*) will reveal an air-fluid level in the right upper quadrant. The lateral decubitus film has the advantage of being easier to interpret and confirms the presence of the associated pleural effusion. The subphrenic abscess that has such definite plain film findings as in the present case (see Fig 4–1, *A–C*) does not usually need further confirmation, but a subphrenic abscess that does not have air under the diaphragm cannot be confirmed by plain film criteria. In such a case, ultrasound or CT confirms the diagnosis. In answer to question 2, all of the procedures listed, except an expiratory chest film, could be useful in the evaluation of a subphrenic abscess. Other patients with abdominal disease that might lead to pleural effusion require careful clinical correlation and evaluation of their abdominal disease. Laboratory evaluation of the pleural fluid is beneficial and often diagnostic; for example, patients with pancreatitis may have extremely elevated levels of amylase in the fluid, and patients with an amebic liver abscess may have parasites in their pleural fluid.[651]

SUMMARY

1. Free pleural fluid should be radiologically confirmed by lateral decubitus films or serial films that show a change in contour.

2. Loculated effusions are difficult to confirm by plain film examination but may be confirmed by ultrasound examination of pleural opacities.

3. The presence of pleural effusion must be carefully correlated with other radiologic findings, both on the chest film and in other organ systems.

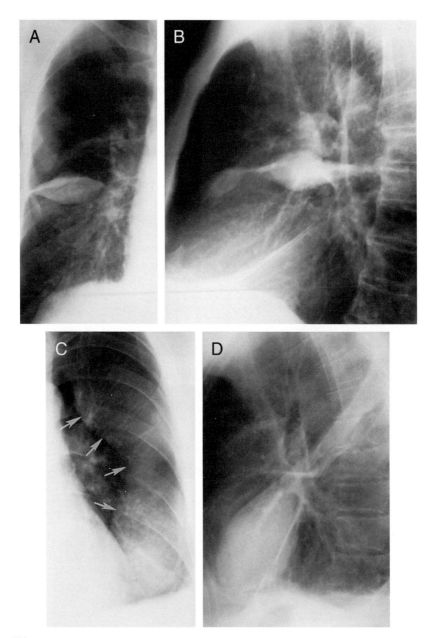

FIG 4–4
A, PA film demonstrates elliptical opacity in the minor fissure. **B,** Lateral film confirms that the opacity is in the minor fissure. This is the characteristic appearance of loculated fluid in the minor fissure. These collections may be more round and are often called pleural pseudotumors. They may be transient and are described as vanishing tumors, especially when they are the result of congestive heart failure. **C,** PA film from another case demonstrates the appearance of fluid in the major fissure. This is less masslike, with the fluid spreading out in the fissure. The medial inferior border *(arrows)* is well circumscribed, with an arch that appears to outline the superior segment of the lower lobe. **D,** Lateral film of the case seen in Fig 4–4, C shows thickening of the entire length of the major fissure.

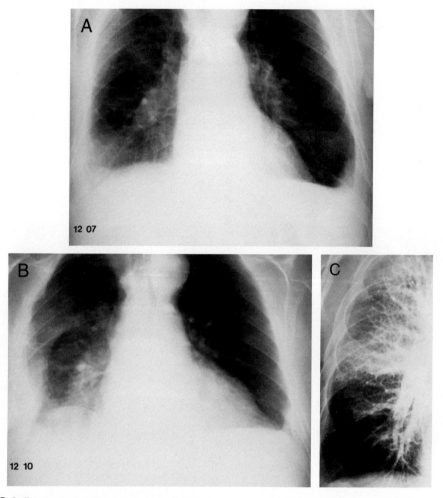

FIG 4–5

A, PA film shows blounting of both costophrenic angles with thickening of the right lateral pleural space consistent with bilateral pleural effusion. **B,** Three days later, the patient complained of bilateral chest pain and developed hemoptysis. Repeat PA film reveals that the right pleural effusion had increased, and thoracentesis reveals bloody pleural effusion. **C,** Pulmonary arteriogram confirmed the suspected diagnosis of pulmonary embolism.

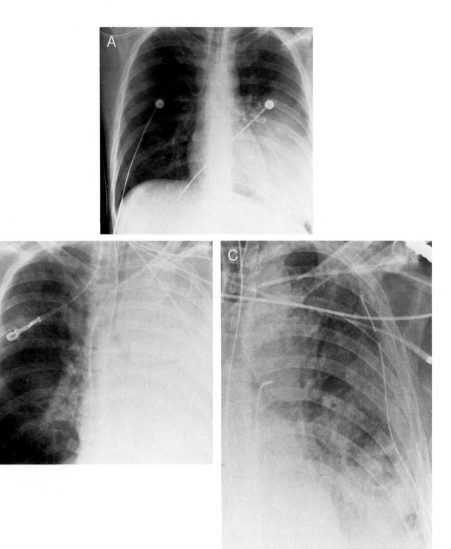

FIG 4–6
A, Left lower lobe pneumonia without pleural fluid. Observe that the diaphragm and the left costophrenic angle are visible. **B,** Film taken 24 hours later shows nearly complete opacification of the left chest. This could be from further pulmonary consolidation, accumulation of pleural fluid, or both. **C,** Film taken after placement of a thoracostomy tube demonstrates the left chest to be less opaque. This resulted from drainage of a large quantity of purulent pleural fluid. The rapid development of a large pleural effusion over a short period of time favors the diagnosis of empyema over parapneumonic effusion.

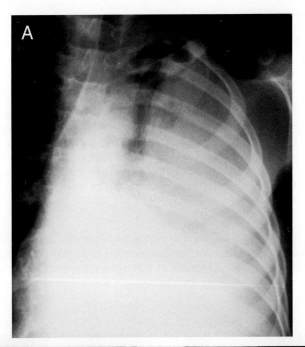

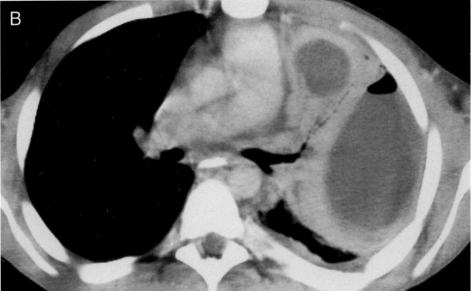

FIG 4–7
A, Patient with clinical and laboratory diagnosis of pneumonia develops an almost completely opaque left hemithorax. The upper medial border of the opacity is suggestive of a
large pleural collection. The upper medial border of the opacity is suggestive of a
large pleural collection. **B,** CT confirms a large multiloculated pleural fluid collection consistent with empyema. The small pneumothorax seen on the plain film and confirmed
with the CT indicates associated bronchopleural fistula.

ANSWER GUIDE

LEGENDS FOR INTRODUCTORY FIGURES

FIG 4–1
A, This posteroanterior chest film demonstrates apparent elevation of the right hemi-diaphragm. **B,** Lateral film shows blunted posterior costophrenic angle, suggesting that apparent elevation seen on PA film may be secondary to pleural effusion. Note the anterior collection of air under the elevated right side of diaphragm *(arrows)*. **C,** Lateral decubitus film confirms presence of pleural fluid *(small arrowheads)* and reveals large air-fluid level below the diaphragm *(large arrowheads)*. The latter finding confirms the diagnosis of subphrenic abscess.

FIG 4–2
Air-fluid level in left costophrenic angle *(arrowheads)* indicates both free fluid and air in pleural space (hydropneumothorax). The combination of multiple pulmonary nodules and pleural effusion is virtually diagnostic of metastases. The primary tumor in this case is osteosarcoma, well known for its association with pneumothorax. (Case courtesy of William Barry, M.D.)

FIG 4–3
Minimal blunting of costophrenic angle *(small arrowheads)* and thickening of minor fissure *(large arrowheads)* suggests the possibility of a small pleural effusion. Additional findings of cardiomegaly and a fine reticular pattern are most suggestive of congestive heart failure.

ANSWERS

   1, c; 2, d; 3, b; 4, c; 5, d.

CHAPTER 5

Pleural Thickening and Pleural Calcification

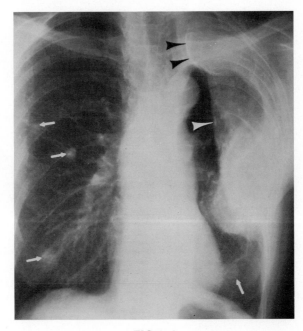

FIG 5–1

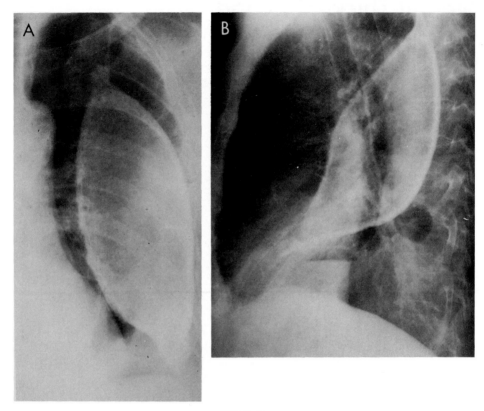

FIG 5–2

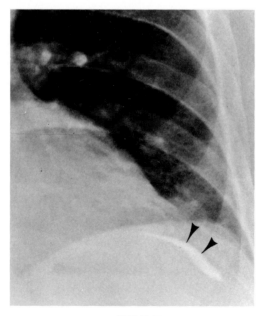

FIG 5–3

QUESTIONS

1. What is the most likely diagnosis for the case illustrated in Figure 5–1?
   a. Mesothelioma.
   b. Metastases.
   c. Tuberculous empyema.
   d. Primary lung cancer.
   e. Lymphoma.
2. The large calcification in Figure 5–2 is most probably caused by:
   a. Mesothelioma of the major fissure.
   b. Asbestosis.
   c. Old healed empyema.
   d. Organizing pneumonia.
   e. Metastases.
3. Basilar interstitial disease is consistent with all of the following, but the observation of pleural calcification in Figure 5–3 confirms the diagnosis of:
   a. Rheumatoid lung.
   b. Scleroderma lung.
   c. Usual interstitial pneumonitis.
   d. Desquamative interstitial pneumonitis.
   e. Asbestosis.

CHART 5–1.
Pleural Thickening

  I. Infection
     A. Empyema (chronic)
     B. Tuberculosis[412]
     C. Aspergillosis (saprophytic form, i.e., fungus ball)[360,402,621]
 II. Neoplasm
     A. Metastases[185]
     B. Diffuse mesothelioma[395,444]
     C. Pancoast's tumor[442]
     D. Leukemia[316]
III. Collagen-vascular (rheumatoid arthritis)
 IV. Trauma (healed hemothorax)
  V. Inhalational diseases
     A. Asbestosis[3,37,197,395,529–531]
     B. Talcosis[154]
 VI. Other
     A. Organization of serous pleural effusion
     B. Sarcoidosis[647]
     C. Splenosis[298]
     D. Mimics (extrathoracic musculature)[97]

CHART 5–2.
Pleural Calcification

  I. Trauma (healed hemothorax)
 II. Infection
      A. Chronic empyema[539]
      B. Tuberculosis
III. Inhalation
      A. Asbestos-related plaques[188,531]
      B. Talcosis[154]

DISCUSSION

The evaluation of pleural thickening requires distinguishing between pleural fluid and true thickening (Chart 5-1). Like pleural effusion, pleural thickening is usually appreciated as a thick white line between the lucency of the lung and the ribs. Lateral decubitus films are frequently necessary for distinguishing free pleural effusion from pleural thickening, but loculated effusions are not as easily distinguished from pleural thickening. This may sometimes be accomplished by comparison with previous films. When the pleural thickening is of recent onset (days to weeks), pleural effusion is the most likely cause of the opacity, whereas if the process has been stable for months to years, it is most probably true pleural thickening. As with pleural masses, ultrasound or CT scanning may be essential for detecting loculated fluid collections when they are surrounded by a pneumonia or within a mass of pleural reaction (Fig 5–4, A and B).

Organizing Effusion

Organization of a pleural effusion is one of the most common causes of pleural thickening. The detection of a small amount of associated pleural effusion may seem unimportant, but is vital for diagnostic thoracentesis.[500] The fluid may be nondiagnostic, but it provides material for culture and cytology. The organizing fibrothorax is definitely less diagnostic, since it usually consists of chronic inflammatory cells and fibrosis. It may be the end result of a variety of bacterial, fungal, and tuberculous pulmonary infections. In such cases, the radiologic finding of pleural thickening is nonspecific, and the radiologic diagnosis usually depends on the characteristically associated pulmonary findings. Apical pulmonary cavities with associated pleural thickening are characteristic of old granulomatous infection such as tuberculosis or histoplasmosis.[412] A strongly reactive skin test may clinch the diagnosis. Another example is the patient with old cystic or cavitary disease who develops a new opacity in the area of one of the old cystic lesions and concomitantly a new area of pleural thickening in the same vicinity. This may be suggestive of aspergilloma, which develops in old cavities and is commonly associated with pleural thickening.[360] As in other cases of inflammatory pleural thickening, the histologic appearance of the pleural disease secondary to aspergilloma is nonspecific. The fungus is not usually identifiable in the pleural reaction.

The less specific appearance of extensive pleural thickening over the bases, with associated parenchymal scars, can best be diagnosed as chronic empyema when a definite history of previous pneumonia is obtained. Some noninfectious causes of pleural effusion, such as rheumatoid disease, occasionally fail to resolve, with the final result of a thick pleural reaction (Fig 5–5).[77] A history of known rheumatoid arthritis may suggest this diagnosis. In addition, positive results of serologic studies for rheumatoid factor may also suggest the diagnosis, particularly if there is a history of thoracic disease prior to the onset of joint disease.

Asbestos-Related Plaques

Asbestos-related pleural plaques are a common cause of pleural thickening.[529,530] They occur along the lateral chest walls or on the diaphragmatic pleura (Fig 5–6, *A* and *B*), sparing the apices and costophrenic angles.[304] High-resolution CT (HRCT) has been advocated for distinguishing these plaques from other causes of pleural thickening.[188] Basilar interstitial disease is occasionally an associated finding that may also be more accurately assessed with HRCT.[3] The diagnosis requires a history of exposure to asbestos for confirmation (see discussion of pleural calcification).

A curious feature of the pleural thickening of asbestos exposure is the tendency for marked parietal pleural thickening and relative sparing of the visceral pleura. This is in contrast to other causes of pleural thickening such as empyema, tuberculosis, and rheumatoid disease. The finding is rarely useful for the radiologist except in those patients who at some time have either spontaneous or iatrogenic pneumothorax (see Fig 5–5).

Neoplasm

As mentioned in the discussion of pleural masses (see Chapter 3), diffuse nodular pleural thickening raises the differential of (1) loculated effusion, (2) metastases, and (3) malignant mesothelioma (Fig 5–7).[140] In such cases the nodular character of the pleural reaction may not be appreciated prior to thoracentesis for removal of associated pleural effusion. Thoracentesis should be done in combination with pleural biopsy, which frequently confirms the diagnosis.

Apical pleural "capping" is a common radiologic appearance[398,495,496] and must not be confused with normal structures such as the subclavian artery, supraclavicular border, sternomastoid muscle, or rib companion shadows.[466] There is a tendency to attribute true pleural thickening to old tuberculosis, but it is often a fibrotic scar of obscure etiology. It is possible to confuse tuberculous pleural thickening with an early Pancoast's tumor (Fig 5–8).[442] Apical lordotic and kyphotic films may confirm the presence of the opacity but rarely add diagnostic information. Coned-down views of the ribs or CT may show bone destruction, which would indicate a neoplastic process, but the absence of bone destruction does not exclude a malignant neoplasm. Radionuclide bone scans are more sensitive than plain film for early bone involvement by a Pancoast's tumor. Comparison with old films that show the apical pleural cap to be stable over a period of years is essentially diagnostic of an old inflammatory process. When the serial films demonstrate a change, it is strongly suggestive of tumor or active infection.

Pleural Calcification

In contrast to the lack of specificity of both pleural effusion and pleural thickening, pleural calcification involves only a brief differential (Chart 5–2) and is frequently a diagnostic finding.

Hemothorax is usually confirmed by a history of significant chest trauma. There may be associated healed rib fractures. Although pulmonary contusion may have accompanied the acute episodes, contusion usually resolves without significant residual effect. Associated parenchymal scarring thus favors a diagnosis other than previous hemothorax.

Chronic empyema is a more common cause of pleural calcification. Calcification was previously considered a sign of an old healed process, but recent CT studies indicate that chronic empyemas may calcify around their periphery while retaining collections of fluid for years.[539]

Occasionally, calcified pleural thickening from empyema does assume unusual or bizarre configurations and may be very extensive. It must be remembered that the interlobar fissures are part of the pleural space and may therefore be involved by an empyema (see Fig 5–2). (Answer to question 2 is *c.*) A careful history will frequently date these pleural reactions to a specific episode of pneumonia. Empyema may also be the result of penetrating injuries such as bullet and stab wounds.

Tuberculosis is no longer a common cause of empyema, but since calcification indicates a long-standing process, tuberculosis is a likely cause of calcified empyema. The pleural reaction is most commonly apical and asymmetric. Associated apical parenchymal scarring, cavities, or even multiple calcified granulomas are virtually diagnostic of tuberculosis. In answer to question 1, the asymmetric apical pleural thickening and calcification along with multiple granulomas (see Fig 5–1) are diagnostic of tuberculous empyema.

Asbestos exposure is a common cause of pleural calcifications measuring less than 3–4 cm (see Fig 5–3). (Answer to question 3 is *e.*) The pleural calcifications resulting from asbestos exposure most commonly affect the domes of the diaphragmatic pleura. They may be extensive and bilateral but are often asymmetric. Noncalcified plaques are the most common finding in patients with asbestos exposure, but they are more difficult to identify on plain film and are less specific than the calcifications. Computed tomographic scans (Fig 5–9, *A* and *B*), especially HRCT, have been shown to be the most sensitive means for detecting minimal pleural changes from asbestos exposure.[3,577] Pleural calcification is not seen in all cases of asbestos exposure, but can lead to one of the most specific appearances in chest radiology.

Talcosis is the result of exposure to a variety of talc mixtures.[154] While pure talc is not very fibrogenic, mixtures of talc with silica or magnesium silicate are very fibrogenic. Both asbestos and tremolite talc contain magnesium silicate. The radiologic findings in this type of talcosis are the same as those in asbestosis.

SUMMARY

1. Distinction of pleural thickening from effusion may be suggested by the configuration and position of the opacity on the upright film (e.g., apical pleural thickening), but comparison with previous films and lateral decubitus films is frequently required for identifying small associated effusions.

2. The most common cause of chronic pleural thickening is organization of an empyema. This may result from bacterial, tuberculous, or fungal infections.

3. Recurrent pleural effusion with development of pleural thickening is one of the more frequent manifestations of rheumatoid disease in the thorax.

4. Diffuse nodular pleural thickening is consistent with diffuse metastases or mesothelioma, but must be distinguished from loculated effusion. Thoracentesis and pleural biopsy are frequently required for making the distinction.

5. Apical pleural thickening is a common observation. Serial films showing that the process is stable are adequate proof of a benign inflammatory process. A change suggests either activity of the inflammatory process or presence of a tumor (e.g., Pancoast's tumor).

6. Apical pleural thickening with rib destruction should be considered neoplastic until proved otherwise.

7. Pleural calcification indicates empyema, tuberculosis, hemothorax, or asbestos exposure.

8. Pleural calcifications over the domes of each hemidiaphragm in combination with pleural thickening are diagnostic of asbestos exposure or talcosis. A history of such exposure should confirm the diagnosis.

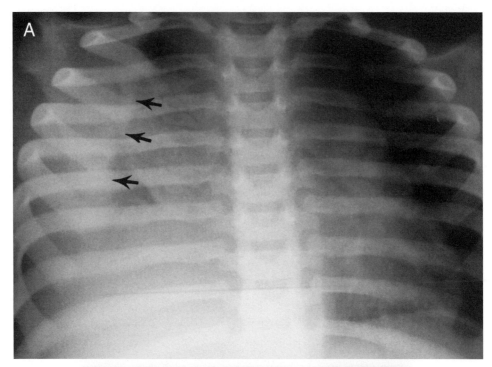

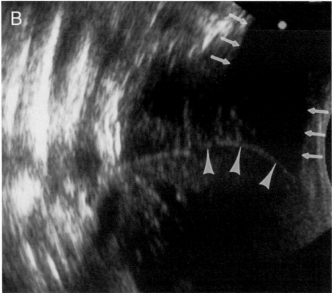

FIG 5–4
A, PA film of a child with extensive pneumonia shows more severe lateral opacification of the right lateral thorax, with a curved line *(arrows)* suggesting a large parapneumonic pleural effusion. **B,** Ultrasound of the right lateral inferior thorax shows a large sonolucent area *(arrows)* above the diaphragm *(arrowheads)*. This is a loculated empyema. Ultrasound or CT guided thoracentesis is important for diagnosis and drainage.

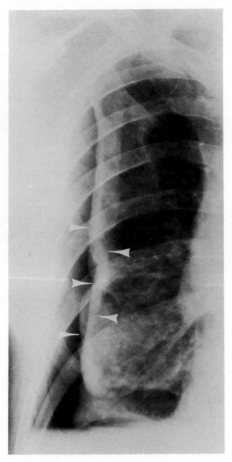

FIG 5–5
This case of rheumatoid pleural thickening *(arrowheads)* illustrates involvement of visceral pleura. Distinction of visceral from parietal pleural thickening is possible only in the presence of pneumothorax. Recall that asbestosis is one of the few causes of pleural thickening that can appear to spare the visceral pleura.

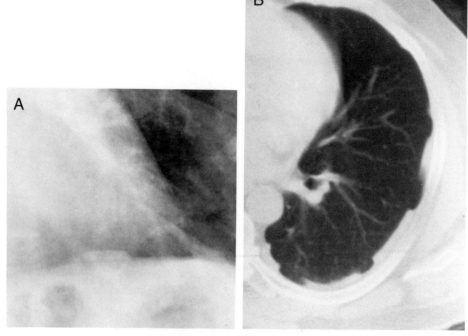

FIG 5–6
A, Asbestos-related plaques typically involve the diaphragmatic pleura. Noncalcified plaques are often difficult to see on plain film. **B,** CT scan of same case reveals plaques on the lateral and posterior pleura to be much more extensive than suspected from the plain film.

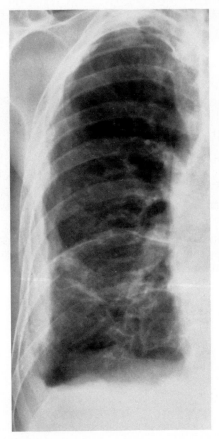

FIG 5–7
This case of diffuse malignant mesothelioma, like the one in Figure 3–10, has produced diffuse unilateral pleural thickening.

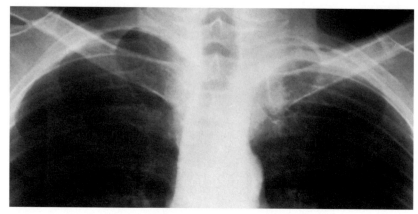

FIG 5–8

Asymmetric apical opacity raises the question of carcinoma vs. pleural scarring. Documentation of a change by comparison with old films should be the first step in evaluation. A recent change indicates either active granulomatous disease (probably tuberculosis) or cancer. In this case the asymmetric pleural thickening was caused by a superior sulcus or Pancoast's tumor.

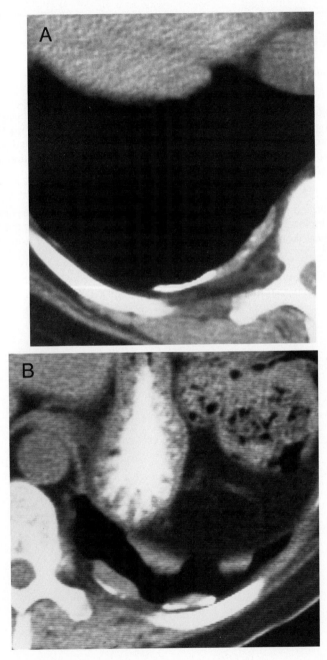

FIG 5–9
A and **B,** Two sections from a CT scan demonstrate calcified and noncalcified pleural plaques typical of asbestos exposure.

ANSWER GUIDE

LEGENDS FOR INTRODUCTORY FIGURES

FIG 5–1
Extensive pleural thickening over left upper lobe has plaques of calcification *(arrowheads)* along its medial border. The location, over the upper lobe, helps eliminate asbestosis from consideration. The additional finding of multiple, calcified pulmonary nodules *(white arrows)* should essentially confirm the diagnosis of old tuberculous empyema. (Answer to question 1 is *c.*)

FIG 5–2
A, Large, calcified opacity might be confused with intrapulmonary mass on the PA film. **B,** Lateral film localizes the abnormality to the major fissure and thus the pleural space. This pleural calcification resulted from old empyema.

FIG 5–3
Pleural calcification *(arrowheads)* should confirm the diagnosis of asbestos exposure. Combination of basilar interstitial disease and pleural calcification is compatible with asbestosis.

ANSWERS

1, c; 2, c; 3, e.

CHAPTER 6

Elevated Diaphragm

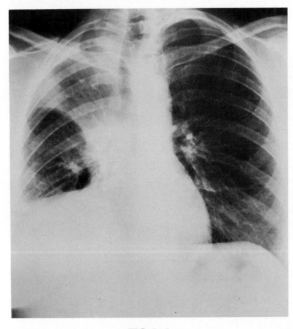

FIG 6–1

QUESTIONS

1. Which of the following diagnoses is most likely in the case illustrated in Figure 6–1?
   a. Subphrenic abscess.
   b. Interposition of the colon.
   c. Atelectasis of the right upper lobe.
   d. Phrenic nerve paralysis.
   e. Right upper lobe pneumonia.
2. Which of the following is least likely to be associated with pleural effusion?
   a. Primary lung tumor.
   b. Interposition of colon.
   c. Subphrenic abscess.
   d. Echinococcal cyst.
   e. Metastasis.
3. Which of the following is not true of phrenic nerve paralysis?
   a. Results in complete loss of motion of the diaphragm at fluoroscopy.
   b. May be secondary to primary lung tumor in the apex.
   c. May be secondary to mediastinal malignant tumor.
   d. Occasionally is idiopathic.
   e. Results in paradoxical motion of the diaphragm.

CHART 6–1.
Elevated Diaphragm

   I. Subpulmonic pleural effusion[30, 63]
  II. Abdominal disease
      A. Subphrenic abscess
      B. Distended stomach
      C. Interposition of the colon
      D. Liver mass (tumor, abscess, echinococcal cyst)
 III. Altered pulmonary volume
      A. Atelectasis
      B. Postoperative lobectomy and pneumonectomy
      C. Hypoplastic lung
  IV. Phrenic nerve paralysis
      A. Primary lung tumor
      B. Malignant mediastinal tumor
      C. Iatrogenic
      D. Idiopathic
   V. Diaphragmatic hernia (foramina of Morgagni, Bochdalek)
  VI. Eventration of the diaphragm
 VII. Traumatic rupture of the diaphragm
VIII. Diaphragmatic tumor,[12] (lipoma,[166] fibroma, mesothelioma, metastasis, lymphoma)

DISCUSSION

Elevation of the diaphragm offers a variety of radiologic challenges. When both sides of the diaphragm are symmetrically elevated, the differential is significantly different from that with unilateral elevation. The most common cause of elevation of both sides of the diaphragm is failure of the patient to inspire deeply. This is frequently voluntary, but may be an indicator of a significant pathologic process. Obesity is probably the most common abnormality resulting in poor inspiratory effect. A similar appearance may be produced by a variety of abdominal conditions, including ascites and large abdominal masses. Bilateral atelectasis may also result in elevation of both sides of the diaphragm, but is usually identifiable by increased opacity in the lung bases. Restrictive pulmonary diseases may likewise result in elevation of both sides of the diaphragm (see Chapter 13 on cicatrizing atelectasis).

Subpulmonic Pleural Effusion

Subpulmonic pleural effusion is an important cause of apparent elevation of the diaphragm.[30, 63] This is most commonly unilateral, but on occasion may be bilateral. The PA film may suggest this diagnosis when the dome of the diaphragm appears to be near the costophrenic angle with an abrupt dropoff (Fig 6–2). The lateral view may help to confirm this impression by demonstrating a posterior meniscus (Fig 6–3). The diagnosis is usually confirmed with lateral decubitus films (Fig 6–4). Caution must be exercised in evaluating a subpulmonic pleural effusion, since pleural effusions may be associated with other significant abnormalities, such as subphrenic abscess, primary lung tumor, and liver masses (including abscesses and echinococcal cysts), that result in true elevation of the diaphragm.

Altered Pulmonary Volume

Atelectasis is a common cause of diaphragmatic elevation and is recognizable by the associated pulmonary opacity. Elevation of the diaphragm is an expected complication of lower lobe, lingula, or middle lobe atelectasis, but is also seen in upper lobe atelectasis (see Fig 6–1). (Answer to question 1 is *c*.) Postoperative volume loss should be easily recognized in cases with rib defects, metallic sutures, and shift of the heart or mediastinum.

Abdominal Diseases

Subphrenic abscess is not a rare cause of unilateral elevation of the diaphragm following abdominal surgery. It is usually accompanied by pleural effusion. Plain films alone confirm the diagnosis when localized collections of air are demonstrated below the diaphragm (see Fig 4–1). Ultrasound is probably the least invasive method for confirming the diagnosis, and it is virtually diagnostic when localized fluid collections are demonstrated below the diaphragm.

Distended abdominal viscera, such as the colon and stomach, may occasionally elevate one side of the diaphragm. Interposition of the colon is a completely benign condition in which the colon is interposed between the liver and the right side of the diaphragm. It may result in elevation of the right side of the diaphragm, but would not be adequate explanation for pleural effusion. (Answer to question 2 is *b*.) Occasionally, large liver masses will elevate the right diaphragm. CT scan with biopsy may be required to confirm the diagnosis.

Phrenic Nerve Paralysis

Phrenic nerve paralysis is another common cause of elevation of one side of the diaphragm. It may be due to a variety of problems, including primary lung tumors, malignant mediastinal tumors, and surgery of the mediastinum. It may even be idiopathic. The combination of a lung or mediastinal mass and elevation of the diaphragm strongly suggests phrenic nerve paralysis. The condition can be confirmed by fluoroscopy, which will reveal paradoxical motion of the diaphragm: as the patient inspires, the paralyzed diaphragm appears to rise. This may be associated with slight flutter and is best demonstrated with the patient in the lateral position. (Answer to question 3 is *a*.) A sniff accentuates diaphragmatic motion and is therefore useful in eliciting paradoxical motion.

Diaphragmatic Hernias

Diaphragmatic hernias through the foramen of Morgagni or Bochdalek may mimic the appearance of elevation of one side of the diaphragm on a single view. However, the lateral view reveals the characteristic anterior location of Morgagni's hernia or posterior location of Bochdalek's hernia. Hiatal hernias should be near the midline and are more likely to be confused with either cavities or masses than with elevation of the diaphragm.

Eventration of the Diaphragm

Eventration of the diaphragm is similar to paralysis but represents an area of weakness and thinning of the diaphragm. With eventration there may be motion of the diaphragm but a smaller excursion between inspiration and expiration. It should not entail a paradoxical movement of the diaphragm. In infancy, eventration may result in elevation of a large portion of the diaphragm. In these cases the entire leaf of the diaphragm may consist of thin fibrous tissue. Elderly patients frequently have localized irregularities of the diaphragm that lead to a lobulated appearance but are of little pathologic significance.

Traumatic Rupture of the Diaphragm

Traumatic rupture of the diaphragm may result in apparent elevation of the diaphragm, particularly when the right side of the diaphragm is injured. In this situation the liver herniates into the right hemithorax and simulates elevation of the diaphragm. This is frequently associated with other signs of chest or abdominal trauma, including multiple fractures. Because of the severity of the injury, it may also be associated with pulmonary contusion and chest wall vascular injury leading to pleural effusion. Rupture of the left side of the diaphragm gives a more characteristic roentgenologic appearance, since the stomach and bowel may herniate into the chest (Fig 6–5). These structures are likely to contain air, so that the patient will appear to have multiple fluid levels in the left side of the chest rather than an elevation of the left hemidiaphragm. When there is a large amount of fluid in these structures, the radiologic appearance may be that of near opacification of the left hemithorax.

Diaphragmatic Tumor

Mesothelioma, fibroma, and lipoma may produce apparent elevation of the diaphragm[12] when the tumor assumes a massive size, but this is an infrequent occurrence. Serial films may confirm growth of the mass. Fluoroscopy should demonstrate respiratory movement and thus help eliminate diaphragmatic paralysis.

SUMMARY

1. Subpulmonic pleural effusion is the problem that most commonly mimics diaphragmatic elevation. It should be distinguished from true diaphragmatic elevation with lateral decubitus films.

2. The most common causes of diaphragmatic elevation are atelectasis, abdominal masses, eventration of the diaphragm, and phrenic nerve paralysis.

3. Abdominal masses, such as subphrenic abscess and liver masses (including tumors, abscesses, and even echinococcal cysts), must be considered in the differential diagnosis of an elevated right hemidiaphragm.

4. Traumatic rupture of the right hemidiaphragm may mimic elevation of the diaphragm by permitting herniation of the liver into the right hemithorax. This diagnosis should be considered when there is a history of significant abdominal or chest trauma and the appearance of a high right hemidiaphragm.

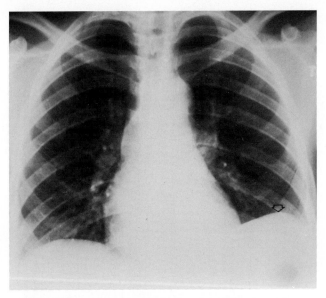

FIG 6–2
Observe that the left hemidiaphragm is not only elevated but domes more laterally *(arrowhead)* than the normal right side, suggesting a subpulmonic pleural effusion.

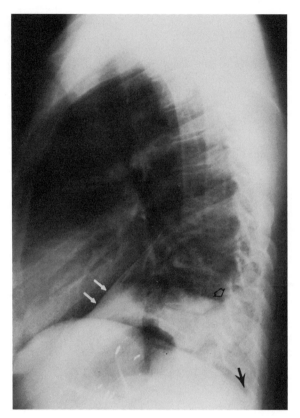

FIG 6–3
Lateral projection film from case illustrated in Figure 6–2 reveals sharp right costophrenic angle *(black arrow)*, but blunting of the left costophrenic angle *(open arrowhead)*. Only the posterior portion of left hemidiaphragm appears elevated; it appears to end at the major fissure *(white arrows)*. This unusual appearance is another clue to a subpulmonic pleural effusion mimicking elevation of the left hemidiaphragm.

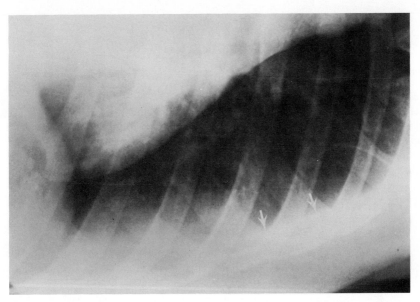

FIG 6–4
Lateral decubitus film from the case illustrated in Figures 6–2 and 6–3 confirms the diagnosis of free pleural fluid. Note opacity between the lung and ribs *(arrows)*.

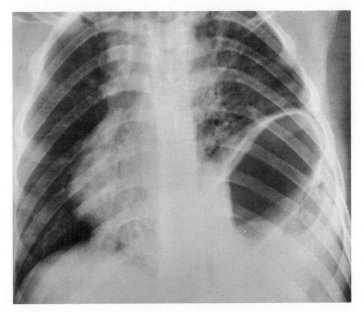

FIG 6–5
This is a common appearance for traumatic rupture of the left hemidiaphragm. The elevated, air-filled stomach following thoracoabdominal trauma should strongly suggest this diagnosis. Also, notice the shift of the mediastinum to the right, indicating a space-occupying abnormality in the lower left thorax.

ANSWER GUIDE

LEGEND FOR INTRODUCTORY FIGURE

FIG 6–1
Elevated right hemidiaphragm in this patient with bronchogenic carcinoma could have resulted from phrenic nerve paralysis, but the film reveals additional findings of right upperlobe atelectasis. Note inxXcreased opacity and elevation of the minor fissure.

ANSWERS

1, c; 2, b; 3, a.

CHAPTER 7

Shift of the Mediastinum

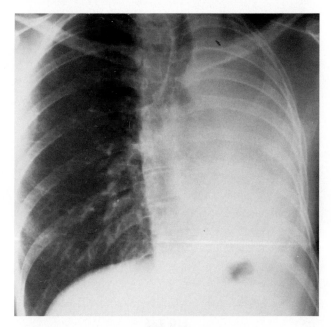

FIG 7–1

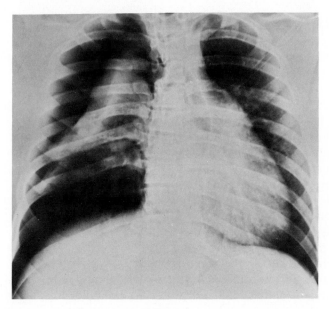

FIG 7–2

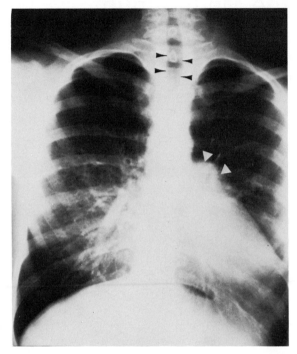

FIG 7–3

QUESTIONS

1. Regarding the case shown in Figure 7–1, which of the following statements is incorrect?
   a. The right lung is hyperinflated.
   b. There is herniation of right lung in front of the ascending aorta.
   c. The left pleural effusion is compressing the left lung.
   d. Endobronchial mass or mucous plug should be considered.
   e. The most significant abnormality may not be visible on this film.
2. Referring to Figure 7–2, indicate which one of the following statements is not true of tension pneumothorax.
   a. Collections of air may mimic the appearance of herniation of lung through the mediastinum.
   b. Shift of the mediastinum may be life threatening.
   c. Air may collect medial to the lung.
   d. Air may collect in the azygoesophageal recess.
   e. There is always complete collapse of the lung.
3. Referring to Figure 7–3, identify which of the following diagnoses would be most likely to result in shift of the heart without shift of the aorta or trachea.
   a. Tension pneumothorax.
   b. Partial absence of the pericardium.
   c. Foreign body in the bronchus.
   d. Lobar emphysema.
   e. Bullous emphysema.

CHART 7–1.
Shift of the Mediastinum

I. Decreased lung volume
  A. Atelectasis
  B. Hypoplastic lung
  C. Postoperative (lobectomy, pneumonectomy)
II. Increased lung volume
  A. Foreign body obstructing large bronchus (common in children)
  B. Bronchiolitis obliterans (Swyer-James syndrome) (rare)
  C. Bullous emphysema
  D. Congenital lobar emphysema (only in infants)[149]
  E. Interstitial emphysema
  F. Bronchogenic cyst (usually in infants)
  G. Cystic adenomatoid malformation (only in infants)
  H. Large masses (pulmonary, mediastinal)
III. Pleural space abnormalities[606]
  A. Large unilateral pleural effusion[378]
  B. Tension pneumothorax
  C. Large diaphragmatic hernias (usually either congenital or posttraumatic)
  D. Large masses
IV. Other
  A. Partial absence of the pericardium (shift of heart)

DISCUSSION

Shift of the mediastinum is identified by displacement of the heart, trachea, aorta, and hilar vessels. Since shift of the mediastinum indicates an imbalance of pressures between the two sides of the thorax, one of the first steps in the evaluation of this problem is to determine which side is abnormal. Associated findings are frequently helpful in making this determination. For example, atelectasis is frequently associated with elevation of the hemidiaphragm and crowding of the ribs, as well as increased opacity of the lung. It is also frequently accompanied by hyperexpansion of the contralateral side of the chest, which is described as compensatory overaeration or emphysema. In the absence of diaphragmatic elevation, the possibility that the hyperexpanded lung is the abnormal one has to be considered; the hyperexpanded lung could be compressing the normal lung with the result of increased opacity on the normal side. The radiologist has two tools for making this determination. The best-known method is the expiratory film, which will demonstrate that air moves freely from the overexpanded side when it is the normal side and will show that the underexpanded lung is essentially unchanged and thus atelectic; in contrast, air trapping in a hyperexpanded lung will be exaggerated. When the patient is unable to cooperate, the best substitute for the expiratory film is the lateral decubitus film. In this procedure the overexpanded side should be down, with the effect of splinting the down side. The radiologic result is similar to that in the expiratory film. An overexpanded side that remains overexpanded in the down position indicates bronchial obstruction with obstructive overaeration. The lateral decubitus film is particularly helpful in a child who has a foreign body in the bronchus. If the overexpanded lung resumes normal size in the down position, the smaller lung can be assumed to be abnormal.

Another method of evaluating shift of the mediastinum is fluoroscopy. In the case of atelectasis that has resulted from an endobronchial mass, deep inspiration will cause the mediastinum to shift more toward the side of the atelectasis, while the diaphragm moves normally on the hyperexpanded side. Fluoroscopic examination will reveal that air trapping causes shifting of the mediastinum away from the lucent side during forced expiration, while the lung that is hyperexpanded to compensate for volume loss on the opposite side will decrease its size normally during expiration.

Decreased Lung Volume

Loss of lung volume is an important cause of shift of the mediastinum. The case shown in Figure 7–1 illustrates shift of the mediastinum caused by a bronchogenic carcinoma arising in the left main bronchus. There is total atelectasis of the left lung with compensatory hyperinflation of the right lung and herniation of lung through the anterior mediastinum. There is no evidence of left pleural fluid. (Answer to question 1 is *c.*) The various types of atelectasis that are considered in Chapter 13 may all result in shift of the mediastinum. It should also be apparent that lobectomy and pneumonectomy are common causes of mediastinal shift. In fact, shift of the heart and mediastinum accounts for much of the thoracic opacity that follows pneumonectomy.

Hypoplastic lung is a rare anomaly resulting in a characteristic radiologic appearance consisting of a small hemithorax with crowding of the ribs, elevation of the hemidiaphragm, shift of the mediastinum, and an absent or very small pulmonary artery to the involved side. In addition to the small or absent hilar pulmonary artery, the peripheral vascularity of the involved lung is primarily bronchial, with small, irregular vessels lacking the normal hilar orientation of pulmonary arteries. This phenomenon is usually referred to as the hypogenetic lung or congenital venolobar syndrome.[665] It is most often seen on the right, and it is frequently associated with dextrocardia and anomalous pulmonary venous return from the right lung to the inferior vena cava. When the anomalous venous drainage is roentgenographically visible as a large vein coursing through the right lung to the inferior vena cava, the so-called scimitar syndrome is said to be present. Signs of decreased size of the lung with shift of the mediastinum or elevation of the diaphragm need not be present to suggest the diagnosis of hypogenetic lung syndrome when the characteristic vascular changes are present (Fig 7–4).

Increased Lung Volume

A foreign body obstructing a mainstem bronchus is a common cause of air trapping in children.[186] This typically leads to a hyperlucent lung with shift of the mediastinum toward the opaque but normal side (Fig 7–5, *A* and *B*). In effect, this is a ball-valve obstruction of the bronchus that permits air to enter the lung but obstructs outflow. Collateral air drift also appears to contribute to the overexpansion. Collateral air drift through the pores of Kohn and canals of Lambert is not a bidirectional process; it only permits air to enter an alveolus and thus contributes to the hyperexpansion distal to a bronchial obstruction. It must be remembered that the interlobar fissures are commonly incomplete, and that collateral pathways between lobes may exist.

Bronchiolitis obliterans[397] is a small airway obstructive disease that is well known for producing the Swyer-James syndrome. This is a radiologic syndrome that consists of a unilateral hyperlucent lung (see Chapter 22). The history frequently reveals a previous viral pulmonary infection. Biopsy has shown these patients to have small airway obstructive disease. Some reports have suggested that these patients do not have significant air trapping; however, there have been instances of considerable air trapping resulting in shift of the mediastinum and herniation of the overexpanded lungs through the mediastinum.

The localized form of bullous emphysema may cause considerable overexpansion of one side of the chest.[185, 186] This usually assumes a characteristic radiologic appearance because of the large avascular areas of the lung and the thin linear opacities that separate the bullae (see Chapter 22).

Congenital lobar emphysema[149] is another entity that causes overexpansion of one lobe and may therefore result in shift of the mediastinum. It has been observed only in infants. The hyperexpanded lobe frequently herniates through the mediastinum and may lead to serious respiratory insufficiency by compressing the normal lung. There is diminished vasculature in the overexpanded lobe, with the result of a large hyperlucency (Fig 7–6). Congenital lobar emphysema most commonly involves an upper lobe, but has been reported in the right middle lobe. It should be easily distinguished from large cystic structures such as cystic adenomatoid malformations and bronchogenic cysts. Both of the latter may become very large, leading to shift of the mediastinum with respiratory compromise, but both are cystic structures that should have well-defined walls. Lobar emphysema should not result in any increased opacities unless the entire lobe is homogeneously filled with fluid. In the latter case, the appearance may mimic a large mass lesion with displacement of the mediastinum. Interstitial dissection of air (interstitial emphysema) is another process that may rarely produce a unilateral expanded lung with shift of the mediastinum. Since the normal vascular markings are outlined with air, there is a pattern of diffuse, course lines (Fig 7–7), which should distinguish interstitial emphysema from lobar emphysema. Unilateral involvement typically occurs as a residual effect of diffuse interstitial emphysema. Interstitial emphysema is a common complication of positive pressure ventilation therapy and should be suspected on the basis of history and serial roentgenograms.

Both bronchogenic cyst and cystic adenomatoid malformation are possible causes of shift of the mediastinum in infants and children. The bronchogenic cyst should present as a solitary structure. The rare cyst that results in shift of the mediastinum is usually air filled. The cyst probably has a connection with the bronchus, which is partially obstructed by a sleeve valve mechanism that permits air to enter but not to leave the cyst. When this results in massive overdistention of the cyst, the mediastinum may be shifted secondarily (Fig 7–8).

Cystic adenomatoid malformation[376] is a more complex foregut anomaly consisting of multiple cystic structures that, like the bronchogenic cyst, may become overdistended with air and appear to herniate through and shift the mediastinum (see Chapter 24).

Masses constitute an infrequent cause of mediastinal shift. When they become large enough to shift the mediastinum, it is usually difficult to determine their precise site of origin (Fig 7–9). Unusually large masses are frequently benign or of low-grade malignancy. It is true that bronchogenic carcinoma often causes shifting of the mediastinum, but the shift is the result of atelectasis rather than a large, bulky mass. In the case of atelectasis, the shift is toward the side of the carcinoma, whereas very large masses shift the mediastinum to the side opposite the mass.

Pleural Space Abnormalities

A massive increase in the content of the pleural space may dramatically compress the lung and shift the mediastinum.[606] This may occur with either fluid or air in the pleural space. Pleural effusion may result in a virtually opaque hemithorax before the mediastinum begins to shift (Fig 7–10) (see Chapter 4). In these cases the underlying lung parenchyma will be completely obscured. Correlation with clinical findings is often helpful in identifying the more common causes of effusion, such as metastases, emphysema, and congestive heart failure.[378] Thoracentesis is the most direct method of establishing the diagnosis. If the entire thorax is filled with fluid without shift of the mediastinum, the mediastinum is probably fixed, which suggests a metastatic tumor, malignant mesothelioma, or extensive fibrosis (as might be seen with fibrosing mediastinitis).

Tension pneumothorax is a medical emergency. It is the result of a leak from the lung into the pleural space. As the patient takes a deep breath, additional air enters the pleural space and the tension is increased. Total collapse of the lung may be a relatively late complication in tension pneumothorax. Often, the first detectable signs of tension are a shift of the mediastinum and depression of the diaphragm (see Fig 7–2). As the pressure increases, there may be displacement of the anterior and posterior junction lines. On the PA film this will have the appearance of a large lucency collecting above the heart. Air may also collect in the azygoesophageal recess behind the heart. This resembles herniation of lung through the mediastinum, except that the lung is collapsed away from the area of lucency. All of the statements in question 2 are true except *e*: There is *not* always complete collapse of the lung. This is especially true in patients with either emphysema or diffuse interstitial disease, which may prevent complete collapse owing to abnormal compliance.

A less common cause of shift of the mediastinum is a large diaphragmatic hernia. In these patients, either the small bowel may be herniated into the chest or, in the case of a right-sided hernia, the liver may be herniated into the right thorax. Both of these abnormalities are usually congenital and, because of their severity, are usually detected in the neonatal period. Herniated bowel produces a bubbly appearance because of the air-containing loops of bowel, while the liver produces an opaque hemithorax.

Another entity that may mimic shift of the mediastinum is partial absence of the pericardium, which results in shift of the heart. This should be suspected when there is a striking shift of the heart in the absence of shift of the trachea, aorta, or other borders of the mediastinum (see Fig 7–3). (Answer to question 3 is *b*.)

SUMMARY

1. Shift of the mediastinum indicates a severe asymmetry of intrathoracic pressures.

2. Pulmonary abnormalities that result in shift of the mediastinum include both increase and decrease in pulmonary volume.

3. Atelectasis is the most common cause of decreased pulmonary volume leading to shift of the mediastinum.

4. Increased lung volume in infancy is most likely due to congenital lobar emphysema or cystic adenomatoid malformation, but interstitial emphysema may be unilateral, resulting in shift of the mediastinum.

5. A foreign body in a bronchus is the most likely cause of air trapping during childhood.

6. Tension pneumothorax is a life-threatening emergency that appears with shift of the mediastinum.

7. Large pleural effusions result in shift of the mediastinum when there is nearly complete opacification of one side of the thorax. The absence of a shift implies fixation of the mediastinum either by tumor or fibrosis or by a combination of atelectasis and effusion.

8. Partial absence of the pericardium permits shift of the heart and may therefore mimic shift of the mediastinum. It is recognized by observing that other mediastinal structures are in a normal position.

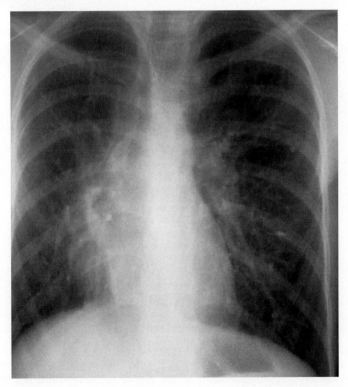

FIG 7–4
PA chest shows shift of the mediastinum to the right. A small right hilum is partially obscured by an overlying anomalous vein from the right upper lobe. This is an example of hypogenetic right lung with scimitar syndrome.

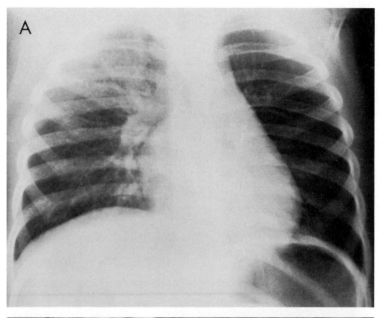

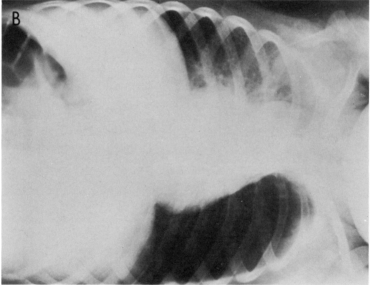

FIG 7–5
A, A young child was admitted with wheezes. The right upper lobe is abnormally
opaque, and the left lung is hyperlucent. Subtle shift of mediastinum to the right is not
diagnostic, since either right upper lobe collapse or air trapping on the left would shift
the mediastinum to the right. **B,** Lateral decubitus film of case illustrated in A (taken
with left side down) emphasizes shift of mediastinum and confirms the presence of air
trapping on the left, virtually confirming the diagnosis of a foreign body in the left
bronchus. (Case courtesy of Jeffrey Blum, M.D.)

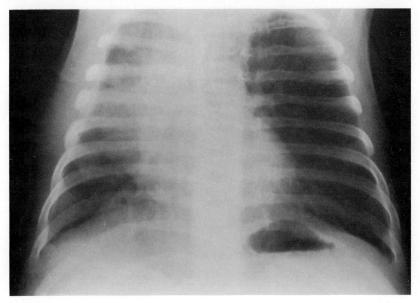

FIG 7–6
Combination of hyperlucent left lung, shift of mediastinum to the right, and flattening of left hemidiaphragm in this newborn infant is essentially diagnostic of congenital lobar emphysema.

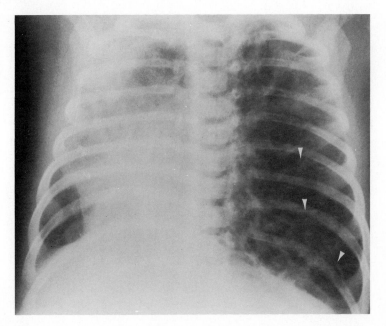

FIG 7–7
This infant had signs of air trapping on the left similar to those seen in Figure 7–5. The additional finding of a coarse reticular pattern *(arrowheads)* is not consistent with un-complicated lobar emphysema. The reticular pattern is the result of normal interstitial and vascular markings, which are accentuated by interstitial emphysema. (Case courtesy of Herman Grossman, M.D.)

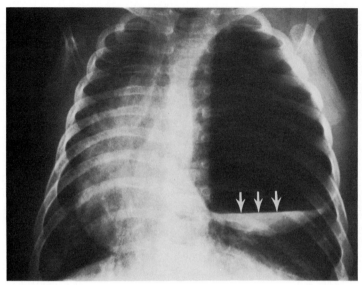

FIG 7–8
Shift of mediastinum to the right and hyperlucency of left side of the chest are similar to the cases illustrated in Figure 7–5 and 7–6. The air-fluid level *(arrows)* indicates the presence of a single large space, incompatible with lobar emphysema. This is a very large bronchogenic cyst.

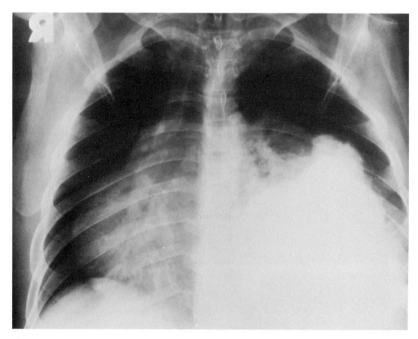

FIG 7–9
Very large calcified mass that has shifted the mediastinum is difficult to identify as a mediastinal mass because of its size. It is a schwannoma arising from the posterior mediastinum. (From Reed JC, Hallet KK, Feagin DS: Neural tumors of the thorax: subject review from the AFIP. *Radiology* 1978;126:9–17. Used by permission.)

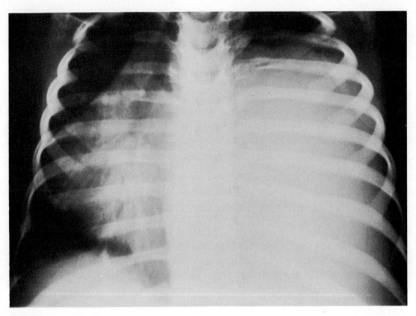

FIG 7–10
Loculated empyema has resulted in large left pleural mass that has shifted the mediastinum.

ANSWER GUIDE

LEGENDS FOR INTRODUCTORY FIGURES

FIG 7–1
Shift of the mediastinum and complete opacification of the left hemithorax are the result of complete atelectasis of the left lung caused by a bronchogenic carcinoma arising in the left main bronchus. Note the shift of the trachea and the heart.

FIG 7–2
Tension pneumothorax is diagnosed by observing shift of the mediastinum or depression of the diaphragm in a patient with pneumothorax. The lung may not be totally collapsed, even in the presence of increasing positive pressure.

FIG 7–3
Shift of heart to the left might suggest mediastinal shift, but the midline position of the trachea *(black arrowheads)* argues against this diagnosis. Prominent left atrial appendage *(white arrowheads)* is typical of partial absence of the pericardium (Case courtesy of James T.T. Chen, M.D.)

ANSWERS

  1, c; 2, e; 3, b.

CHAPTER 8

Widening of the Mediastinum

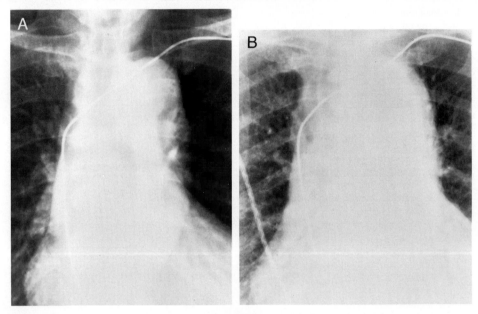

FIG 8–1

QUESTIONS

1. Referring to Figure 8–1, *B*, indicate which is the most likely diagnosis in this patient with chest pain. Figure 8–1, *A* was taken 13 months before the patient's presentation.
   a. Bronchogenic carcinoma.
   b. Lymphoma.
   c. Transection of the aorta.
   d. Dissecting aortic aneurysm.
   e. Lipomatosis.
2. Which of the following statements about mediastinal hematomas are true?
   a. Often obscure the aortic arch and descending aorta.
   b. May indicate aortic transection.
   c. May be caused by vertebral fractures.
   d. May occur when sternal fractures injure internal mammary vessels.
   e. All of the above.

CHART 8–1.
Widening of the Mediastinum

  I. Radiographic technique
   A. Magnification (AP supine film, low-volume inspiration)
   B. Lordotic position[278]
 II. Vascular structures (nontraumatic)
   A. Tortuous atherosclerotic dilatation of aorta
   B. Aneurysm
   C. Aortic dissection[296]
   D. Coarctation of aorta[667]
   E. Congenital left superior vena cava (SVC) with absent right SVC[637]
III. Trauma
   A. Hematoma
      1. Transection of aorta[666]
      2. Venous and arterial tears
      3. Sternal fractures
      4. Vertebral fractures (thoracic and lower cervical spine)[125]
      5. Postoperative
      6. Malposition of vascular catheters (also the cause of hydromediastinum[267])
 IV. Neoplasms
   A. Lymphoma
   B. Primary bronchogenic carcinoma (small cell tumors)
   C. Metastases
  V. Inflammation
   A. Mediastinitis
      1. Perforated esophagus (Boerhaave's syndrome, carcinomas)
      2. Tracheobronchial rupture (traumatic)[179]
      3. Iatrogenic[52] (postoperative, endoscopic)
      4. Pneumonias
      5. Tuberculosis[653]
      6. Coccidioidomycosis
      7. Histoplasmosis[157, 645]
      8. Actinomycosis
      9. Fibrosing or sclerosing mediastinitis[322, 390]
   B. Granulomatous adenopathy
      1. *Mycobacterium avium-intracellulare* (in patients with acquired immune deficiency syndrome [AIDS][328])
      2. Tuberculosis[290]
      3. Coccidioidomycosis
   C. Extension of extrathoracic infections
      1. Pharyngeal abscess
      2. Abdominal abscess
      3. Pancreatitis or pancreatic pseudocyst
 VI. Lipomatosis[280, 464, 590]
   A. Cushing's syndrome
   B. Corticosteroid therapy
   C. Obesity
   D. Normal variant
VII. Other
   A. Chylomediastinum[179] (thoracic duct obstruction or iatrogenic laceration)
   B. Mediastinal edema (allergic)[179]
   C. Penetrating trauma (stab wound)
   D. Achalasia

DISCUSSION

Diffuse mediastinal widening is a common observation on the PA film. It is more difficult to identify confidently on a supine AP film because of magnification and crowding of normal vascular structures by the splinting effect on the patient's chest. In addition, the lordotic projection distorts and magnifies the superior mediastinum.[278] This is a common problem in the patient who is unable to voluntarily make a deep inspiratory effort, and it is a serious consideration in the emergency department or an intensive care unit in which the critically ill patient must be evaluated with portable supine radiographs.

Determining the cause of the mediastinal widening is even more difficult than recognizing the presence of an abnormality, especially in older patients with atherosclerotic vascular disease that leads to tortuosity of the aorta and great vessels. Patients who have had cardiac or vascular surgery are easily recognized by the radiographic identification of surgical clips and metal sutures, but this may further confuse the evaluation of mediastinal widening. These patients may have both tortuous vessels and postoperative abnormalities, including hematomas during the acute convalescent period and, later, mediastinal scarring. A mass lesion that develops subsequent to mediastinal or cardiac surgery may be obscured by postoperative changes.

The plain film analysis must begin with the identification of as many normal structures as possible, including the ascending aorta, aortic arch, descending aorta, aortic pulmonary window, trachea, paratracheal stripes, carina, mainstem bronchi, and paraspinous stripes. Failure to visualize these landmarks requires an explanation and may be an indication for additional procedures including CT, MRI, or even angiography.

Vascular Structures

Aortic and vascular tortuosities are most often the result of atherosclerotic disease and are very frequent in elderly patients. Dilatation of the ascending aorta is observed in patients with severe hypertension and may also result from aortic stenosis. The tortuous aorta must be distinguished from aortic aneurysms, aortic dissection, and even mass lesions (Fig 8–2, *A–C*). When the entire aorta is extremely dilated and tortuous, the abnormality may be regarded as a long fusiform aneurysm.

Dissection of the aorta results from an intimal tear followed by intramural hematoma. Complete dissection occurs when there are multiple tears permitting blood to flow through the aortic wall and creating a false lumen. The patient may be asymptomatic, but typically presents with retrosternal chest pain, syncope, and signs of peripheral vascular arterial occlusion.

The most frequent plain film findings in dissection of the aorta include mediastinal widening and enlargement of the aortic arch and descending aorta (see Fig 8–1, *A* and *B*). Other findings may include enlargement of the ascending aorta, blurring of the aortic arch, soft tissue opacity lateral to calcification in the aortic arch, deviation of the trachea or a nasogastric tube, a wide paraspinal stripe, and pericardial and pleural effusions. The finding of widening of the mediastinum and aortic arch should be followed by CT[255] or MRI[207] in patients who are clinically stable. Aortography is preferred for those patients who are hemodynamically unstable and are candidates for emergency surgery. It provides precise anatomic detail and permits application of the DeBakey classification, in which type I dissections start at the aortic root and extend to the descending aorta and are often associated with aortic insufficiency; type II dissections involve only the ascending aorta and sometimes the brachiocephalic vessels; and type III dissections arise near the origin of the left subclavian artery and extend down the descending aorta.

Trauma

Transection of the aorta is one of the most urgent diagnoses to be considered following major trauma. The reported plain film findings include mediastinal widening (greater than 8.5 cm), a mediastinal-width/chest-width ratio (greater than 25%), a wide right paratracheal stripe (>5 mm), a left apical cap, deviation of a tracheal or nasogastric tube to the right, and pleural effusion (Fig 8–3, *A*). These are all signs suggestive of mediastinal hemorrhage, but they are not specific for aortic transection. A CT scan may occassionaly make the correct diagnosis of aortic transections (Fig 8–3, *B*), but more often it confirms the presence of a mediastinal hematoma without revealing the source of bleeding. Furthermore, CT may be time consuming and entail dangerous delay. Aortography (Fig 8–4, *A* and *B*) should be performed as soon as possible in patients suspected of having an aortic rupture on the basis of the plain film criteria previously described or on the basis of clinical suspicion.

Mediastinal hematomas following acute trauma have been well documented as resulting from injuries to structures other than the aorta, including internal mammary vessels and the superior vena cava, and fractures of the sternum, posterior ribs, and thoracic and lower cervical vertebrae (Fig 8–5, *A* and *B*). While these findings may explain the source of a mediastinal hematoma, they do not exclude the possibility of associated aortic injury and should therefore not be used as a reason to avoid aortography.

Neoplasms

Mediastinal tumors are expected to produce discrete masses, but neoplasms that involve multiple lymph node groups may cause diffuse mediastinal widening. This type of tumor dissemination results from lymphomas and from metastases of primary lung cancer and distant primaries. It is particularly common with poorly differentiated primary tumors such as small cell undifferentiated tumors. Such extensive nodal involvement may also be seen with metastases from retroperitoneal tumors and even from testicular tumors, particularly seminomas.

Hodgkin's lymphoma frequently involves mediastinal lymph nodes (Fig 8–6). When the involvement is extensive, the massive nodes may diffusely widen the mediastinum. The tumor should regress following chemotherapy, but the nodes may be replaced by extensive fibrosis that may leave residual mediastinal widening. This is most often recognized by identification of the paramediastinal reticular opacities that result from mediastinal fibrosis. Occasionally, the postradiation change may appear to become more prominent over a short period, requiring further consideration of recurrent tumor vs. radiation-induced change. Increasing opacity from the radiation effect on the mediastinum might be further evaluated with an MR scan, which has been reported to be useful for identifying viable tumor in the midst of postradiation scarring.

Infections

Mediastinal infection may take the form of diffuse mediastinitis or abscess (Fig 8–7). These two may even coexist. Acute infections may enter the mediastinum by direct extension from a nasopharyngeal abscess, subphrenic abscess, pancreatic pseudocyst, pneumonia, or empyema. Infection may also result from spontaneous esophageal perforation (Boerhaave's syndrome), rupture of an esophageal carcinoma, iatrogenic esophageal perforation from endoscopy, or dilatation of an esophageal stricture. Perforation of either the esophagus or the tracheobronchial tree also causes mediastinal emphysema, which will often precede the mediastinitis and may be the initial cause of mediastinal widening. Mediastinitis has been reported as an infrequent but serious complication of cardiovascular surgery. [52]

Granulomatous infections, including tuberculosis,[653] coccidioidomycosis, and histoplasmosis, may also produce diffuse mediastinitis (Fig 8–8, *A* and *B*). While mediastinal adenopathy is a common manifestation of primary tuberculosis, diffuse involvement of the mediastinal nodes by tuberculosis is rare except in patients who are immunologically compromised. Histoplasmosis is the most common cause of chronic mediastinitis and fibrosis.[645] This typically produces a smooth, tapered mediastinal widening that is most severe in the right superior mediastinum and often leads to superior vena caval obstruction.[152] In contrast, superior vena caval obstruction by a tumor is caused by a lobulated mass that may be demonstrated in a superior vena cavogram or CT scan. Additionally, histoplasmosis may cause pulmonary venous and arterial obstruction leading to cor pulmonale and death.[646]

Lipomatosis

Mediastinal lipomatosis is a benign cause of diffuse mediastinal widening (Fig 8–9),[209, 464, 590] and may suggest the diagnosis of diffuse mediastinal adenopathy. Some signs that help to suggest this diagnosis include (1) a large mediastinum without indentation on the trachea, (2) smooth contours of pleural lines, and (3) a prominent epicardial fat pad. While fat appears similar to soft tissue when compared with the opacity of the aerated lung on a plain film, the diagnosis of lipomatosis should be easily confirmed with a CT scan.[288] The condition will cause an attenuation intermediate between that of the normal soft tissue structures of the mediastinum and the lower attenuation of the aerated lung. Mediastinal lipomatosis may result from Cushing's syndrome, corticosteroid therapy, or exogenous obesity, or it may be a normal variant.

SUMMARY

1. Acute posttraumatic mediastinal widening with loss of definition of the aortic arch or descending aorta should be considered suspicious for aortic transection.

2. Atherosclerotic tortuosity of the aorta is very common in the elderly. A change in aortic size or definition is suggestive of dissection. This diagnosis may be confirmed with contrast-enhanced CT, MRI, or aortography.

3. Tortuosities of the aorta and great vessels may obscure mediastinal masses.

4. Neoplasms that involve mediastinal nodes may diffusely widen the mediastinum.

5. Mediastinitis may result from bacterial and granulomatous infections, esophageal perforation, and extension of extrathoracic abscesses.

6. Lipomatosis is a benign cause of mediastinal widening.

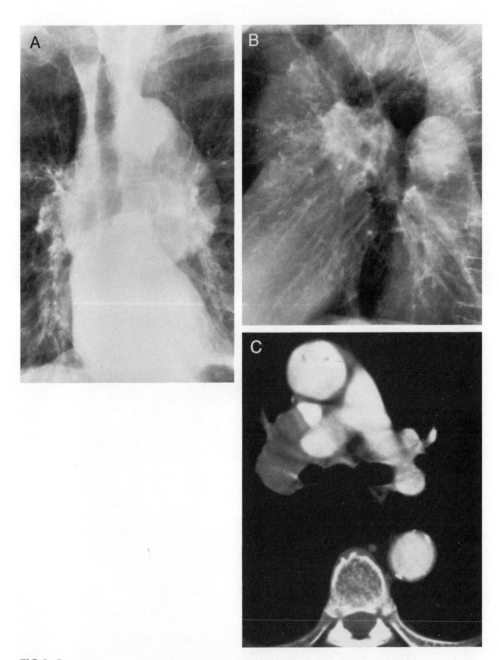

FIG 8–2
A, Large tortuous aorta must be distinguished from aneurysm and could obscure a mass in the mediastinum or either hilum. **B,** Lateral view reveals dilated ascending aorta and acute tortuosity of the descending aorta. Also note the increased opacity of the hila projected between the aortic opacities. **C,** Contrast-enhanced CT scan, performed to exclude the diagnosis of aneurysm, confirmed the thoracic aorta to be very tortuous with an upper abdominal aneurysm (not shown). The scan also confirmed right hilar adenopathy caused by small cell carcinoma.

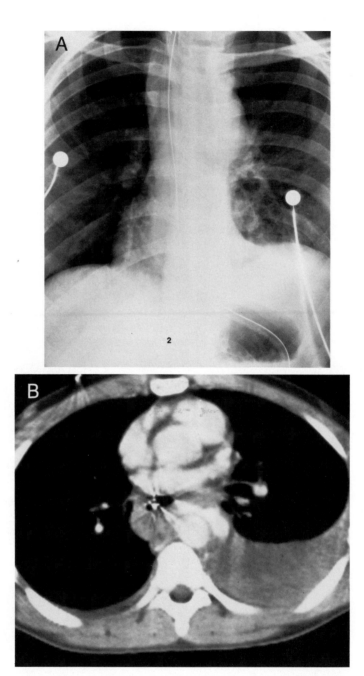

FIG 8–3
A, This motor vehicle accident victim developed a wide mediastinum and left subpulmonic pleural effusion, with deviation of a nasogastric tube to the right. **B,** Contrast-
enhanced CT scan shows a large left effusion and extraluminal contrast medium around
the descending aorta, indicating aortic transection.

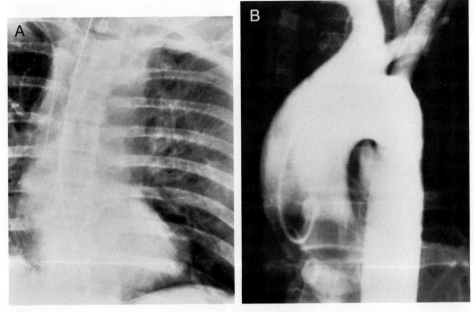

FIG 8—4
A, Wide mediastinum, loss of definition of the aortic arch and descending aorta, left apical pleural cap, and deviation of a nasogastric tube and trachea are indications for aortography. **B,** Aortogram confirms the suspected transection of the aorta.

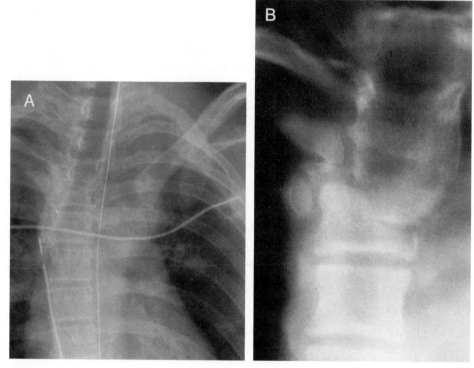

FIG 8–5
A, Wide mediastinum, loss of definition of the aortic arch, and apical cap indicate mediastinal hematoma, but this patient had a normal aortogram. **B,** Tomogram of upper thoracic spine better demonstrates the fracture dislocation that caused the mediastinal
hematoma.

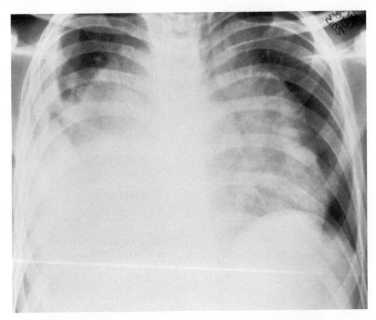

FIG 8–6
Hodgkin's lymphoma may diffusely widen the mediastinum by massively infiltrating multiple lymph node groups. Metastases, particularly from small cell tumors, may also produce this appearance. This patient also has a large, malignant right pleural effusion.

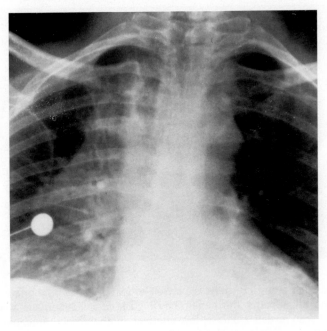

FIG 8–7
Acute mediastinitis from extrathoracic infections should be suspected from the clinical presentation. This patient has a retropharyngeal abscess. An admission film taken 5 days earlier was normal.

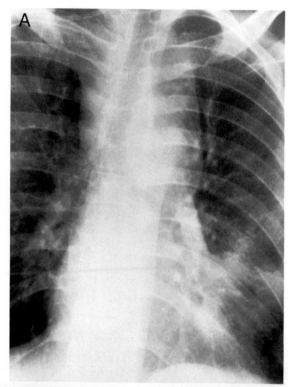

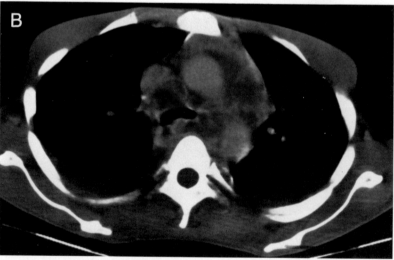

FIG 8–8
A, Primary granulomatous infections are a well-known cause of pulmonary consolidation and mediastinal adenopathy. This patient has lingular consolidation and a wide mediastinum. **B,** CT scan reveals a diffuse, low-attenuation abnormality spreading through the soft tissues of the mediastinum. This is acute tuberculous mediastinitis. (Case courtesy of Thomas L. Pope, Jr., M.D.)

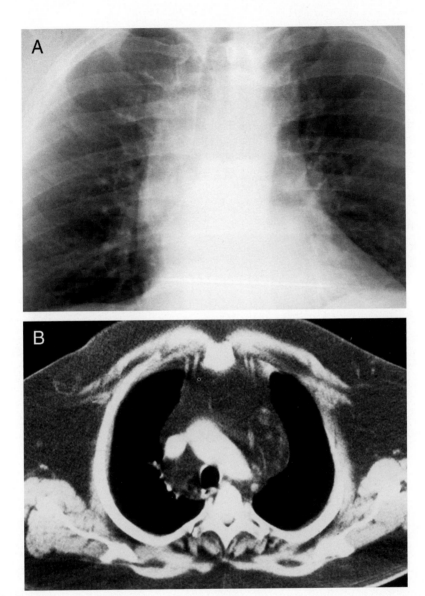

FIG 8–9
A, Mediastinal lipomastosis is a benign fatty infiltration that may diffusely widen the mediastinum. The fat is intermediate in opacity and may not obscure normal soft tissue structures such as the aorta. Note that the left mediastinal pleural interface with the lung is lateral to the aorta. **B,** CT confirms the diagnosis of mediastinal lipomatosis.

ANSWER GUIDE

LEGENDS TO INTRODUCTORY FIGURES

FIG 8–1
A, Tortuous aorta accounts for wide mediastinum. Observe the sharply defined aortic arch and descending aorta. **B,** This film was taken 13 months later. The patient presented with acute chest pain. The widening of the aorta has increased as a result of aortic dissection.

ANSWERS

1, d; 2, e.

CHAPTER 9

Anterior Mediastinal Mass

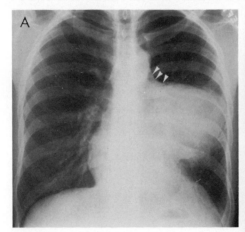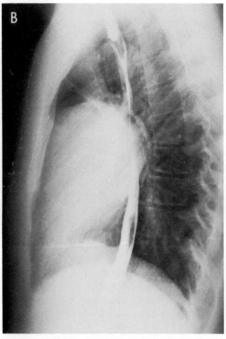

FIG 9–1

QUESTIONS

1. Referring to Figure 9–1, *A* and *B* (PA and lateral-projection chest films in a 20-year-old man), indicate which of the following diagnoses is most likely.
    a. Goiter.
    b. Thymoma.
    c. Teratoma.
    d. Cystic hygroma.
    e. Pericardial cyst.
2. Which of the following tumors is most likely to spread contiguously and is unlikely to metastasize to distant sites?
    a. Malignant thymoma.
    b. Thyroid carcinoma.
    c. Malignant teratoma.
    d. Lymphoma.
    e. Thymic carcinoid.
3. Which of the following is least likely to calcify?
    a. Substernal thyroid.
    b. Thymic cyst.
    c. Thymoma.
    d. Dermoid Cyst.

CHART 9–1.
Anterior Mediastinal Mass

I. Thymic lesions[508]
   A. Thymoma (benign and malignant)[416]
   B. Thymic cyst[670]
   C. Thymolipoma[507, 601]
   D. Lymphoma
   E. Thymic hyperplasia
   F. Thymic carcinoid tumor[49]
II. Teratoid lesions
   A. Dermoid cyst
   B. Teratoma (benign and malignant)[352]
   C. Embryonal cell carcinoma
   D. Choriocarcinoma
   E. Seminoma[275]
III. Thyroid
   A. Goiter
   B. Adenoma
   C. Carcinoma
IV. Lymph nodes[80]
   A. Lymphoma (both Hodgkin's and non-Hodgkin's)
   B. Metastases
   C. Benign lymph node hyperplasia
   D. Angioblastic lymphoid adenopathy
   E. Sarcoidosis[39] and granulomatous infections (rare)
V. Cardiovascular
   A. Epicardial fat pad
   B. Aneurysm of ascending aorta[570]
   C. Aneurysm of sinus of Valsalva[447, 494]
   D. Dilated superior vena cava
   E. Pericardial cyst[163]
   F. Cardiac tumors
   G. Traumatic false aneurysm of common carotid artery[545]
VI. Cysts
   A. Cystic hygroma (lymphangioma)[373]
   B. Bronchogenic cysts
   C. Extralobar sequestration
   D. (See thymic and teratoid lesions, above)
VII. Other
   A. Neural tumors of vagus or phrenic nerves[439, 483]
   B. Paraganglioma (chemodectoma and pheochromocytoma)[483]
   C. Hernia of the foramen of Morgagni[41]
   D. Parathyroid adenoma,[549] adenocarcinoma
   E. Primary bone tumors and metastases to the sternum
   F. Lipoma,[209, 352] lipomatosis[280]
   G. Hemangioma[118]
   H. Pancreatic pseudocyst[317]

CHART 9–2.
Inlet Lesion from the Neck into the Superior Mediastinum

I. Thyroid masses
II. Cystic hygroma
III. Lymphoma
IV. Metastases

CHART 9–3.
Right Cardiophrenic Angle Mass

   I. Epicardial fat pad
  II. Pericardial cyst (mesothelial cyst)
 III. Aneurysm
  IV. Dilated right atrium
   V. Diaphragmatic lesion
  VI. Other anterior mediastinal masses (Chart 9–1)
 VII. Primary lung mass
VIII. Hernia of the foramen of Morgagni

DISCUSSION

The anterior mediastinum contains the thymus, lymph nodes, vessels, and fat. There is considerable variation in the normal width of the mediastinum on the PA film and in the size and opacity of the retrosternal clear space on the lateral film. These variations result from differences in the shape and size of vessels and fat content.[339] When there is minimal anterior fat, both lungs extend in front of the ascending aorta, pressing all four layers of pleura together to form the anterior junction line. Masses are visible on the PA and lateral films when they displace the mediastinal pleura and alter the normal mediastinal contour. Visibility is mainly determined by the interface of the mass with the aerated lung, but soft tissue masses that are surrounded by fat may appear as minimally visible opacities that often require CT for confirmation.[258]

Once the presence of a mediastinal mass has been confirmed, precise localization of the mass is the most important aspect of plain film evaluation. Strict anatomic divisions of the mediastinum are not easily translated to the lateral chest film. The anatomy texts divide the mediastinum into four compartments: superior, anterior, middle, and posterior. When this division is applied to the lateral chest film, we should consider a fifth compartment corresponding anatomically to the posterior gutter. These anatomic divisions of the mediastinal compartments were established before the development of chest radiology. Felson [162] was one of the first to recognize the cumbersome nature of applying anatomic definitions to the lateral chest film and devised a simplified method based on easily identifiable radiologic landmarks. He divided the anterior and middle compartments by drawing a line from the intersection of the anterior border of the trachea with the sternum to intersect the diaphragm. This line follows the posterior border of the heart and the inferior vena cava. A second line, 1 cm posterior to the anterior border of the vertebral bodies, is used to separate the middle from the posterior mediastinum (Fig 9–2). This method of dividing the mediastinum is not anatomically precise, but it is much less cumbersome to apply to the lateral chest film and thus improves the radiologist's ability to accurately describe the location of a mediastinal mass.

Thymic Lesions

Thymomas are among the most common primary tumors of the anterior mediastinum. They characteristically present as a well-circumscribed mass that frequently appears to touch the sternum without being flattened by the compressing effect of the heart and great vessels. This resistance to flattening results in the so-called sulcus sign, which indicates that the mass is very firm.

Thymomas occur most frequently in patients ranging from 45 to 50 years of age. They are infrequently encountered in young adults and are rarely seen in patients younger than age 20. While the well-circumscribed mass seen in Figure 9–1 is a typical radiographic appearance for a thymoma, the patient's age of 20 is not typical. A thymoma is therefore possible but not the most likely diagnosis based on the patient's age.

Myasthenia gravis is the most common clinical syndrome to be associated with thymoma; 15% of patients with this condition have a thymoma, and approximately 40% of patients with a thymoma have myasthenia gravis. Because of this strong clinical association, CT has been advocated as a screening procedure for detection of thymomas in patients with myasthenia gravis[416] (Fig 9–3, A–C). Other autoimmune disorders that have been linked with thymomas include acquired hypogammaglobulinemia, red cell hypoplasia, aplastic anemia, and Cushing's syndrome. Other reported associations include systemic lupus erythematosus, rheumatoid arthritis, polymyositis, hyperthyroidism, and Sjögren's syndrome.

Differentiation of benign from malignant thymomas is a challenge for the radiologist, surgeon, and pathologist. This distinction is not usually based on histologic features, but rather is made by observing evidence of local invasion. Well-encapsulated thymomas are usually benign, but any evidence of local invasion suggests malignancy. Malignant thymomas spread contiguously, invading other mediastinal structures, pleura, and lung. (Answer to question 2 is a.) It is not unusual for a malignant thymoma to spread around the pleura and cause multiple pleural masses that resemble malignant mesothelioma. Like mesothelioma, thymomas rarely metastasize to distant sites. In a patient with an anterior mediastinal mass, the presence of hematogenous metastases should suggest another diagnosis, such as teratoma, thymic carcinoma, or lymphoma.

Other abnormalities arising from the thymus include thymolipoma, thymic cyst, lymphoma, thymic carcinoma, and thymic carcinoid tumors.[49, 508] Thymolipoma is a benign tumor with both thymic remnants and fat.[507] These masses are very soft and conform to the shape of surrounding structures. They may simulate an elevated diaphragm or enlarged heart. A right-sided mass makes the cardiac contour appear symmetric, with the appearance suggesting cardiomegaly or even a large pericardial effusion. The diagnosis of a mixed fatty and soft tissue tumor may be confirmed with CT (Fig 9–4, A and B). A thymic cyst is also benign and has a plain film appearance that is indistinguishable from that of a thymoma. CT should confirm low-attenuation fluid and thus suggest a thymic cyst. Thymic carcinomas are rare tumors that arise from the epithelial portions of the thymus. A variety of cell type carcinomas include squamous, small cell, mucoepidermoid, adenocystic, clear cell, and sarcomatoid carcinomas. These tumors probably account for the cases in which a thymoma appears to spread by hematogenous metastasis, and they may be mistaken for metastases from distant primary tumors. There are no associated syndromes. Thymic carcinoid tumors are identical to thymomas in radiologic appearance but have substantial histologic, clinical, and prognostic differences. These tumors are thought to arise from neural crest cells, unlike thymomas of epithelial origin. There are no reported cases of carcinoid syndrome, but 40% of patients with thymic carcinoid tumors have Cushing's syndrome, and 19% of these tumors have been associated with multiple endocrine neoplasia syndromes, including hyperparathyroidism resulting from either parathyroid adenoma or hyperplasia. Thymic carcinoid tumors have not been reported to have an association with myasthenia gravis, hypogammaglobulinemia, red cell aplasia, megaesophagus, or collagen vascular disease. They may be locally invasive, like thymoma, but they tend to be more aggressive. They are more likely to cause superior vena caval obstruction and they frequently metastasize to distant sites.

Teratoid Lesions

Teratoid lesions also present in the middle to lower portion of the anterior mediastinum.[275] These masses tend to be midline structures and, like thymomas, are frequently found between the sternum and the heart and great vessels. Teratomas contain elements from all three germ layers with soft tissue, fat, cystic fluid collections, and calcification. When they contain either sebaceous or fatty materials, they are softer than the solid thymomas and tend to flatten against the sternum. The sulcus between the mass and the sternum that may be seen on the lateral film in thymomas is therefore less often encountered in the teratoid lesions. CT may demonstrate a characteristic fat-fluid level in cystic teratomas[191] and MR usually reveals a mixed signal pattern (Fig 9–5). Calcification is another feature that might be expected to be helpful in identifying these entities, but plain film identification of teeth and bones, as often occurs in dermoid cysts in the pelvis, is rare in mediastinal teratomas and dermoid cysts. A rim of calcification in the wall of a cystic structure may be seen in a dermoid cyst, but it is also seen in thymic cysts and aneurysms. Other causes of calcification in anterior mediastinal masses include mesenchymal tumor, goiter (Fig 9–6, A and B) and treated lymphomatous nodes (Fig 9–7). (Answer to question 3 is c.)

Lymphadenopathy

Lymphoma is another important consideration in cases such as that of the 20-year-old man whose films are shown in Figure 9–1. Lymphoma arises in both the thymus and the lymph nodes and is the most common primary neoplasm of the mediastinum. Lymphomas may present as well-circumscribed masses and may be indistinguishable from thymic and teratoid lesions. However, the radiologic signs of malignancy and the differences in the routes of malignant spread are important considerations in the evaluation of anterior mediastinal masses. The only reliable signs that suggest malignancy are signs of spread. Lymphoma is well known for its radiologic appearance: a mass that appears well circumscribed on the frontal view but ill defined on the lateral view (Fig 9–8, A and B). The lateral film may reveal complete obliteration of the normal retrosternal clear space and silhouetting of normal structures, such as the ascending aorta, by a poorly marginated mass that involves multiple nodes and thymus. The more occult infiltrating lymphomas may not have the expected appearance of a discrete mass on the frontal film, but may only alter a mediastinal pleural contour. This appearance may also be explained by the tendency for lymphoma to be locally invasive, although other tumors, including thymomas and teratomas, may also be locally invasive. Both lymphoma and thymoma may spread into the lung, leading to loss of definition of the borders of the mass (Fig 9–9, *A* and *C*). They may even follow the interstitium of the lung, producing a reticular pattern like that seen in patients with lymphangitic spread of a carcinoma. Involvement of other node groups, as with hilar adenopathy (Fig 9–10), may provide a clue for distinguishing lymphoma from the other anterior mediastinal tumors.

Other causes of adenopathy include metastases from other primary tumors—particularly from lung and breast cancer—and granulomatous diseases. Tuberculosis, fungi, and sarcoidosis are common causes of mediastinal adenopathy, but these diseases rarely present with anterior mediastinal adenopathy in the absence of middle mediastinal or hilar adenopathy.

Inlet Lesions

Once the mass is localized to the anterior mediastinum, its precise location must be considered. Thyroid masses, for example, almost always appear as inlet lesions (Fig 9–11), and may even be associated with a palpable neck mass. They may therefore appear to extend above the clavicles, in contrast to masses that arise from the anterior mediastinum. They also tend to displace the trachea posteriorly. Thus, a mass that appears to extend through the inlet of the thorax from the neck, and which deviates the trachea, suggests a thyroid mass. Occasionally, a thyroid mass may be evident posterior to the trachea with anterior deviation of the trachea, and may thus present in a more posterior location. Careful clinical correlation is essential. An inlet lesion in a child with an associated neck mass is more likely to be a cystic hygroma (lymphangioma). In this instance, physical examination may reveal a soft neck mass and confirm the diagnosis. Ultrasound, CT, or MRI should confirm the cystic character of the lesion. Lymphoma rarely manifests as an inlet lesion, but it should be considered when there are palpable neck or supraclavicular lymph nodes instead of a definite thyroid mass.

Cardiophrenic-Angle Mass

The right cardiophrenic angle is another location that suggests a more limited diagnosis (Chart 9–3). The epicardial fat pad or lipoma is the most common cause of a mass in this area. It is frequently possible to appreciate that the mass is less opaque than the heart but obviously more opaque than the surrounding lung. If there is any doubt about the diagnosis, examination of previous films will usually confirm the impression of the fat opacity and show that the mass has not changed in size or configuration. A word of caution is required, however, since fat pads occasionally increase in size. It is well known that there may be growth of fatty tissue in response to treatment with corticosteroids. It is therefore necessary to correlate the radiologic observation of an enlarging mass in this area with the clinical history. In the absence of an obvious reason for the growth, it sometimes becomes necessary to consider further evaluation. Another method of confirming that the opacity is fat is to measure the attenuation coefficient by CT, but such an expensive approach is rarely necessary.

The right cardiophrenic angle is the most common location for a pericardial cyst, which should be of tissue opacity, in contrast to the fat pad. However, either lesion may be seen in the left cardiophrenic angle. Both ultrasound and CT may be reliable for confirming the cystic nature of the lesion, but CT offers the added advantage of being able to distinguish fat, as previously mentioned. Hernias of the foramen of Morgagni also occur in this location and are best confirmed by CT or sometimes barium studies of the GI tract.

Aneurysm

A vascular lesion (aneurysm) must be considered if a mediastinal mass cannot be shown to be separate from the aorta.[447] In the past, angiography has provided the only method for excluding the diagnosis of aneurysm, but CT with vascular enhancement or MRI clearly defines the aorta[108, 255] and provides a less-invasive technique for excluding the diagnosis of aneurysm. Magnetic resonance imaging avoids the risk involved in using contrast medium and may become the procedure of choice.[207] Rarely, these anterior aneurysms have been reported to compress the right pulmonary artery and have been diagnosed from the levophase of a pulmonary arteriogram.[673]

SUMMARY

1. Localization within the anterior mediastinum to the inlet strongly suggests a thyroid lesion in an adult or cystic hygroma in a child.

2. Anterior mediastinal masses must be distinguished from the aorta. This may require special procedures, including CT, MRI, or arteriography.

3. Thymomas are most commonly seen after age 40, whereas lymphoma and teratomas are commonly seen in young adults. Lymphoma also has a second peak incidence in the elderly.

4. Malignant thymomas spread contiguously and essentially never beyond the thorax, in contrast to lymphoma and teratomas, which may involve multiple organ systems.

5. The presence of bones or teeth is diagnostic of a teratoid lesion, but this is a rare finding, in contrast to the presence of these structures in dermoid cysts that occur in the pelvis.

6. Rimlike calcifications are not rare but have limited diagnostic value.

7. Lymphoma commonly presents with a mass that is ill-defined on the lateral projection, probably because of its tendency to spread through the mediastinum by infiltration or by involvement of multiple node groups.

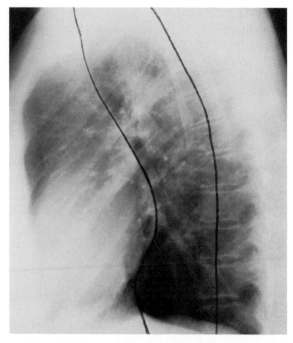

FIG 9–2
This simplified division of the mediastinum was first described by Felson. Anterior border of the trachea and posterior borders of the heart and inferior vena cava form the line for dividing anterior from middle compartments. A line drawn 1 cm posterior to the anterior border of vertebral bodies divides the middle and posterior compartments.

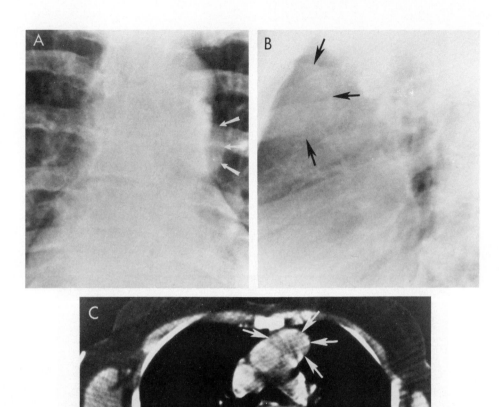

FIG 9–3
A, PA chest film of patient with myasthenia gravis reveals a subtle opacity *(arrows)* on the left in the aortic-pulmonary window. **B,** Lateral film shows a minimally visible opacity *(arrows)* in the anterior mediastinum. **C,** CT scan confirms the presence of a mass *(arrows)* to the left of the ascending aorta. Thoracotomy documented the presence of an anterior mediastinal thymoma.

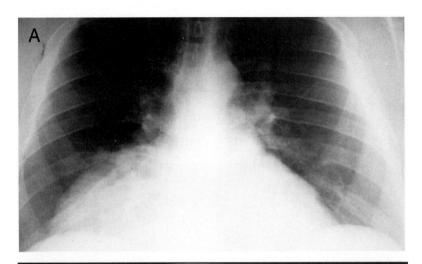

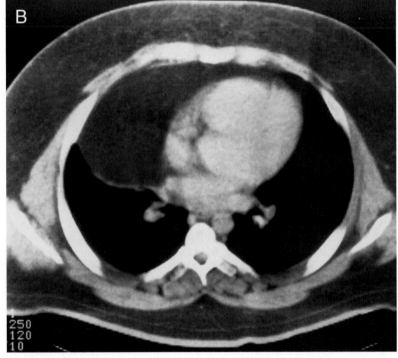

FIG 9–4
A, PA film demonstrates a large, well-circumscribed mass filling the right cardiophrenic angle. This has obliterated the right heart border and gives the appearance of a symmetric heart shape. This even resembles the "water bottle appearance" that is associated with large pericardial effusions. **B,** CT reveals a large fat-density mass consistent with thymolipoma.

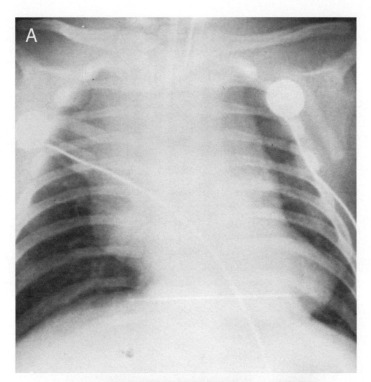

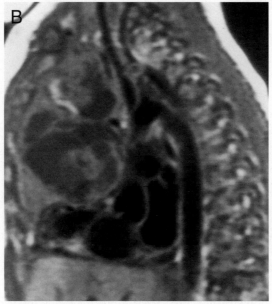

FIG 9–5
A, PA film of a young child demonstrates a large anterior mediastinal mass. Teratoma is the most likely diagnosis in a child. **B,** T$_1$-weighted sagittal MR image of the mass shows a mixed signal pattern that is a typical MR appearance for a teratoma. Observe the compression of the heart and great vessels. (From Link KM, Samuels LJ, Reed JC, et al: *Magnetic resonance imaging of the mediastinum. J Thorac Imaging* 1993; 8(1):34–53. Used by permission.)

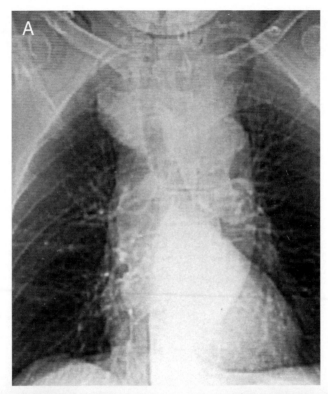

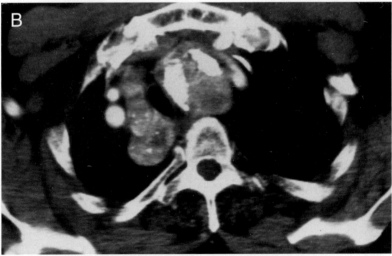

FIG 9–6
A, This large superior mediastinal mass deviates the trachea to the right and extends above the clavicles. This appearance is strongly suggestive of goiter. Calcification is frequently present but may not be obvious on the plain film. **B,** CT is most sensitive for detecting calcification and confirms that the mass arises from the thyroid. This is useful in order to rule out nodal masses and thyroid carcinoma. The presence of calcification confirms the diagnosis of a benign goiter.

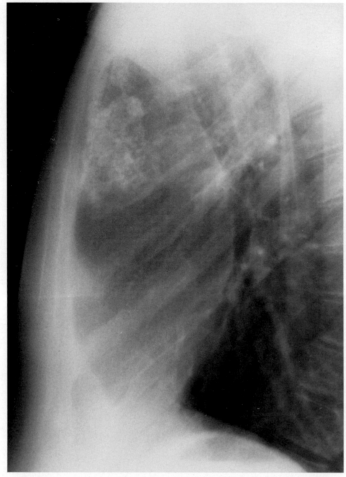

FIG 9–7
This lateral film demonstrates the typical appearance of calcified lymph nodes, which are the late result of lymphoma that was treated with radiation.

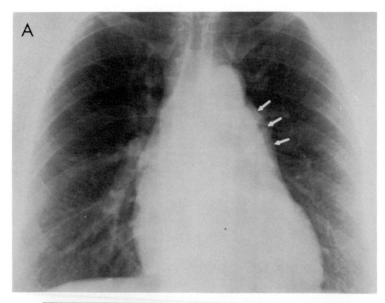

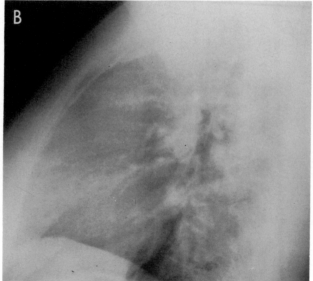

FIG 9–8
A, Opacity projected over left hilum has a sharp lateral border *(arrows).* **B,** Lateral film from the case in **A** shows ill-defined opacity obscuring the ascending aorta. The opacity fills in the normal retrosternal clear space. This is a common radiologic appearance of lymphoma in the anterior mediastinum.

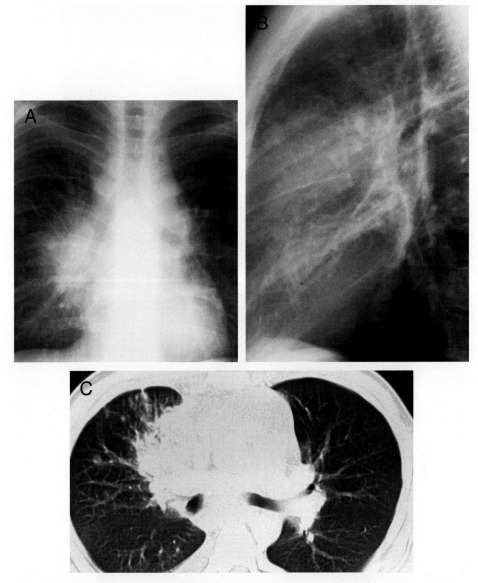

FIG 9–9
A, PA film demonstrates a large mass involving the aorticopulmonary window on the left and the right paratracheal area and projecting over the right hilum. **B,** Lateral film confirms a large, poorly marginated opacity in the anterior mediastinum. **C,** CT scan with lung windows reveals irregular linear opacities extending from the mass into the right lung and additional contiguous lung nodules. This is lymphoma that has spread into the adjacent lung.

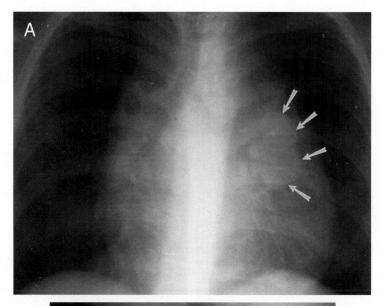

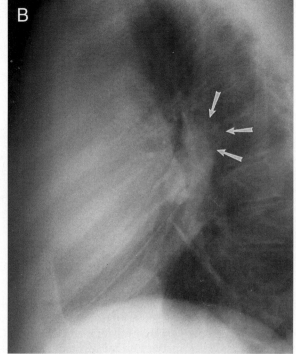

FIG 9–10
A, PA film shows widening of the mediastinum and left hilar adenopathy *(arrows)*.
B, Lateral film confirms that a large mass is filling the retrosternal clear space and veri-
fies the presence of lobulated hilar nodes *(arrows)*. This combination is most suggestive
of lymphoma.

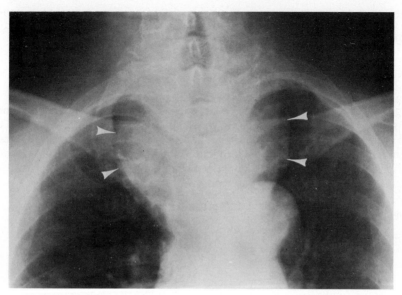

FIG 9–11
A typical location and appearance for intrathoracic goiter. Note that the mass crosses the midline *(arrowheads).*

ANSWER GUIDE

LEGENDS FOR INTRODUCTORY FIGURES

FIG 9–1
A, Large mass obscures the left heart border and is therefore in an anterior position. Tapered superior borders *(arrows)* indicate an extrapulmonary location. The tapered border results from the mediastinal mass pushing the two layers of pleura laterally. **B,** Lateral projection film confirms the anterior location. Young age of patient (20 years) favors correct diagnosis of teratoma over thymoma, but lymphoma cannot be radiologically eliminated.

ANSWERS

1, c; 2, a; 3, c.

CHAPTER 10

Middle Mediastinal Mass

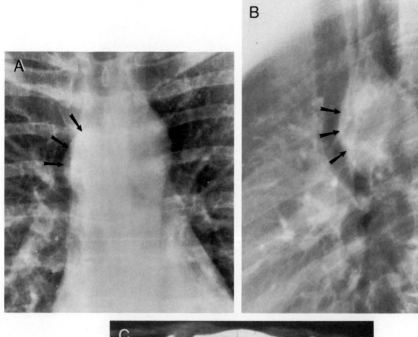

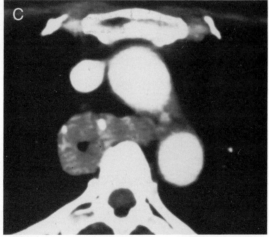

FIG 10–1

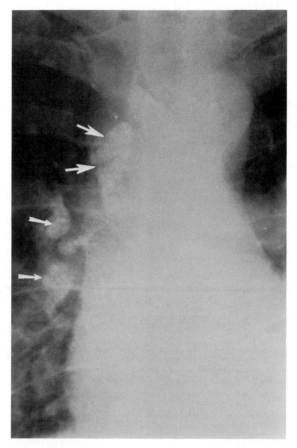

FIG 10–2

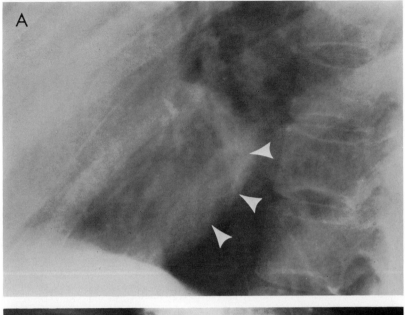

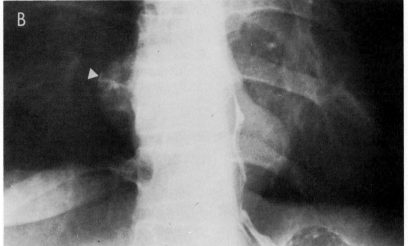

FIG 10–3

QUESTIONS

1. Which one of the following is the most likely diagnosis for the case illustrated in Figure 10–1?
   a. Lymphoma.
   b. Metastases.
   c. Primary tuberculosis.
   d. Sarcoidosis.
   e. Leiomyoma of the esophagus.

2. Referring to Figure 10–2, which of the following diagnoses may result in calcified middle mediastinal masses?
   a. Histoplasmosis.
   b. Tuberculosis.
   c. Sarcoidosis.
   d. Silicosis.
   e. All of the above.
3. The most likely diagnosis in the asymptomatic young male patient in Figure 10–3, *A* and *B* is
   a. Bronchogenic cyst.
   b. Leiomyoma of the esophagus.
   c. Carcinoma of the esophagus.
   d. Lymphoma
   e. Neurenteric cyst.

CHART 10–1.
Middle Mediastinal Masses

I. Neoplastic adenopathy
  A. Metastasis, including lesions derived from lung primaries[399]
  B. Lymphoma (Hodgkin's)[171]
  C. Leukemia[41]
  D. Angioimmunoblastic lymphadenopathy[314]
  E. Kaposi's sarcoma (in AIDS patients)[119, 328]
II. Inflammatory adenopathy
  A. Tuberculosis[349, 412, 413]
  B. Histoplasmosis[104, 390, 645]
  C. Blastomycosis (rare)[474]
  D. Coccidioidomycosis
  E. Sarcoidosis[39]
  F. Viral pneumonia (particularly measles[383] and cat scratch fever)
  G. AIDS[328]
  H. Infectious mononucleosis[274]
  I. Pertussis pneumonia[153]
  J. Amyloidosis[271]
  K. Plague[565]
  L. Tularemia[515]
  M. Drug reaction[258, 523]
  N. Giant lymph node hyperplasia (Castleman's disease)[626]
  O. Connective tissue disease (mixed, rheumatoid, and lupus)[218]
  P. Bacterial lung abscess[505]
  Q. *Mycobacterium avium-intracellulare* (in AIDS patients)[328]
III. Inhalational disease adenopathy[186]
  A. Silicosis
  B. Coal-worker's pneumoconiosis
  C. Berylliosis
IV. Duplication cysts
  A. Bronchogenic or respiratory cyst (includes tracheal and some esophageal cysts)[487]
  B. Enteric cyst
  C. Extralobar sequestration (including esophageal lung)[256]
V. Primary tumors
  A. Carcinoma of the trachea
  B. Bronchogenic carcinoma[195, 564]
  C. Esophageal tumor
    1. Benign (leiomyoma)[552]
    2. Malignant (carcinoma, leiomyosarcoma)

(Continued.)

Chart 10–1   (cont.)

   D. Mesothelioma
   E. Granular cell myoblastoma of trachea (rare)[532]
VI. Vascular lesions
   A. Aneurysms
   B. Distended veins (e.g., superior vena cava, azygous vein, esophageal varices[28, 345])
   C. Hematoma
   D. Primary angiosarcoma (pulmonary artery)
   E. Left superior vena cava
   F. Aberrant right subclavian artery
   G. Right aortic arch
VII. Other
   A. Hiatal hernia
   B. Esophageal diverticulum
   C. Dilated esophagus (achalasia)
   D. Thyroid[34] and parathyroid[325] masses that extend into the mediastinum
   E. Cystic hygroma (lymphangioma)

DISCUSSION

The evaluation of a middle mediastinal mass requires careful consideration of the normal structures found in the middle mediastinum.[99, 261, 467, 468, 534, 567] The middle mediastinum in this instance does not correspond precisely with the classic anatomic description of the middle mediastinum. Rather, it is the area between the anterior border of the trachea and posterior border of the heart and a line drawn 1 cm posterior to the anterior border of the vertebral bodies. This area includes the trachea, bifurcation of the trachea, arch of the aorta, great vessels, pulmonary arteries, esophagus, and numerous paratracheal and peribronchial nodes.

The causes of a middle mediastinal mass can be divided into four broad categories: lymphadenopathy, primary tumors, vascular lesions, and duplication cysts. When the various causes of lymphadenopathy are taken together, it is clearly the most common cause of a middle mediastinal mass.

Middle mediastinal lymphadenopathy is most reliably identified by the detection of a mass in an area that is known to have a specific lymph node, for example, a subcarinal, right paratracheal, azygous, or ductal node (Fig 10–4). Since many of the processes that will be considered involve multiple nodes in the same area, there is a strong but not invariable tendency for mediastinal adenopathy to result in the appearance of a lobulated mass. The causes of middle mediastinal adenopathy greatly overlap the causes of hilar adenopathy, a condition that further contributes to the lobulated appearance of the masses.

Neoplasms

Neoplastic involvement of middle mediastinal lymph nodes is usually metastatic.[399] It must be emphasized that primary bronchogenic carcinoma of the lung most often metastasizes to the middle mediastinal nodes.[564] In fact, nodal metastases frequently constitute the bulk of the mass produced by carcinomas that arise in the mainstem bronchi. Metastases from peripheral lung tumors and even distant primaries may also produce metastatic deposits in the middle mediastinum[105] (Fig 10–5).

The problem of detecting small mediastinal masses and masses that are deep in the mediastinum with minimal contact with the lung, such as subcarinal masses (Fig 10–6, A–C), is similar in all three compartments of the mediastinum. Both CT and MRI[628] are very sensitive methods for detecting small mediastinal masses and are of particular value in staging lymphomas and carcinomas, which have a tendency to metastasize to mediastinal nodes. The two techniques are especially useful in detecting nodal metastases from primary lung carcinoma and local extensions of esophageal carcinoma.[258, 431, 541, 572]

Lymphoma, and particularly Hodgkin's lymphoma, is another important cause of middle mediastinal adenopathy.[171] Lymphoma may be confined to the middle mediastinum, but it frequently involves the anterior mediastinal and hilar nodes. Chronic lymphocytic leukemia is a less common hematologic malignancy to involve the middle mediastinal nodes, but as many as 25% of patients with leukemia are reported to have mediastinal adenopathy in the late stages of their disease. Like lymphoma, the adenopathy that occurs in patients with leukemia is often not confined to the middle mediastinum, but involves the bronchopulmonary (hilar) nodes as well.

The diagnosis of a neoplastic condition is frequently suggested by clinical information. A patient who is being followed up for a known primary carcinoma elsewhere, and who develops a middle mediastinal mass, should be assumed to have a metastatic lesion until it is proved otherwise. A primary lung tumor should be suspected in patients who have associated hemoptysis and a history of smoking. Patients with primary lung tumors frequently have other indirect radiologic signs of the tumor, including atelectasis or obstructive pneumonia. These signs of an obstructing lesion are helpful for distinguishing primary bronchogenic tumors from metastases, since endobronchial metastases are infrequent (see Chapter 13). On the other hand, associated pulmonary opacities and even atelectasis are unreliable features for distinguishing a primary bronchogenic tumor from lymphoma. Both types of tumor may invade the pulmonary interstitium locally, with a resultant ill-defined perihilar opacity that may be associated with a mediastinal mass. This is best known in the case of small cell carcinoma, which can completely mimic the appearance of lymphoma in the chest because of its early metastases to the regional lymph nodes. Small cell carcinoma[67] may even produce massive mediastinal adenopathy before the primary tumor is radiologically detectable.

Calcification of lymph nodes that are enlarged by tumor is very rare. It is reported to occur as a result of bone-forming metastases from malignant bone tumors (osteosarcoma). Calcification has also been observed to develop in nodes affected by Hodgkin's disease after treatment with radiation therapy.[60] In both cases, serial films and the history should permit a correct diagnosis.

Inflammatory Diseases

A large variety of inflammatory lesions (Chart 10–1) may result in middle mediastinal adenopathy. Like the neoplastic processes, these diseases commonly cause associated bronchopulmonary adenopathy. Careful correlation of clinical and laboratory information is usually required for their diagnosis.

Primary tuberculosis may present with hilar or mediastinal adenopathy.[64, 290, 653] There is frequently an associated exudative pneumonitis with the radiologic appearance of a localized or even lobar consolidation. This combination of a localized air space consolidation, particularly in the middle or lower lobe, with either hilar or mediastinal adenopathy in a child is a classic radiologic presentation of primary tuberculosis. The adenopathy results from the formation of tuberculoid, caseating granulomas in the lymph nodes. This reaction may resolve completely or heal by fibrosis and calcification. It is therefore a common cause of mediastinal nodal calcification. Although primary tuberculosis is usually expected to occur in children, this combination of localized air space consolidation and mediastinal adenopathy may occur in any age group.[64]

The age at onset of primary tuberculosis closely follows geographic distribution. In areas in which tuberculosis is endemic, the age at onset is younger, whereas in areas in which the disease is no longer common, the first exposure and therefore the initial infection may occur at a later age. For example, in eastern Asia, adults would not typically sustain the onset of primary tuberculosis, while in the United States or Canada the incidence of primary tuberculosis in adults is greater simply because the number of adults previously exposed to tuberculosis is relatively small.

Histoplasmosis is another common cause of middle mediastinal adenopathy. Indeed, the adenopathy in histoplasmosis may be more dramatic, with bulkier nodes, than that in tuberculosis. The incidence of histoplasmosis as a cause of middle mediastinal masses probably exceeds that of tuberculosis in those areas of the world in which histoplasmosis is endemic. The radiologic features of lymphadenopathy secondary to histoplasmosis are nonspecific. There is, however, an even higher incidence of calcification in lymph nodes that are enlarged by histoplasmosis granulomas. Skin testing for tuberculosis and histoplasmosis frequently enables a distinction to be made between these two causes of mediastinal node enlargement or calcification. Fibrosing mediastinitis[161] may be either idiopathic or a late and rare complication of histoplasmosis that may produce diffuse widening of the mediastinum with superior vena caval obstruction.[152] Pulmonary artery occlusion is also a rare late sequela of histoplasmosis.[646]

Other fungal infections, including coccidioidomycosis and blastomycosis, cause mediastinal adenopathy less frequently, although radiologically, both of these infections may mimic primary tuberculosis. Coccidioidomycosis is particularly well known for this presentation in endemic areas in the desert of the southwestern United States (Fig 10–7). Blastomycosis rarely causes either hilar or mediastinal adenopathy. Rabinowitz et al.[474] reported that only 3 of 51 cases had definite hilar adenopathy.

Sarcoidosis is another common cause of middle mediastinal adenopathy that often has a characteristic radiologic appearance. This appearance is characteristic because of the propensity for sarcoidosis to involve the bronchopulmonary nodes symmetrically in addition to causing middle mediastinal adenopathy. The middle mediastinal adenopathy in sarcoidosis is frequently asymmetric, with predominant involvement of the right paratracheal lymph nodes. The frequency of left-sided paratracheal adenopathy may be greater than suspected because of the difference in the anatomy of the mediastinum; that is, left paratracheal lymph nodes may be enlarged but not readily appreciated because of the arrangement of the aorta and great vessels that produce the left lateral border of the mediastinum. Middle mediastinal adenopathy without hilar adenopathy is highly atypical in sarcoidosis—in fact, so atypical that a patient with middle mediastinal nodes who is believed to have sarcoidosis should have a very careful review of all available histologic material, and the sizes of these histologic specimens should be considered to exclude the possibility of a small, sarcoidlike reaction around a malignant tumor such as lymphoma.

Viral pneumonias, particularly measles pneumonias,[383] have also been associated with lymphadenopathy. The combination of pulmonary opacities with adenopathy must be distinguished from primary tuberculosis and the fungal infections previously described. In contrast to primary tuberculosis, this presentation of viral infection is almost always restricted to the pediatric age group. The diagnosis of viral pneumonia with adenopathy should be suspected on the basis of clinical presentation. An acute febrile response with leukocytosis during an epidemic of viral infection supports the diagnosis. Confirmation requires laboratory tests, including serologic studies and frequently viral cultures.

Infectious mononucleosis[274] is another entity that resembles a viral infection. In contrast to the viral pneumonias, which may mimic primary tuberculosis, infectious mononucleosis does not usually produce a significant pneumonic process. There are only rare reports of a fine interstitial pneumonitis caused by this disease. However, widespread lymphadenopathy is a common observation in infectious mononucleosis and occasionally involves the middle mediastinum or the hilum. Laboratory confirmation of the diagnosis is essential to exclude early lymphocytic malignancy, a more common cause of middle mediastinal adenopathy. Splenic enlargement is frequent in patients with infectious mononucleosis, but it also occurs with lymphoma and sarcoidosis. Associated splenomegaly is therefore not specific, but narrows the differential to these three possibilities.

The diagnosis of inhalational diseases that produce adenopathy is generally straightforward. Silicosis and coal-worker's pneumoconiosis are well-known causes of both hilar and mediastinal adenopathy and will be considered together. The adenopathy in both silicosis and coal-worker's pneumoconiosis is almost invariably associated with the pulmonary disease, which will be discussed in the chapters on fine nodular patterns, fine reticular interstitial disease, honeycomb lung, and masses. In both diseases, silica particles appear to be picked up by pulmonary macrophages and transported to the lymph nodes. There the silica excites a granulomatous and later a fibrotic reaction that enlarges the nodes. Calcification of the nodes is a late result of this reaction. There is a well-described but unexplained tendency for the calcification to appear in the periphery of the nodes, leading to the distinctive radiologic appearance described as eggshell calcification. Eggshell calcification was once considered to be a diagnostic finding of silicosis, but a similar appearance has been observed rarely as a late finding in sarcoidosis and tuberculosis. In answer to question 2, all of the listed entities may result in calcified mediastinal nodes.

Berylliosis is a rare disease that produces a granulomatous reaction very similar to that of sarcoidosis. The adenopathy is due to the accumulation of granulomas in the nodes. Berylliosis typically involves both the hilar and the mediastinal lymph nodes and is often associated with either a diffuse nodular or reticular pulmonary pattern also resembling that of sarcoidosis. Even histologic distinction of the reactions of berylliosis and sarcoidosis may be impossible. The diagnosis is usually suspected because of a history of exposure, and it is confirmed by spectrographic examination of wet tissue.

AIDS-related Adenopathy

Lymphadenopathy is a common occurrence in patients infected with the HIV virus. The most likely cause of the adenopathy is determined by the stage of the infection, which is closely related to the CD4 cell count. In early HIV infection, while the CD4 count is in the 300 to 500 range, patients may clinically present with persistent generalized lymphadenopathy (PGL).[585] Biopsy of nodes in patients with PGL reveals reactive lymph node hyperplasia. Although this is a common cause of axillary and inguinal adenopathy, occurring in 50% of patients with AIDS, it is not a common cause of mediastinal adenopathy. PGL may account for nodes that are detectable with CT in the range of 1 to 1.5 cm, but it is not a likely cause of adenopathy that is detectable by plain film. Kuhlman et al.[328] reported that extensive adenopathy is most likely the result of mycobacterial infections, Kaposi's sarcoma, non-Hodgkin's lymphoma, fungal infection, or drug hypersensitivity. As the CD4 count decreases below 300, tuberculosis, lymphoma, and Kaposi's sarcoma are more likely causes of mediastinal adenopathy.[387, 581] *Mycobacterium avium intracellulare* (MAI) and Kaposi's sarcoma become more likely causes of mediastinal adenopathy after the CD4 has dropped below 200 (Fig 10–8, *A* and *B*). Additionally, the observation of mediastinal adenopathy may be important in the differentiation of pneumocystis carinii pneumonia (PCP) from tuberculosis. PCP and tuberculosis are both causes of diffuse lung disease in patients with CD4 counts less than 200, but adenopathy is a rare manifestation of PCP, though a common finding in patients with tuberculosis.

Vascular Abnormalities

Enlargement of the great vessels often has a radiologic appearance simulating that of a mediastinal mass.

Aneurysm must be ruled out when a mediastinal opacity is indistinguishable from the shadow of the aorta. Aneurysms are encountered in the anterior, middle, and posterior mediastinum. Fluoroscopy is generally of little value in distinguishing masses from aneurysms, since masses adjacent to the aorta commonly appear to pulsate because of transmitted pulsation. The most conventional method of confirming the diagnosis of aortic aneurysm is aortography; however, CT with contrast enhancement provides a less invasive method for diagnosing aneurysm, and MRI avoids the risk of toxicity induced by contrast medium (Fig 10–9).[207]

Distention of normal veins, in particular the azygous vein and superior vena cava, may occasionally be confused with a mass. The distinction of an enlarged azygous node from a distended azygous vein may be done by comparing flat and upright films that document a change in size, or a Valsalva maneuver that shows the opacity to decrease in size. The latter phenomenon may be observed at fluoroscopy or documented with films (Fig 10–10, *A* and *B*).

Transection of a great vessel following rapid deceleration injury to the chest may produce a false aneurysm with the appearance of a mediastinal mass. The appearance of a mediastinal mass after significant chest trauma should nearly confirm the diagnosis, but arteriography is necessary to fully confirm the diagnosis and localize the transection. More commonly, rupture of a great vessel results in diffuse mediastinal widening. Extensive hemorrhage into the mediastinum also obscures the aortic arch, and frequently dissects extrapleurally over the apex of the lung. Apparent asymmetric apical pleural thickening after chest trauma is therefore a clue to a significant vascular injury. When the pleura is lacerated, there will be associated intrapleural bleeding. In these cases aortography is an emergency procedure.

Primary Tumors

With the exception of lymphoma, primary tumors in the middle mediastinum are infrequent. As previously indicated, the mediastinal masses that result from bronchogenic carcinoma metastasize to the regional lymph nodes.

Primary carcinoma of the trachea, a rare tumor, is easily missed on the initial chest film since it may produce only a contour abnormality with tracheal narrowing. In the later stages it may produce a paratracheal mass. In such cases, radiologic distinction of an intrinsic mass from an extrinsic mass compressing the trachea may be difficult. Computed tomography[198] is most useful for outlining the contour of the mass. A nodular irregular defect in the trachea indicates an intrinsic mass and nearly confirms the diagnosis of primary tumor. Final confirmation requires bronchoscopy and biopsy. Less common endotracheal masses include carcinoid, granuloma, papilloma, metastasis, lipoma, fibroma, and amyloid tumor. A history of stridor is often elicited in patients with an endotracheal mass.

Esophageal carcinomas are typically seen as constricting lesions of the esophagus with symptoms of dysphagia long before there is a significant mass effect. It is therefore unusual to identify a primary carcinoma of the esophagus as a middle mediastinal mass. One middle mediastinal finding that has been observed in esophageal tumor is thickening of the paratracheal stripe (Fig 10–11). This finding has also been seen in other constricting lesions of the esophagus, and may represent either inflammatory infiltrate or spread of the tumor in the paraesophageal tissues. Leiomyoma[552] is a primary esophageal tumor that is more likely to present as a mediastinal mass. The tumor grows in the wall of the esophagus and may displace the esophagus, producing a large, bulky mass before symptoms of obstruction become significant (see Fig 10–1, A–C). (Answer to question 10–1 is e.)

Mesothelioma is another primary tumor that occasionally mimics a middle mediastinal mass. This tumor arises from the pleura of the mediastinum on the medial aspect of the lung. Although not a true mediastinal tumor, it has the radiologic appearance of such a tumor because of its location. Biopsy is required to make this diagnosis. The radiologist's role is to identify the mass.

Duplication Cyst

Duplication cysts of foregut origin are relatively rare causes of intrathoracic masses, but the middle mediastinum is their most common location (Fig 10–12). The dorsal foregut gives rise to the esophagus, while the tracheobronchial tree is derived from the ventral foregut. This probably explains the frequency of a middle mediastinal location for the foregut cyst.

Bronchogenic or respiratory cysts arise from the trachea, mainstem bronchi, or esophagus.[487] They are identified histologically by their characteristic respiratory epithelium, the presence of seromucous glands, and cartilage plates (Fig 10–13). The cartilage plates are the most diagnostic feature of these cysts. Some cysts with a respiratory epithelium have actually been dissected from the wall of the esophagus and may thus be named esophageal cysts on the basis of their location, while their histologic appearance is that of a bronchogenic cyst. These cysts have also been reported to extend below the diaphragm.[11]

The most common radiologic appearance of a duplication cyst is that of a homogeneous opacity. The most common location of the cyst within the mediastinum is around the area of the carina, but such cysts may also be paratracheal and even retrocardiac. Duplication cysts rarely communicate with either the tracheobronchial tree or esophagus, but when communication is established, the fluid in the cyst may drain out, leaving a cystic structure. Infrequently, a thin rim of calcification develops in the wall of the cyst (see Fig 10–3, *B*). This feature is a reliable indication of the cystic character of the lesion. (Answer to question 3 is *a*.) However, distinguishing these cysts from solid masses is not usually possible by plain film radiography, and ultrasound is not useful because of interference from bone and aerated lung. Computed tomography can reliably identify some of these cysts as fluid-filled structures when the fluid is of low attenuation[208, 329] (Fig 10–14, *A–C*). However, numerous authors have reported cases in which the cysts are filled with high-attenuation material that resembles a solid mass on CT scan. Magnetic resonance imaging is more reliable for determining the cystic character of these lesions[628] (Fig 10–15, *A–C*).

Enteric cysts are radiologically very similar to bronchogenic cysts. They also appear as homogeneous opacities, occasionally in the middle mediastinum but are more commonly posterior (see Chapter 12).

Extralobar sequestration is a rare cause of a middle mediastinal mass. It is a complex foregut anomaly that contains multiple cysts. The cyst linings resemble both alveoli and bronchioles. When this lesion is closely related to the esophagus, the phenomenon is often called esophageal lung. The extralobar sequestration should have an anomalous feeding vessel identifiable by vascular studies. In the past, the diagnosis has not been suspected preoperatively, and most extralobar sequestrations have not been examined angiographically.

SUMMARY

1. Lymphadenopathy is the most common cause of a middle mediastinal mass. The azygous, subcarinal, ductus, and paratracheal nodes are located in the middle mediastinum.

2. Middle mediastinal masses that result from bronchogenic carcinoma are regional nodal metastases.

3. Lobar consolidation in combination with mediastinal adenopathy is a classic radiologic appearance for primary tuberculosis.

4. Lymph node calcification generally indicates an old inflammatory process such as tuberculosis, histoplasmosis, silicosis, or, rarely, sarcoidosis. Lymphomatous nodes sometimes calcify after radiation. There are also rare reports of bone-producing metastases to mediastinal nodes. The neoplastic cause of calcified nodes should be readily suspected when the clinical presentation is considered.

5. The middle mediastinum is a common location for aortic aneurysm. Masses that are not easily distinguishable from the aorta should be studied by aortography, CT with contrast enhancement, or MRI to rule out this diagnosis.

6. Carcinoma of the trachea, a rare cause of a middle mediastinal mass, is easily missed on the initial x-ray film, but it should be sought when there is a history of wheezing.

7. Esophageal tumors typically produce symptoms of obstruction before there is an appreciable mediastinal mass.

8. Bronchogenic cyst most commonly presents as a smooth, homogeneous, middle mediastinal mass in an asymptomatic young patient.

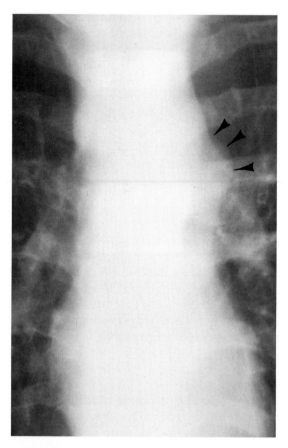

FIG 10–4
A convex opacity between the arch of the aorta and the left pulmonary artery *(arrowheads)* should always be regarded as abnormal. This is the typical appearance of an enlarged ductus node in the aorticopulmonary window. In this case, the diagnosis is Hodgkin's lymphoma.

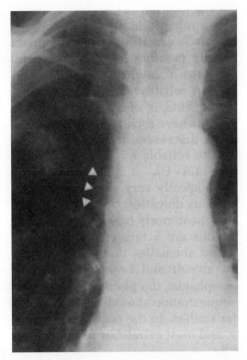

FIG 10–5
Right upper lobe nodule in combination with azygous node enlargement *(white arrow-heads)* suggests the differential of mediastinal adenopathy. Adenopathy is the most common cause of middle mediastinal masses. The enlarged lymph node in this patient with a peripheral carcinoma of the lung is evidence of spread of the tumor to regional lymph nodes.

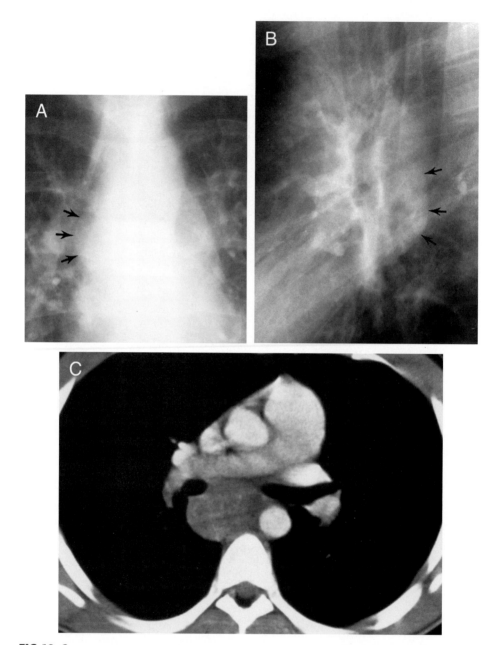

FIG 10–6
A, A large subcarinal mass is deep in the mediastinum, with only one interface with the lung *(arrows)*. Even a very large mass in this location may be subtle on the frontal film. **B,** Lateral film reveals a large opacity that appears to project inferior to the hilum and posterior to the heart. It has a posterior interface with the lung, resulting in a partial sharp border *(arrows)*. **C,** Contrast-enhanced CT confirmed a large subcarinal soft tissue mass consistent with nodal enlargement. Biopsy confirmed histoplasmosis as the cause of the mass.

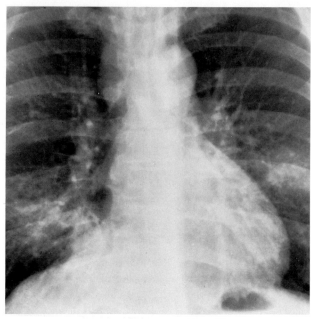

FIG 10–7
Pulmonary opacities with hilar or mediastinal adenopathy are classic for active granulomatous disease. This patient had recently traveled in the desert of California. The right paratracheal adenopathy and bilateral lower lobe opacities resulted from coccidioidomycosis.

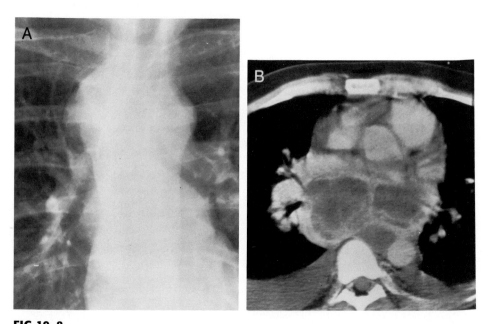

FIG 10–8
A, This patient with AIDS has a large right-sided paratracheal mass that is continuous with a mass of subcarinal nodes. **B,** CT scan confirms a collection of large middle mediastinal nodes with central necrosis. There are also bilateral pleural effusions. Biopsy revealed a mixture of Kaposi's sarcoma and *Mycobacterium avium-intracellulare.*

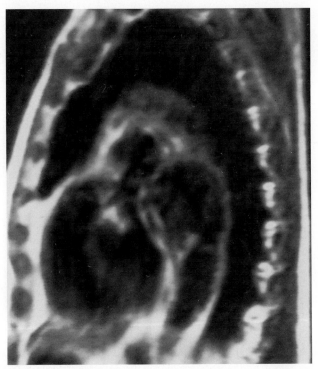

FIG 10–9
Sagittal MR scan is diagnostic of a large aneurysm of the descending aorta.

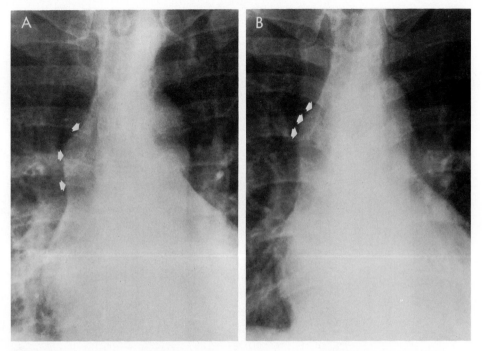

FIG 10–10
A, Opacity in the azygous area resembles the appearance of the azygous node seen in Fig 10–5. **B,** Repeated examination during Valsalva maneuver demonstrated reduction in size of opacity. It is therefore the azygous vein.

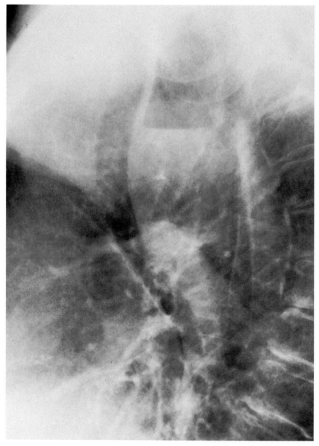

FIG 10–11
Carcinoma of the esophagus caused obstruction with an air-fluid level in the dilated proximal esophagus. Thickening of the posterior tracheal stripe is another indication of carcinoma of the esophagus.

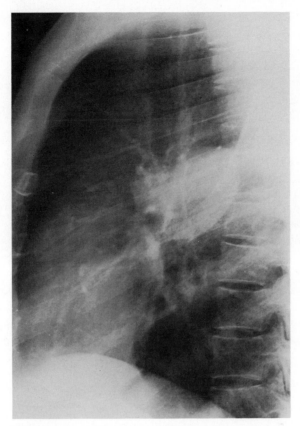

FIG 10–12
Most common location for a bronchogenic cyst.

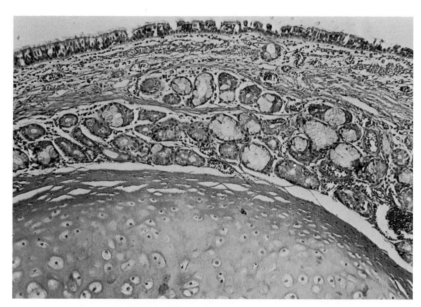

FIG 10–13
Histologic diagnosis of bronchogenic cyst is made from presence of respiratory epithelium, seromucinous glands, and cartilage plates. Cartilage plates are the most diagnostic
feature.

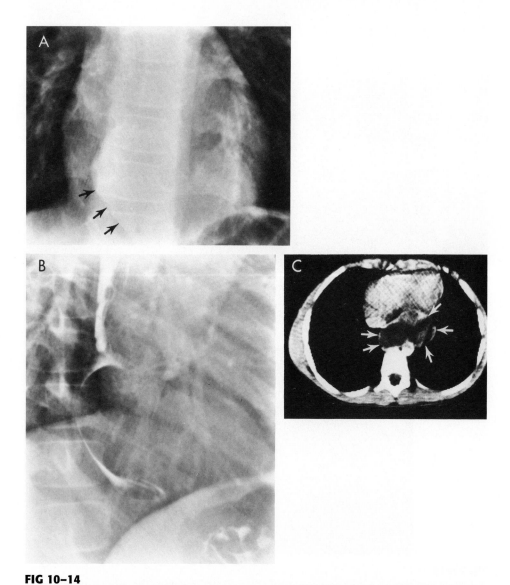

FIG 10–14
A, PA chest film demonstrates a mass crossing the midline posterior to the heart. Note the tapered inferior border *(arrows),* indicating a mediastinal location. **B,** Lateral barium swallow film confirms the presence of a middle mediastinal lesion deviating the esophagus. The appearance suggests that the lesion may be arising from the wall of the esophagus. **C,** CT scan reveals low-attenuation material filling the lesion *(arrows).* This is consistent with a fluid-filled esophageal duplication cyst.

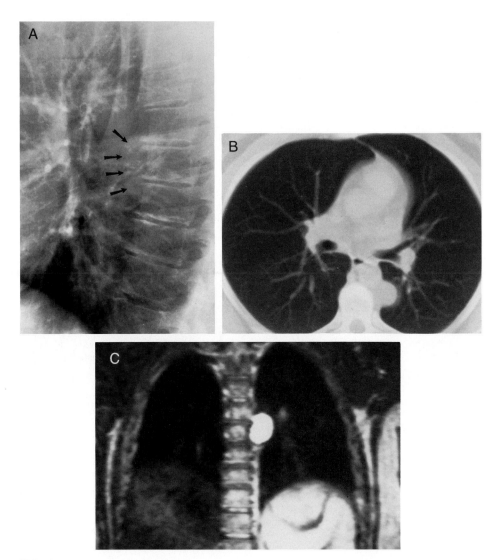

FIG 10–15
A, Lateral film reveals a soft tissue opacity *(arrows)* that overlaps the arbitrary line that divides the middle and posterior mediastinal compartments. **B,** CT scan suggested that this was a homogeneous soft tissue mass in contrast with the cystic lesion seen in Figure 10–13,C. **C,** T_2-weighted coronal MR scan reveals a bright white lesion, indicating that it is a fluid-filled cystic structure. This is a bronchogenic cyst.

ANSWER GUIDE

LEGENDS FOR INTRODUCTORY FIGURES

FIG 10–1
A, PA film demonstrates right paratracheal opacity *(arrows).* **B,** Lateral film shows the opacity to be posterior to the trachea *(arrows)* and to indent the posterior wall of the trachea. **C,** CT scan reveals the soft tissue mass to contain calcifications, surround the esophagus *(central lucency),* and extend across the mediastinum. This is a leiomyoma of the esophagus.

FIG 10–2
Calcified lymph nodes in middle mediastinum *(large arrows)* often occur in combination with hilar nodes *(small arrows)* and virtually always indicate a granulomatous process. Exceptions are usually suspected on the basis of history (i.e., treated lymphoma or new calcifications in patients with osteosarcoma).

FIG 10–3
A, Bronchogenic cyst typically occurs in the middle mediastinum *(arrowheads).* It may arise from either the tracheobronchial tree or the esophagus. This retrocardiac position would not be a likely location for adenopathy, and an esophageal lesion should therefore be suspected. Other esophageal masses (e.g., carcinoma) rarely produce a mass of this size. **B,** PA view of bronchogenic cyst seen in **A** reveals the mass to cross the midline, with an extrinsic impression on the barium-filled esophagus. At surgery, it was found to be attached to the esophagus wall. The thin rim of calcification *(arrowhead)* is a further clue to its cystic nature.

ANSWERS

1, e; 2, e; 3, a.

CHAPTER 11

Hilar Masses

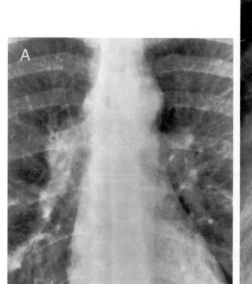

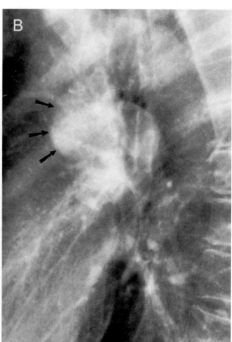

FIG 11–1

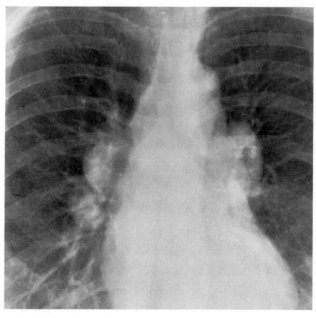

FIG 11–2

QUESTIONS

1. The most likely cause of unilateral hilar enlargement in the adult in Figure 11–1, *A* and *B* is:
   a. Bronchogenic cyst.
   b. Lymphadenopathy.
   c. Large right pulmonary artery.
   d. Pulmonary varix.
   e. Aneurysm of the descending aorta.
2. The most likely cause of the bilateral hilar enlargement in the asymptomatic young adult in Figure 11–2 is:
   a. Metastasis.
   b. Primary tuberculosis.
   c. Sarcoidosis.
   d. Lymphoma.
   e. Histoplasmosis.

CHART 11–1.
Hilar Masses

  I. Large pulmonary arteries (pulmonary arterial hypertension)
     A. Left-sided heart failure, mitral stenosis,[87] and left atrial myxoma
     B. Emphysema[388] (see Chapter 22)
     C. Chronic interstitial lung disease (see Chapter 19)
     D. Pulmonary embolism (acute and chronic)[174, 649]
     E. Portal hypertension[93]
     F. Metastatic tumor emboli
     G. Idiopathic pulmonary hypertension (plexogenic pulmonary arteriopathy)
     H. Cardiac shunts
        1. Ventricular septal defect
        2. Atrial septal defect
        3. Patent ductus arteriosus
        4. Truncus arteriosus
        5. Transposition of great vessels
 II. Unilateral hilar adenopathy
     A. Neoplasm
        1. Bronchogenic carcinoma[564]
        2. Metastasis[399]
        3. Lymphoma
     B. Inflammation
        1. Tuberculosis[412, 413]
        2. Fungal infection (histoplasmosis,[104] coccidioidomycosis,[392] blastomycosis,[474])
           (rare in cryptococcosis)[20, 217]
        3. Viral infections (atypical measles)[153]
        4. Infectious mononucleosis (rare)[274, 341]
        5. AIDS[328]
        6. Drug reactions [259, 523] (phenytoin [Dilantin])
        7. Sarcoidosis (infrequent)
        8. Bacterial lung abscess[505]
III. Bilateral hilar adenopathy
     A. Neoplasm
        1. Lymphoma
        2. Leukemia[41] (chronic lymphocytic leukemia)
        3. Metastasis
        4. Primary bronchogenic carcinoma (usually asymmetric)

(Continued.)

CHART 11–1.   (cont.)

   B. Inflammation
      1. Sarcoidosis[39, 654]
      2. Occupational diseases: silicosis
   C. Collagen-vascular diseases
      1. Lupus (rare)
      2. Polyarteritis nodosa
      3. Mixed
IV. Duplication cysts (bronchogenic cysts)[487]

DISCUSSION

The first problem in the evaluation of a hilar mass is its recognition.[85] The radiologic findings in the case of a hilar mass are increased opacity or alteration in the configuration of the hilum. Since increased opacity of the hilum is the most common presentation of a hilar mass, comparison with the opposite hilum is one of the most reliable methods for detecting a subtle hilar mass. It is important to note whether the increased opacity blends imperceptibly with the normal pulmonary artery shadows and thus obscures their borders or whether the pulmonary arteries are easily identified in addition to the suspected opacity. When the borders of the pulmonary arteries are clearly identifiable, it must be assumed that the mass is discrete and either anterior or posterior to the hilum. The contour of the pulmonary artery is visible because of adjacent aerated lung. When aerated lung is either filled or displaced, the border of the pulmonary artery will no longer be detected. An area of increased opacity either anterior or posterior to the hilum has no effect on the air adjacent to the pulmonary artery and therefore no effect on its visibility. Felson[162] described this phenomenon as the "hilum overlay sign" (Fig 11–3, *A* and *B*). In such cases, the lateral film is usually adequate for verifying that the abnormality is not in the hilum.

Once it has been ascertained that a hilum is abnormal, the next step in evaluating a hilar mass is to determine whether the mass is an enlarged vascular structure or a solid mass. This requires detailed understanding of the anatomy of the hilum in at least the PA and lateral projections (Fig 11–4, *A* and *B*). As mentioned earlier, the hilar shadows in both projections are produced mainly by the right and left pulmonary arteries. The left pulmonary artery is very characteristic in its appearance on the PA film, creating an opacity above the left mainstem bronchus and continuing as an opacity that appears to be lateral to the large bronchi. In a normal subject, the lateral border of the main pulmonary artery should be smooth. On the lateral view film, the left pulmonary artery courses over the origin of the left upper lobe bronchus, which is seen as a circle on edge. The left pulmonary artery descends behind the bronchus. On the PA film, the right pulmonary artery casts a shadow that is mainly lateral to the bronchus intermedius and largely inferior to the right upper lobe bronchus. Like the left pulmonary artery, the major portion of the descending right pulmonary artery has a smooth contour. This large, smooth portion of the right pulmonary artery parallels the bronchus intermedius. It must be emphasized that both pulmonary arteries are branching structures that result in multiple, superimposed opacities. In the lateral view, the right pulmonary artery is seen on end, with its superior portion superimposed over the origin of the left pulmonary artery and its inferior portion anterior and slightly inferior to the circular origin of the left upper lobe bronchus.

Pulmonary veins can best be distinguished from arteries by tracing the course of the vessels, keeping in mind that the veins converge on the left atrium inferior to the hilum. With one exception, the pulmonary veins do not make a major contribution to the hilar shadows.[40] This is most easily appreciated on the lateral film. The lower lobe veins can be readily observed crossing the arteries and converging on the left atrium. The exception is that on the PA film, the upper lobe veins tend to be lateral to the arteries and may be identified especially on the right, when their shadows are observed to cross the hilar arteries in a downward direction. The right upper lobe vein characteristically enlarges in left-sided heart failure.

Pulmonary Arterial Hypertension

Pulmonary arterial hypertension is a major cause of bilateral hilar enlargement (Fig 11–5). Heart failure on the left side is the most common cause of heart failure on the right and therefore a common cause of pulmonary arterial hypertension. This is all preceded by pulmonary venous hypertension, and left heart failure therefore differs significantly from most of the other causes of pulmonary artery hypertension that will be described in this chapter. Congestive heart failure and mitral stenosis both result in enlargement of the upper lobe vessels and constriction of the lower lobe vessels, or cephalization. Cephalization[479] is rapidly followed by interstitial edema as the intravascular pressure exceeds the osmotic and interstitial pressures that normally maintain fluid in the vascular compartment. The radiologic result is increased markings (a fine reticular pattern) and blurring of the margins of pulmonary vessels, which may be accompanied by enlargement of the hila, the main pulmonary artery, and the right ventricle. Failure to appreciate pulmonary arterial enlargement secondary to pulmonary venous hypertension is usually the result of cardiac rotation. Because of the increased markings, this radiologic appearance of pulmonary arterial hypertension is in sharp contrast to the appearance of all other causes of pulmonary artery hypertension.

The loss of normal arterial tapering results in an abrupt change in caliber between the proximal pulmonary arteries and the peripheral pulmonary arteries. There is marked enlargement of the proximal vessels[84] and abrupt tapering or loss of the peripheral vessels. Measurements of the right descending pulmonary artery (>16 mm) and left descending pulmonary artery (>18 mm) in width correlate well with an elevated pulmonary arterial pressure (>20 mm Hg).[388] Other radiologic clues to the diagnosis of pulmonary artery hypertension include enlargement of the main pulmonary artery and enlargement of the right ventricle. The main pulmonary artery produces a bulging, rounded shadow that projects over the left pulmonary artery on the PA film. On the lateral film, enlargement of the right ventricle and main pulmonary artery has the effect of filling in the retrosternal clear space. Oblique films may confirm this impression. These are routinely taken in two projections. The first is the right anterior oblique projection, which is made at a 45-degree angle. This film is readily identified by hanging it on the viewbox in such a way that the stomach bubble is on the patient's left. When viewed in this projection, the contour of the heart is such that the left atrium makes up the posterior border of the heart and is easily evaluated by displacement of the esophagus. More important, the right ventricle, which does not produce a contour on the normal PA and lateral films, makes up the anterior contour of the heart inferiorly, while superiorly the anterior contour is formed by the main pulmonary artery. The oblique view is therefore an excellent view for evaluating right ventricular and main pulmonary artery enlargement. The left anterior oblique projection is made at a 60-degree angle. The film should be placed on the viewbox with the patient's stomach to the left. This projects the right ventricle anteriorly—that is, away from the spine—so that the anterior border of the heart is formed by the right ventricle and pulmonary artery.

Identification of the anterior segmental bronchus leading to either upper lobe may be helpful in evaluating suspected pulmonary arterial hypertension. When the bronchus is seen on end, it appears as a ring shadow. The segmental pulmonary artery is adjacent to the bronchus. In the normal patient, the size of this artery is slightly larger than that of the bronchus when seen on end. When the anterior segmental artery is more than twice the caliber of the anterior segmental bronchus, pulmonary arterial hypertension can be inferred. A change in the size of a segmental artery over a short time interval may provide a good clue to the diagnosis of pulmonary arterial hypertension secondary to congestive heart failure (Fig 11–6, *A* and *B*).

Chronic lung disease is a major cause of pulmonary artery hypertension. Therefore, identification of other signs of lung disease may be the key to the correct diagnosis of pulmonary arterial hypertension. In the case of emphysema, the presence of large avascular areas surrounded by thin lines that indicate bullous lesions is helpful in making the diagnosis. The other radiologic signs of emphysema are discussed in Chapter 22. In addition to emphysema, chronic restrictive interstitial diseases from a variety of causes, including idiopathic fibrosis, scleroderma, sarcoidosis, and cystic fibrosis, may cause pulmonary arterial hyertension (see Chapter 19).[18]

Pulmonary embolism is another major cause of pulmonary arterial hypertension related to lung disease.[174] Acute massive pulmonary embolism may produce radiologic signs of pulmonary arterial hypertension with marked prominence of the hilar vessels, obliteration of the peripheral vessels, and right-sided heart enlargement. The diagnosis of chronic pulmonary emboli may be suggested by a clinical history of recurrent episodes of pleuritic chest pain and hemoptysis associated with thrombophlebitis, but frequently the history is less dramatic. The diagnosis is often verified only by pulmonary arteriography.

Metastatic tumor emboli are rarely diagnosed premortem. Increasing size of the proximal pulmonary arteries may be the only plain film finding. Radionuclide lung scans are reported to show multiple small peripheral defects. Since these emboli are usually very small, they do not produce the segmental and lobar defects expected with thromboemboli. In addition, pulmonary arteriograms typically reveal small, tortuous vessels typical of pulmonary arterial hypertension, and fail to demonstrate the very small tumor emboli. Because of the severe pulmonary arterial hypertension, pulmonary arteriography is a high-risk procedure in patients with tumor emboli. The diagnosis is confirmed by lung biopsy.

Congenital heart disease is another major cause of pulmonary arterial hypertension. It is most commonly secondary to severe left-to-right shunts that remain undiagnosed and untreated for a long time. These include ventricular and atrial septal defects, patent ductus arteriosus, and, less frequently, the admixture lesions: transposition of the great vessels and truncus arteriosus. These heart lesions are usually suspected from clinical signs, particularly when characteristic murmurs are detected. The ventricular septal defect, atrial septal defect, and patent ductus arteriosus are acyanotic lesions until the pulmonary arterial hypertension becomes severe enough to reverse the shunts. This is in contrast to the admixture lesions, which are a cause of early cyanosis. Definitive diagnosis of the cardiac causes of pulmonary hypertension is best made by cardiac catheterization.

The remaining cause of pulmonary arterial hypertension is referred to as idiopathic, or primary.[498] The diagnosis is reached by exclusion. Of the causes of pulmonary arterial hypertension considered in this chapter, chronic pulmonary emboli are the most difficult to distinguish from primary idiopathic pulmonary hypertension. Only the characteristic plexiform arterial changes seen in histologic sections of the lung permit the definitive diagnosis of idiopathic pulmonary arterial hypertension[623] (plexogenic pulmonary arteriopathy).

Hilar Adenopathy

The contour of the hilum must be carefully evaluated in order to distinguish hilar lymphadenopathy from pulmonary artery enlargement. As suggested earlier, a diffuse, smooth enlargement of the pulmonary arteries with abrupt tapering of peripheral vessels is characteristic of pulmonary artery enlargement. This is in contrast to the appearance of lumpy, nodular hila that is typical of hilar adenopathy (see Fig 11–1). The description makes the problem appear simple, but many cases present a diagnostic dilemma. These cases often require either CT with intravenous contrast or MRI. Computed tomography provides excellent discrimination of hilar nodes from pulmonary vessels (Fig 11–7). Since MRI is sensitive to the blood flow through the pulmonary arteries, it provides a clear distinction of pulmonary vessels from any surrounding soft tissue opacity nodes.

Unilateral Hilar Adenopathy

The vast majority of cases of hilar adenopathy will be of either inflammatory or neoplastic origin. Many of these cases will have associated middle mediastinal adenopathy with involvement of subcarinal, azygous, ductus, or paratracheal lymph nodes. Therefore, this differential overlaps considerably with the differential of middle mediastinal masses.

Bronchogenic carcinoma is the most common neoplastic cause of hilar adenopathy. It should be emphasized that the presence of a hilar mass secondary to peripheral bronchogenic carcinoma is an indication of metastatic spread to the hilar nodes.[564] The majority of central primary carcinomas produce endobronchial masses that may spread along the wall of the bronchus or occlude the bronchus, resulting in atelectasis. These endobronchial masses may produce a minimal mass effect prior to involving the regional hilar lymph nodes. The detection of hilar adenopathy in a case of primary bronchogenic carcinoma is extremely important in staging the tumor and is a primary indication for CT in the evaluation of a known primary lung tumor. These regional metastases are usually unilateral in their early phases. When they become extensive, they may involve the mediastinal nodes and later evolve to bilateral hilar adenopathy. In these advanced cases, the adenopathy continues to be asymmetric, particularly in some left-sided tumors, which may metastasize to the right paratracheal nodes. The very undifferentiated small cell tumor or oat cell carcinoma is notorious for this radiologic presentation.

As indicated in Chapter 10, distant primary tumors may metastasize to the mediastinal nodes with some frequency, but true hilar involvement with no mediastinal involvement is unusual, with the occasional exception of metastatic renal cell carcinoma.[105,352] This is in contrast to lymphomas, and particularly Hodgkin's lymphomas, which may present with asymmetric hilar adenopathy and only minimal mediastinal involvement.

In addition to the strong probability of tumor in patients who have asymmetric hilar enlargement, we must remember that infectious diseases are also seen in association with hilar adenopathy. Primary tuberculosis is notorious for producing asymmetric hilar enlargement as well as mediastinal adenopathy. In the past, primary tuberculosis was considered a childhood disease. This is still true in areas of the world where primary tuberculosis is endemic, but in the continental United States, a large population who are well into their adult years are at risk for primary tuberculosis (Fig 11–8). The diagnosis is frequently confirmed at biopsy, since the risk for tumor is so much greater. Tuberculosis in patients with advanced AIDS resembles primary tuberculosis with hilar and mediastinal adenopathy. Other causes of granulomatous inflammation, in particular such fungi as *Histoplasma,* are also well known for producing asymmetric hilar adenopathy. These two diagnoses are radiologically confirmed only when they lead to the development of hilar lymph node calcification. In this instance, the hilar lymph nodes may be essentially replaced by calcium. Other causes of hilar lymphadenopathy include viral pneumonias (in particular measles), infectious mononucleosis, silicosis, and drug reactions. These entities all require careful clinical correlation. Silicosis is possibly the easiest to confirm when a history of exposure is obtained and the lymph nodes are calcified. The calcification may even assume a characteristic appearance, with a thin rim of calcification.

Bilateral Hilar Adenopathy

Sarcoidosis produces the classic example of bilateral hilar adenopathy (Fig 11–2).[39] (Answer to question 2 is *c.*) In contrast to all of the causes of hilar adenopathy that have been considered so far, the adenopathy of sarcoidosis is typically bilateral, symmetric, and frequently associated with mediastinal (paratracheal and ductus) node enlargement. This cause of hilar adenopathy often assumes such a characteristic radiologic appearance that both radiologists and clinicians will lean strongly toward it as the diagnosis. Even when the patient is asymptomatic, it is prudent to obtain a biopsy for confirmation. Although it is rare, bilateral symmetric hilar adenopathy resembling the appearance of sarcoidosis can result from lymphoma and even chronic lymphocytic leukemia (Fig 11–9).

Sarcoidosis frequently involves the supraclavicular nodes, the liver, and the interstitium of the lung. The interstitium of the lung may be extensively involved with minimal granulomas that are too small for radiologic detection but which may be easily detected on transbronchial biopsy. Therefore, transbronchial biopsy may be a good method for confirming the diagnosis of sarcoidosis, even in the absence of radiologically demonstrable interstitial disease.

Bilateral hilar adenopathy may occasionally be associated with other radiologic abnormalities such as a fine nodular interstitial pattern; large, multifocal, ill-defined opacities; confluent opacities suggestive of pulmonary edema; diffuse interstitial reticular disease; and even pleural effusion. Its combination with these must be carefully evaluated. Both sarcoidosis and lymphoma may result in such combinations. Of the combinations, bilateral symmetric hilar adenopathy with pleural effusion is perhaps the least common presentation of sarcoidosis. No more than 3% of patients with sarcoidosis are reported to have significant pleural effusion. Therefore, the presence of pleural effusion should be an additional reason for biopsy confirmation of the diagnosis of sarcoidosis. In fact, the presence of pleural effusion with asymmetric hilar adenopathy could support a number of diagnoses, including carcinoma of the lung, metastases from a distant site, lymphoma, tuberculosis, and, least likely, sarcoidosis.

Calcified bilateral hilar nodes could be the result of treated lymphoma, but they are almost always the result of chronic granulomatous diseases. Histoplasmosis and tuberculosis are the most common causes of hilar and mediastinal nodal calcifications. The calcifications are usually amorphous and scattered throughout the nodes. Infrequently, peripheral or so-called "egg-shell" calcifications are seen in enlarged nodes that have resulted from silicosis or, less frequently, sarcoidosis (Fig 11–10).

SUMMARY

1. The most common radiologic manifestation of a hilar mass is increased opacity of the hilum.

2. Contour abnormalities are extremely important in distinguishing pulmonary artery from hilar lymph node enlargement. Computed tomography or MRI may be essential to distinguish hilar adenopathy, particularly when the abnormality is minimal.

3. The differential for pulmonary artery enlargement is the same as for pulmonary arterial hypertension and includes both primary lung and cardiac diseases.

4. Most cases of hilar enlargement represent unilateral or bilateral hilar adenopathy. Hilar enlargement is frequently associated with middle mediastinal adenopathy. The most common causes for unilateral hilar enlargement are primary carcinoma of the lung, metastases, lymphoma, and infections, including tuberculosis and fungal infection.

5. The most common cause of bilateral symmetric hilar adenopathy is sarcoidosis; however, both metastatic disease and lymphoma may mimic it radiologically. Patients who have bilateral hilar adenopathy and significant systemic symptoms must be rigorously evaluated to eliminate these two alternative possibilities.

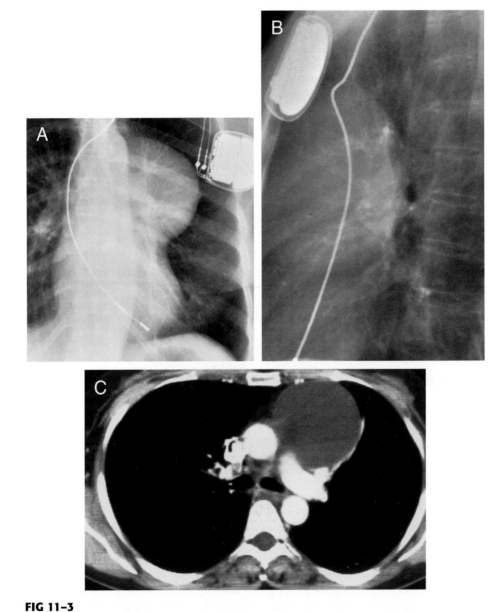

FIG 11–3
A, This large mass has a well-circumscribed lateral border, which is tapered at both the superior and inferior margins. The mass projects over the left hilum but does not obscure the pulmonary artery. This combination of findings indicates that this cannot be a hilar mass. **B,** Lateral film confirms that the mass is anterior to the hilum. **C,** Contrast-enhanced CT confirms that the mass arises anterior to the hilum and displaces the pulmonary artery posteriorly. The low attenuation further indicates that it is not a solid mass. This is a large thymic cyst.

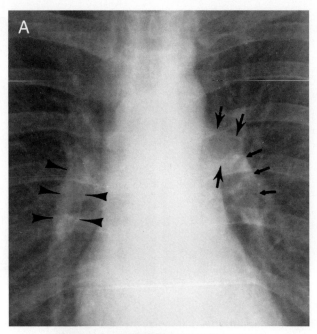

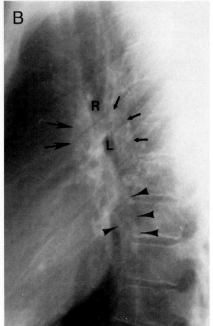

FIG 11–4
A, Arrows outline the normal pulmonary arteries. Right pulmonary artery *(arrowheads)* is lateral to the bronchus intermedius. Left pulmonary artery *(large arrows)* passes posteriorly over the left upper lobe bronchus. The lateral border of the left hilum is formed by the descending left lower lobe artery *(small arrows)*. **B,** Normal appearance of the right pulmonary artery on lateral view is indicated with large arrows. Right upper lobe bronchus is marked with *R*. Course of the left pulmonary artery, crossing over left main bronchus *(L)* is outlined with small arrows. Arrowheads identify confluence of lower lobe pulmonary veins.

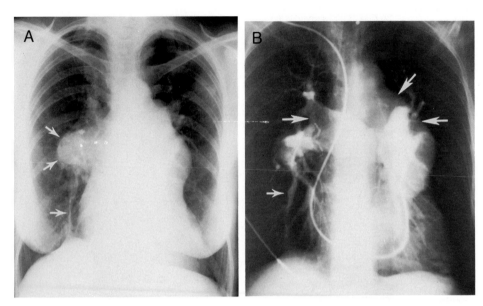

FIG 11–5
A, Bilateral enlargement of proximal pulmonary arteries *(arrows)* with abrupt tapering of peripheral vessels indicates pulmonary arterial hypertension. Linear opacity *(lower arrow)* extending from the hilum to the diaphragm is a scar from a prior infarct. This is pulmonary arterial hypertension secondary to recurrent pulmonary embolism. **B,** Pulmonary arteriogram confirms that hilar opacities represent massively enlarged proximal pulmonary arteries. (From Chen JTT: *Essentials of Cardiac Roentgenology.* Boston, Little Brown, 1987. Used by permission.)

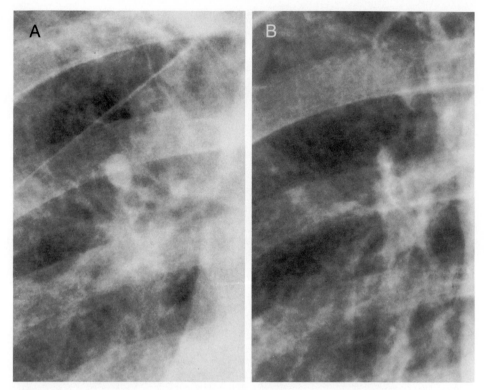

FIG 11–6
A, This segmental artery is larger than its companion bronchus, indicating increased pulmonary arterial pressure in a patient with congestive heart failure. **B,** After treatment, the same segmental artery has returned to normal size.

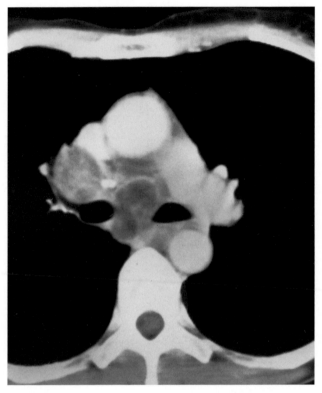

FIG 11–7
Contrast-enhanced CT scan from the case seen in Figure 11–1 shows well-defined soft tissue opacity nodes adjacent to the enhanced pulmonary arteries.

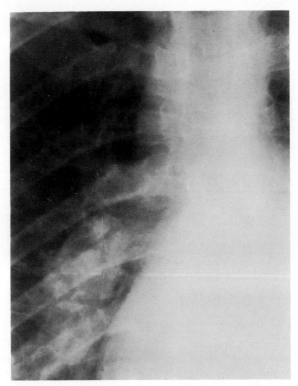

FIG 11–8
Tuberculosis is a well-known cause of asymmetric hilar adenopathy. Note right hilar en-largement in this case of primary tuberculosis. Diagnosis is readily suspected in a pedi-atric patient, but it required biopsy to rule out tumor in this adult.

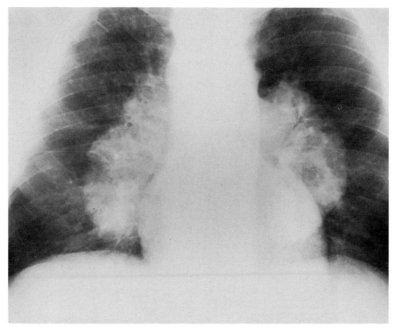

FIG 11–9
Hematologic malignancies, including lymphoma and leukemia, are common causes of middle mediastinal masses. This patient with a late stage of chronic lymphocytic leukemia has extensive hilar adenopathy.

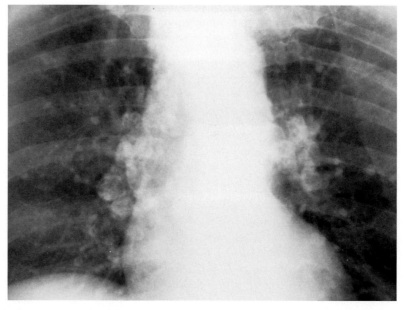

FIG 11–10
These enlarged bilateral hilar nodes are calcified with a unique pattern of calcification. This rimlike peripheral calcification has been described as "egg-shell" and is seen in patients with sarcoidosis and silicosis. This patient has silicosis.

ANSWER GUIDE

LEGENDS FOR INTRODUCTORY FIGURES

FIG 11–1

A, Unilateral enlargement of the right hilum is typical of hilar adenopathy. Note that lobulated opacity blends with the borders of the pulmonary artery. Left pulmonary artery is normal. **B,** Lateral film confirms area of increased opacity, with sharp anterior border *(arrows)*, in the upper portion of the hilum. This hilar adenopathy is the result of metastases to regional nodes from small cell carcinoma of the lung.

FIG 11–2

Lobulated appearance of both hila with normal peripheral vascularity is characteristic of bilateral hilar adenopathy. Normal peripheral vascularity is an important radiologic finding that excludes pulmonary hypertension as a cause of hilar enlargement. This is a classic example of sarcoidosis with bilateral hilar adenopathy. In addition, note enlarged ductus node between aortic arch and top of left pulmonary artery.

ANSWERS

1, b; 2, c.

CHAPTER 12

Posterior Mediastinal Mass

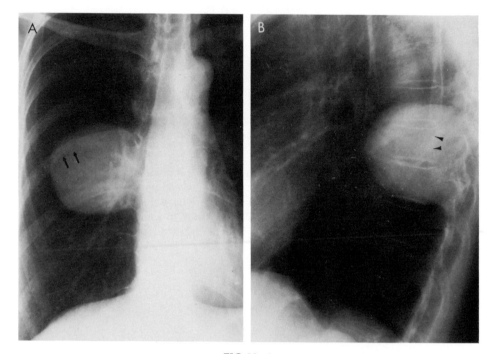

FIG 12–1

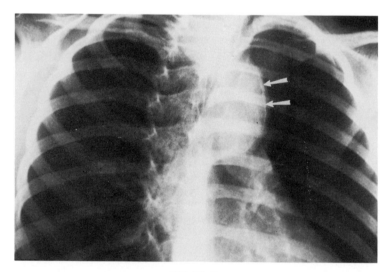

FIG 12–2

QUESTIONS

1. Which of the following diagnoses are most likely in the case illustrated in Figure 12–1, *A* and *B?*
   a. Neuroblastoma.
   b. Paraspinous abscess.
   c. Schwannoma.
   d. Paraganglioma.
   e. Neurenteric cyst.
2. Which of the following neural tumors is most likely in a 6-year-old patient?
   a. Ganglioneuroma.
   b. Neurofibroma.
   c. Ganglioneuroblastoma.
   d. Schwannoma.
   e. Chemodectoma.
3. Referring to Figure 12–2, which of the following is most likely to have a peripheral rim of calcification?
   a. Neurenteric cyst.
   b. Ganglioneuroblastoma.
   c. Neuroblastoma.
   d. Ganglioneuroma.
   e. Neurofibroma.
4. Rib spreading and erosion of multiple ribs is most typically seen in which of the following?
   a. Neurofibroma.
   b. Schwannoma.
   c. Hemangioma.
   d. Neuroblastoma.
   e. Chemodectoma.

Match the following descriptions with the list of diagnoses that might cause a posterior mediastinal mass:

5. Congenital hereditary spherocytosis
6. Alcoholism with elevated amylase level
7. Asymptomatic bilateral hilar adenopathy
8. Hemivertebra

a. Sarcoidosis
b. Neurenteric cyst
c. Extramedullary hematopoiesis
d. Pancreatic pseudocyst

CHART 12–1.
Posterior Mediastinal Masses

I. Neoplasms
   A. Neural tumors[483]
      1. Ganglion series tumors (neuroblastoma, ganglioneuroblastoma, ganglioneuroma)
      2. Nerve root tumors (schwannoma, neurofibroma, malignant schwannoma)
      3. Paragangliomas (chemodectoma, pheochromocytoma)
   B. Metastases
   C. Lymphomas[68,373]
   D. Mesenchymal tumors (fibroma, lipoma, muscle tumors, leiomyoma[220])
   E. Hemangiomas[118]
   F. Thyroid tumors
   G. Vertebral tumors (osteoblastoma and giant cell tumor)   *(Continued.)*

CHART 12–1 (cont.).

II. Inflammation
    A. Paraspinous abscess (tuberculosis and staphylococcus)
    B. Mediastinitis[157,179]
    C. Lymphoid hyperplasia
    D. Sarcoidosis[39]
III. Vascular lesions
    A. Aneurysm of the descending aorta[294,491]
IV. Trauma
    A. Traumatic aneurysm
    B. Hematoma[179]
    C. Loculated hemothorax
    D. Traumatic pseudomeningocele[145]
V. Developmental lesions
    A. Enteric cysts[487]
    B. Neurenteric cysts[487]
    C. Bronchogenic cysts[487]
    D. Extralobar sequestration
VI. Abdominal diseases
    A. Bochdalek's hernia (thoracic kidney)[372]
    B. Pancreatic pseudocyst or abscess[317]
    C. Retroperitoneal masses (teratomas, sarcomas, and metastases)
VII. Other
    A. Loculated pleural effusion (empyema)
    B. Lateral meningocele[352]
    C. Lipoma and lipomatosis[280]
    D. Extramedullary hematopoiesis[275,305]
    E. "Pseudomass" of the newborn[8]

DISCUSSION

This discussion follows the divisions of the mediastinum described by Felson. The middle and posterior compartments of the mediastinum are divided by a line that follows the curvature of the spine and is located 1 cm posterior to the anterior border of the vertebral bodies. Therefore, most of the masses that are considered herein might be classified by other authors as posterior gutter masses. Very large masses often extend into the anatomic posterior mediastinum. It may be difficult to determine the origin of a very large mass and therefore to appreciate that it did arise in the posterior gutter.

Neural Tumors

The neural tumors constitute the largest group of posterior mediastinal and posterior gutter masses.[74,365] These tumors are derived from nerve roots, intercostal nerves, and sympathetic ganglia. Nerve root tumors are either schwannomas or neurofibromas. The sympathetic ganglion tumors include the neuroblastomas, ganglioneuroblastomas, and ganglioneuromas. The paragangliomas, including chemodectoma and pheochromocytoma, are infrequent causes of posterior mediastinal masses.[483]

Schwannomas are derived from the sheath of Schwann, which forms the connective tissues of the nerve root. There are no nerve cells in a schwannoma. This is in contrast to the true neurofibroma, which contains both Schwann cells and nerve cells. Prior to 1955, distinction between these two tumors was not generally made. This resulted in the concept that neurofibromas are the most common cause of posterior mediastinal masses. The schwannomas are much more common than true neurofibromas and are the most common of all the neural tumors. Most schwannomas and neurofibromas are benign tumors; the very rare malignant nerve root tumor is classified as a malignant schwannoma regardless of the presence of nerve cells in the tumor.

The neuroblastomas are highly malignant, undifferentiated, small round cell tumors that originate from the sympathetic ganglia. In contrast, the ganglioneuromas, which are also derived from the sympathetic ganglia, are completely benign.[132] Mature connective tissue that resembles the connective tissues of schwannomas is one of the primary tissues in ganglioneuromas. The presence of mature ganglion cells is the histologic feature that distinguishes schwannomas from ganglioneuromas. Ganglioneuroblastomas are mixed cell tumors that contain not only mature, well-differentiated ganglion cells, but also connective tissues and undifferentiated round cells. In other words, ganglioneuroblastomas have features of both ganglioneuromas, which are completely benign, and neuroblastomas, which are highly malignant. These tumors do have a better prognosis than the neuroblastomas, but must be regarded as malignant tumors. It is true, however, that cases of spontaneous maturation have been observed. Cushing and Wolbach described a case that matured from a neuroblastoma to a completely differentiated ganglioneuroma,[110] but this is unfortunately a very rare event.

The radiologic presentation of most neural tumors is a homogeneous, opaque mass in the posterior mediastinum. A small percentage of these tumors contain calcification.[136,483] This calcification should be evenly distributed through a mass when the lesion is viewed in both the PA and lateral projections. The calcification often assumes a speckled pattern and may vary considerably in quantity (Fig 12–3, A and B).

There is a striking difference between the shape of nerve root tumors and tumors of the ganglion series.[74,483,604] Eighty percent of nerve root tumors appear as round masses (Fig 12–1, A and B), whereas 80% of the ganglion series tumors appear as vertically oriented, elongated masses (Fig 12–4). An additional feature that is helpful in distinguishing these masses is a tapered border, which suggests a ganglion series tumor. In contrast, the round nerve root tumors tend to have a sulcus, which may indicate a more lateral position. This may suggest that the tumor is arising from the intercostal nerve. In Chapter 2, schwannoma was mentioned as a possible cause of a chest wall mass (see Fig 12–1, A and B). (Answer to question 1 is c.)

A variety of bone abnormalities may be observed with the neural tumors, including rib spreading, erosion, and destruction. Neural foramina enlargement indicates extension of the mass into the neural canal (Fig 12–5, A and B). This is often described as a "dumbbell" lesion.[148] Patients with neural foramina enlargement typically have neurologic deficits caused by compression of the spinal cord.[5] This complication most often results from the benign nerve root tumors, but it may also occur when a large neuroblastoma extends posteriorly.[33] The slow-growing benign tumors tend to erode bone, whereas the malignant tumors invade and destroy bone. The erosion caused by a benign tumor may lead to a scalloped sclerotic defect in the posterior aspect of the vertebral body. Rib spreading is associated with a very large mass and most frequently results from a malignant tumor. Scoliosis is likewise seen with very large masses, both benign and malignant (Fig 12–6).

Age is the most important clinical feature in the differential diagnosis of posterior mediastinal masses. In patients less than 1 year old, a posterior mediastinal mass is almost certainly a neuroblastoma. After 10 years of age, neuroblastomas are rare. The ganglioneuroblastomas typically occur in children between 1 and 10 years of age; ganglioneuromas typically occur in the 6- to 15-year age group. All of the ganglion series tumors are relatively infrequent in adults, although ganglioneuromas are observed in persons up to age 50. In contrast, the schwannomas and neurofibromas are infrequent in childhood, occurring most frequently in the third and fourth decades.[483] (Answer to question 2 is *c.*)

Neurofibromatosis (von Recklinghausen's disease) may also be associated with posterior mediastinal masses.[404] As many as 30% of patients with true neurofibromas may have neurofibromatosis. As mentioned earlier, the overall incidence of malignancy in the nerve root tumors is very low, but there is a trend to malignant transformation in patients with von Recklinghausen's disease. Schwannomas and ganglioneuromas have also been reported in this group of patients, but the association is less frequent. Ganglioneuromas more commonly occur as isolated posterior mediastinal masses.

Lymphadenopathy

Lymphadenopathy should not be overlooked as a cause of posterior mediastinal masses. Bronchogenic carcinoma may metastasize to the posterior lymph nodes and should be considered in the presence of other signs of a primary tumor, such as atelectasis or hilar or paratracheal masses. The mass may be quite large and involve both the middle and posterior compartments. Lymphoma[373] is another important cause of posterior mediastinal adenopathy and must be considered in patients with systemic symptoms, including weight loss and low-grade fever. The additional finding of associated hilar adenopathy in these patients could be strongly suggestive of lymphoma. On the other hand, the combination of a paraspinous mass and bilateral symmetric hilar adenopathy in an asymptomatic patient raises the possibility of sarcoidosis. Bein et al.[39] reported a 2% incidence of paraspinous masses in patients with sarcoidosis. Often the differentiation of sarcoidosis from lymphoma can be made by considering the clinical presentation of the patient. In lymphoma it is unlikely for a patient to have extensive hilar and mediastinal adenopathy and remain asymptomatic, while the patient with sarcoidosis may typically be asymptomatic. (Answer to question 7 is *a.*)

Paraspinous Abscess

Tuberculosis is the classic cause of paraspinous abscess, but other bacterial infections—particularly *Staphylococcus*—must be considered in the differential diagnosis of a posterior gutter mass. Tuberculosis and staphylococcal infections may cause spondylitis with destruction of the end plates of the vertebral bodies and the intervertebral disk space. There may also be compression deformity of the vertebral bodies, which in cases of tuberculosis is described as Pott's deformity of the spine. The bone changes of bacterial and tuberculous spondylitis may be minimal and sometimes are not detectable by plain film, requiring CT or MR. The absence of bone destruction does not eliminate the possibility of spondylitis. The subligamentous tuberculous abscess causes a paraspinal soft tissue mass without the expected bone destruction. Clinical correlation and comparison with previous films may occasionally suggest this diagnosis. For example, serial films that reveal the appearance of a mass over a period of a few weeks, during which time the patient has fever and night sweats, strongly suggest tuberculous paraspinous abscess (Fig 12–7, *A* and *C*).

Duplication Cysts

Duplication cysts[487] are rare and typically occur in the mediastinum. The classic location for the bronchogenic cyst is the middle compartment, while the enteric and neurenteric cysts are more typically found in the posterior compartment. The enteric and neurenteric cysts are histologically indistinguishable. These cysts are lined by a gastric epithelium that secretes gastric juices. Because of this epithelium, the masses tend to be large and symptomatic. In contrast to bronchogenic cysts, which usually occur as an asymptomatic mass in young adults, enteric and neurenteric cysts typically appear in children. A neurenteric cyst is distinguishable from an enteric cyst by being accompanied by vertebral body abnormalities, including hemivertebra and butterfly vertebra. On occasion the mass may actually have to be dissected from the vertebral body. It is important to realize that the vertebral body abnormality may occur cephalad to the mass. Calcification may occur in the wall of these cystic structures and is useful in distinguishing a cyst from such neural tumors as neuroblastoma or ganglioneuroblastoma (see Figs 12–2 and 12–8). (Answer to question 3 is *a*; Answer to question 8 is *b*.)

Aneurysm

Aneurysm is another important cause of a posterior mediastinal mass. Oblique views may be helpful in evaluating posterior mediastinal masses, since the mass can sometimes be clearly distinguished from the shadow of the descending aorta, thus excluding the possibility of aneurysm. When the mass is indistinguishable from the aorta, the possibility of an aneurysm must be considered, particularly in older age groups. Curvilinear calcification similar to that seen in the wall of the cyst may also occur in the wall of an aortic aneurysm. Therefore, a posterior mediastinal mass with curvilinear calcification in a 20-year-old patient most likely represents an enteric cyst, while the same radiologic presentation in a 70-year-old patient most likely represents an aneurysm. The diagnosis should be confirmed by angiography (Fig 12–9, *A* and *B*), a CT scan with contrast enhancement (Fig 12–10, *A–C*), or MRI.[207]

Abdominal Diseases

Bochdalek's hernia must be considered as the cause of a posterior mediastinal mass when the mass is continuous with the contour of the diaphragm. The most common structures to herniate through the diaphragm are retroperitoneal fat and kidney.[356] An intravenous pyelogram will often confirm this diagnosis (Fig 12–11).

Pancreatic pseudocyst[317] is an infrequent cause of either a middle or a posterior mediastinal mass. It is likely to have associated pleural effusion. Pancreatic pseudocyst should be suspected when a mass develops over a short period in a patient with the clinical diagnosis of pancreatitis. A history of alcoholism with recurrent pancreatitis and laboratory test results demonstrating elevated amylase levels strongly support the diagnosis. (Answer to question 6 is *d*.)

Teratomas and seminomas that present as primary mediastinal tumors produce anterior mediastinal masses and are not expected in the posterior mediastinum. However, these germinal tumors also present as primary testicular neoplasms that may metastasize to the retroperitoneal nodes. Extension of a retroperitoneal mass into the chest will produce the radiologic appearance of a posterior paraspinous mass (Fig 12–12, *A–D*).

Other

Lateral meningocele[352] is another rare cause of a mediastinal mass and, like the nerve root tumors, may have the additional radiologic feature of enlarged neural foramina. The diagnosis should be considered in patients with neurofibromatosis, and is confirmed by MRI (Fig 12–13).

Occasionally, other rare tumors, including mesenchymal tumors and hemangiomas, which cannot now be diagnosed by radiologic criteria, may be encountered. The diagnosis of these tumors is made only by histologic examination of the mass. However, the ability to detect subtle variations in opacity and gross features of masses has dramatically improved with the use of CT scanning. For example, the fatty tumors such as lipoma and hibernoma, which could not be diagnosed by plain film criteria, may now be recognized by detecting the low opacity of fat with a CT scan. Steroid-induced mediastinal lipomatosis may be suspected when a patient on steroid therapy develops paraspinous masses. Studies by Streiter et al.[590] illustrate how this diagnosis may be confirmed by CT.

Extramedullary hematopoiesis is an infrequent cause of a posterior mediastinal mass and should be considered in patients with a hereditary anemia. In fact, it may cause multiple or lobulated masses. Other associated abnormalities may include distinctive bone changes, such as enlargement of the ribs from longstanding increased activity of the marrow. Associated splenomegaly may provide another radiologic clue to the diagnosis. (Answer to question 5 is *c*.)

SUMMARY

1. The most common cause of a posterior mediastinal mass is a neural tumor.

2. Nerve root tumors, schwannoma, and neurofibroma most commonly occur in adults and are benign.

3. Neuroblastoma and ganglioneuroblastoma are malignant ganglion series tumors and most commonly occur in children.

4. Calcification throughout a mass is most suggestive of a ganglion series tumor. It cannot be used to distinguish benign from malignant tumors.

5. A thin rim of calcification around the periphery of an apparent mass suggests either an aneurysm or a cyst.

6. Rib erosion of a single rib with sclerosis of the rib border, as described in Chapter 2, is compatible with a benign tumor, but spreading of multiple ribs with erosion or destruction suggests a malignant ganglion series tumor.

7. The vertebral anomalies of hemivertebrae or butterfly vertebrae, with a posterior mediastinal mass, are diagnostic of a neurenteric cyst.

8. Paraspinal abscess with intervertebral disk destruction is classic for tuberculosis, but the bone abnormality may be minimal to absent.

9. The gross morphologic features of a posterior mediastinal mass may appear to be nonspecific, but when careful analysis of these features is combined with the clinical presentation of the patient, we should be able to make a precise diagnosis in most cases. Differences in opacity that result from subtle gross differences may now be detected with CT scans and should further improve the diagnostic ability of the radiologist.

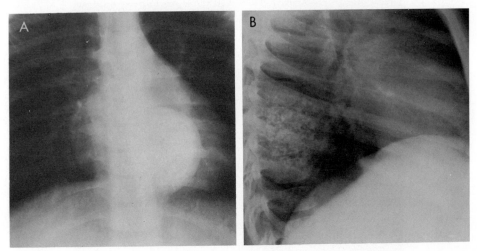

FIG 12–3
A, Distribution of calcium through the mass indicates a solid mass. This is a ganglioneuro-blastoma. **B,** Lateral projection film from case illustrated in **A** confirms the distribution of calcium throughout a solid mass. (From Reed JC, Hallet KK, Feagin DS: Neural tumors of the thorax: subject review from the AFIP. *Radiology* 1978; 126:9–17. Used by permission.)

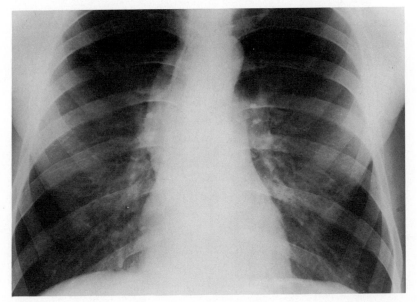

FIG 12–4
Elongated, tapered, homogeneous posterior mediastinal mass has the typical appearance for a ganglion series tumor. It is a ganglioneuroma. (From Reed JC, Hallet KK, Feagin DS: Neural tumors of the thorax: subject review from the AFIP. *Radiology* 1978; 126:9–17. Used by permission.)

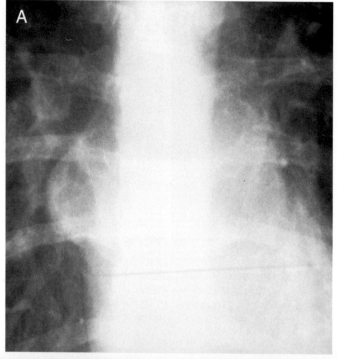

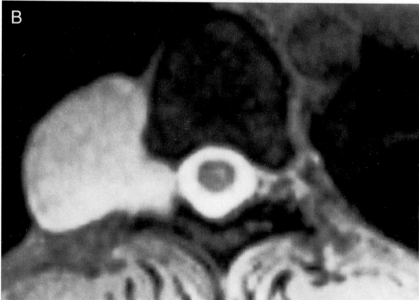

FIG 12–5
A, PA film of schwannoma shows a well-circumscribed right paraspinal mass with
tapered borders, indicating a mediastinal origin. The mass is minimally visible on the lateral view and projects over the spine, consistent with a posterior mediastinal mass.
B, This T$_2$-weighted gradient echo MR image reveals a high signal mass with extension
through the neural foramen. This is a common presentation for a nerve root tumor and
was surgically confirmed to be a schwannoma.

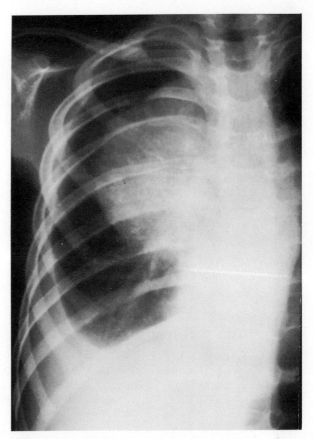

FIG 12–6
Large ganglioneuroblastoma has eroded and spread multiple ribs. Pleural effusion is an additional sign suggesting malignancy. (From Reed JC, Hallet KK, Feagin DS: Neural tumors of the thorax: subject review from the AFIP. *Radiology* 1978; 126:9–17. Used by permission.)

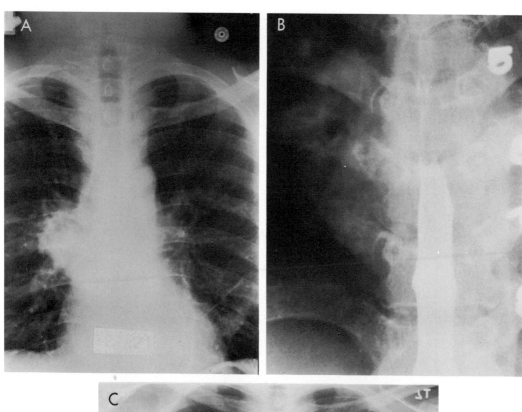

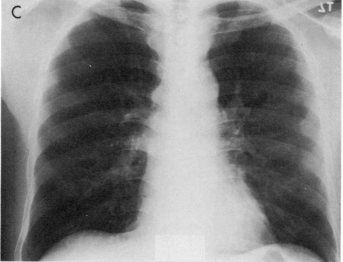

FIG 12–7
A, Elongated, tapered mass resembles a neural tumor. **B,** Myelogram from case illustrated in **A** reveals complete block at the level of the mass. This would be compatible with a neural tumor that has extended through the neural foramina, similar to that seen in Fig 12–5. **C,** Film taken 2 months earlier reveals that a mass has developed over a short period of time. This eliminates the possibility of a slow-growing benign tumor such as a schwannoma or neurofibroma. This is a tuberculous abscess.

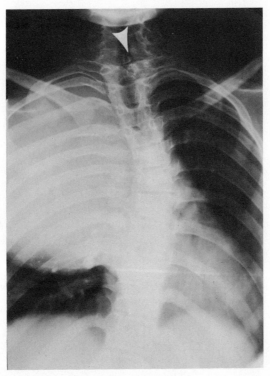

FIG 12–8
Very large mass has associated skeletal abnormalities that provide the clue to diagnosis.
Scoliosis may be associated with a variety of very large posterior mediastinal masses and
is therefore not diagnostic. A diagnostic finding is the hemivertebra *(arrowhead)* in the
cervical spine. This is a neurenteric cyst. (From Reed JC, Sobonya RE: Morphologic analysis of foregut cysts in the thorax. *AJR* 1974; 120:851–860. Used by permission.)

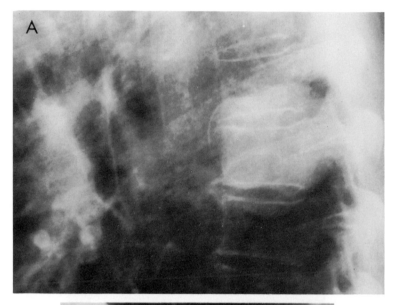

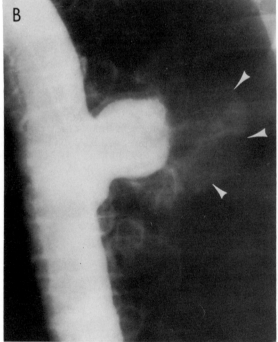

FIG 12–9
A, Thin rim of calcification around the periphery of this mass might resemble that seen in Figure 12–2. Calcification rules out a solid mass and could be seen with either a cyst or an aneurysm. **B,** Aortogram from case illustrated in **A** confirms the diagnosis of aortic aneurysm. The aneurysm is filled with thrombus *(arrowheads).*

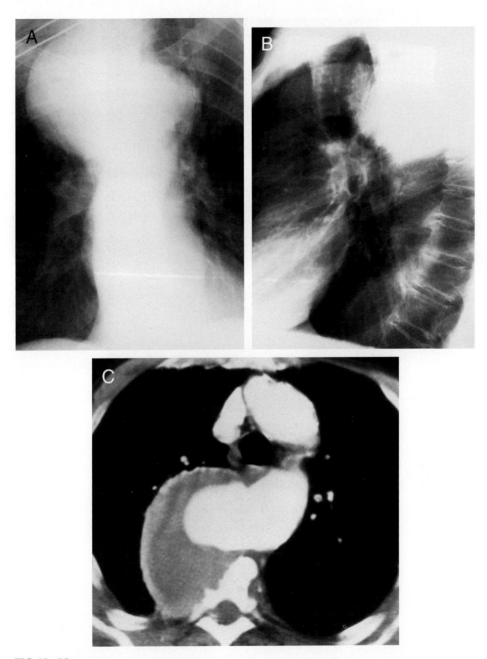

FIG 12–10
A, Large superior mediastinal opacity projects to the right and requires consideration of aneurysm vs. a mass. This is above the ascending aorta, which is the most likely origin for a right-sided aneurysm, but it is adjacent to an enlarged aortic arch. **B,** Lateral film shows the opacity to be posterior and to project over the posterior portion of the aortic arch. **C,** Contrast-enhanced CT confirms a large aneurysm with thrombus and erosion of the vertebral body.

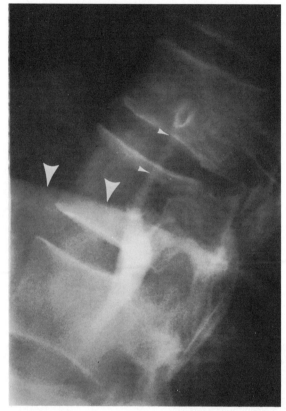

FIG 12–11
Intravenous pyelogram shows that kidney extends above the diaphragm *(large arrow-heads)*. Note the superior pole calyces *(small arrowheads)*. This is an example of Bochdalek's hernia.

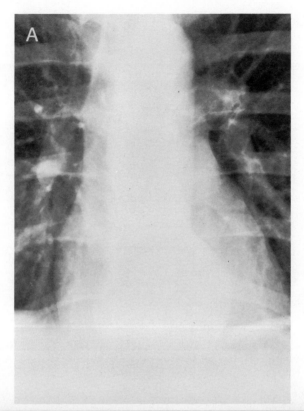

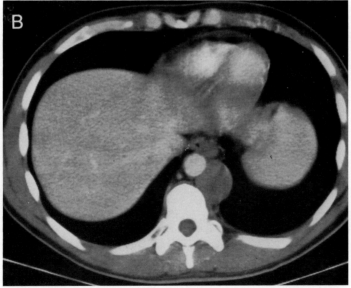

FIG 12–12
A, Metastatic testicular carcinoma caused this smooth, well-circumscribed retrocardiac mass with a tapered superior border. This appearance is similar to that of a ganglioneuroma. **B,** CT scan at the level of the mass confirmed a homogeneous paraspinous mass that extended anteriorly around the arota. **C,** Additional CT sections taken above the level of the paraspinous mass revealed involvement of additional para-aortic nodes. The aorta is surrounded by enlarged nodes. **D,** Abdominal CT scan revealed a much larger mass of nodes surrounding the aorta. Testicular ultrasound examination detected the primary tumor.

(Continued.)

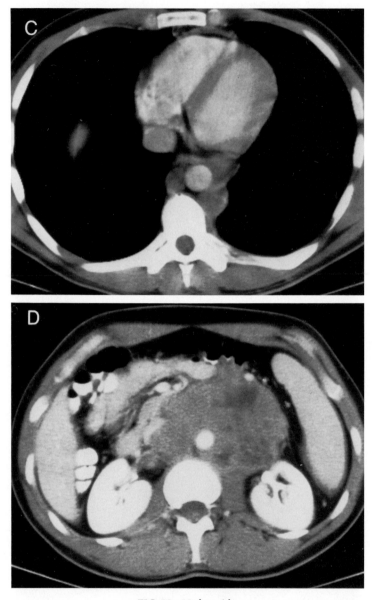

FIG 12–12 (cont.).

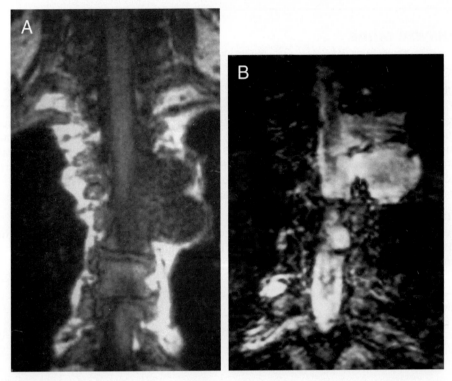

FIG 12–13
A, T_1-weighted coronal MR scan of patient with left paraspinal opacity detected on plain film. Patient is known to have neurofibromatosis. There is a low signal abnormality surrounded by high signal mediastinal fat. **B,** T_2-weighted coronal MR shows a high signal pattern, indicating that the abnormality is fluid filled and confirms the diagnosis of meningocele. (From Reed JC: Schwannoma. Chest Disease (Fifth Series) Test and Syllabus. American College of Radiology 1996; 213–236. Used by permission.)

ANSWER GUIDE

LEGENDS FOR INTRODUCTORY FIGURES

FIG 12–1

A, Homogeneous round mass eroding inferior surface of a posterior rib *(arrows)* illustrates typical radiologic appearance of a nerve root tumor in the posterior mediastinum. This is a schwannoma. (From Reed JC, Hallet KK, Feagin DS: Neural tumors of the thorax: subject review from the AFIP. *Radiology* 1978; 126:9–17. Used by permission). **B,** Lateral projection film from case illustrated in **A** confirms posterior location of mass. Note posterior erosion of the vertebral body *(arrowheads),* indicating extension of the mass through the neural foramina. This is often described as a "dumbbell" mass.

FIG 12–2

Peripheral rim of calcification in posterior mediastinal mass reveals cystic character of the lesion. Enteric and neurenteric cysts typically occur in the posterior compartment. (From Reed JC, Sobonya RE: Morphologic analysis of foregut cysts in the thorax. *AJR* 1974; 120:851–860. Used by permission.)

ANSWERS

1, c; 2, c; 3, a; 4, d; 5, c; 6, d; 7, a; 8, b.

PART II

PULMONARY OPACITIES

CHAPTER 13

Atelectasis

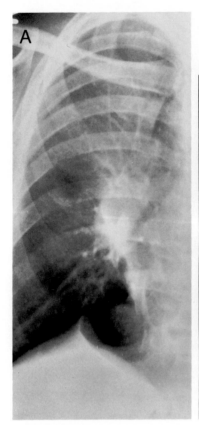
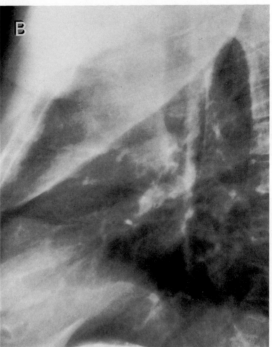

FIG 13–1

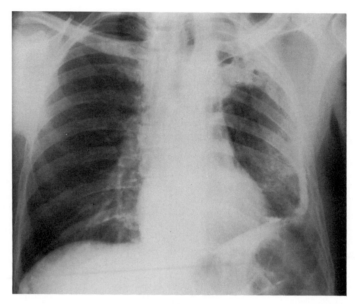

FIG 13–2

QUESTIONS

1. Which of the following abnormalities are present on the films in Figures 13–1, *A* and *B?*
   a. Right upper lobe atelectasis.
   b. Juxtaphrenic peak.
   c. Displacement of the major fissure.
   d. Right middle lobe atelectasis.
   e. All of the above.
2. Which one of the following is the most common cause of atelectasis?
   a. Metastasis.
   b. Bronchial carcinoid.
   c. Lymphoma.
   d. Squamous cell carcinoma.
   e. Sarcoidosis.
3. The case illustrated in Figure 13–2 is an example of which of the following types of atelectasis?
   a. Compressive.
   b. Obstructive.
   c. Cicatrizing.
   d. Relaxation.
   e. Adhesive.

Match the following types of atelectasis with the disease entities listed in the right column.

4. Obstructive ____   a. Pulmonary embolism
5. Compressive ____   b. Bronchial carcinoid
6. Passive ____   c. Radiation pneumonitis

7. Cicatrizing   ____
8. Adhesive   ____

d. Tuberculosis
e. Pneumothorax
f. Bullous emphysema
g. Asthma

CHART 13–1.
Atelectasis

I. Large airway obstruction
  A. Tumor
    1. Bronchogenic carcinoma[257]
    2. Bronchial carcinoid[226,555]
    3. Metastasis[42,99,122,540]
    4. Lymphoma[130,526]
    5. Less frequent (lipoma, granular cell myoblastoma)[226,532,602]
  B. Inflammatory
    1. Tuberculosis (endobronchial granuloma, broncholith,[620] bronchial stenosis)
    2. Sarcoidosis, endobronchial granuloma (rare)[265]
  C. Other
    1. Large left atrium
    2. Foreign body (including malpositioned endotracheal tube)
    3. Amyloidosis[271]
    4. Wegener's granulomatosis[377]
    5. Bronchial transection[334,617]
II. Small airway obstruction: predisposing factors
  A. Mucus plugs[205]
    1. Severe chest or abdominal pain (particularly in the postoperative patient)
    2. Respiratory depressant drugs (e.g., morphine)
    3. Asthma[456]
    4. Cystic fibrosis
  B. Inflammatory[510]
    1. Bronchopneumonia
    2. Bronchitis
    3. Bronchiectasis
III. Compressive atelectasis[186]
  A. Peripheral tumor
  B. Extensive interstitial disease (e.g., sarcoidosis, lymphoma)[484]
  C. Air trapping in adjacent lung (e.g., bullous emphysema, lobar emphysema, interstitial emphysema, bronchial obstruction by foreign body)[186]
IV. Passive atelectasis pleural space–occupying processes[186]
  A. Pneumothorax
  B. Hydrothorax, hemothorax
  C. Diaphragmatic hernia
  D. Pleural masses (e.g., metastases, mesothelioma)
V. Adhesive atelectasis[186]
  A. Respiratory distress syndrome of the newborn
  B. Pulmonary embolism[596]
  C. Intravenous injection of hydrocarbon
VI. Cicatrization atelectasis[186]
  A. Tuberculosis
  B. Histoplasmosis
  C. Silicosis
  D. Scleroderma
  E. Idiopathic pulmonary fibrosis (usual interstitial pneumonia, desquamative interstitial pneumonia)
  F. Radiation pneumonitis (late phase)[362,405,512]

DISCUSSION

Evaluation of the patient with suspected atelectasis should begin with a consideration of the radiologic signs of atelectasis: (1) increased opacity, (2) crowding and reorientation of pulmonary vessels,[469] (3) displacement of fissures,[282] (4) elevation of the diaphragm, (5) displacement of the hilus, (6) crowding of ribs, (7) compensatory overinflation of the normal lung, (8) shift of the mediastinum, (9) cardiac rotation,[310] (10) bronchial rearrangement,[642] and (11) juxtaphrenic peak.[120] On occasion, the change in position of an abnormal structure such as a calcified granuloma may also provide additional clues to the diagnosis.[503] As with other pulmonary problems, the radiologic signs of atelectasis are variable, ranging from nonspecific signs such as increased opacity to specific signs such as displacement of the fissures and a shift of the mediastinum.[310] Perhaps the most specific sign is displacement of the fissures, indicating a loss of volume in a specific lobe. Elevation of the minor fissure with anterior displacement of the major fissure indicates right upper lobe atelectasis (Figs 13–3, A–C). Right middle lobe atelectasis causes a combination of increased opacity that silhouettes the right heart border, inferior displacement of the minor fissure, and an anterior shift of the lower portion of the major fissure (Figs 13–4, A and B). Right lower lobe atelectasis causes increased opacity in the lower thorax without silhouetting of the right heart border. There is an inferior and medial shift of the major fissure. Remember, the major fissure is not normally seen on the PA film, but the shift that results from right lower lobe atelectasis often causes the fissure to become visible on the PA film (Fig 13–5).

Left upper lobe atelectasis causes a poorly marginated left perihilar opacity that appears to be separated from the mediastinal border by a hyperlucency or air-cresent (Luftsichel) that highlights the aortic arch. Compensatory overaeration of the superior segment of the left lower lobe accounts for the hyperlucency that is interposed between the mediastinum and the opaque upper lobe (Fig 13–6, A). Left upper lobe atelectasis assumes a very characteristic appearance on the lateral film, with an anterior opacity that is sharply marginated posteriorly by the displaced major fissure, which is displaced anteriorly (Fig 13–6, B). Because of compensatory overinflation of the right upper lobe, which may give the appearance of herniating across the midline, the opacity of the atelectic left upper lobe does not obliterate the retrosternal clear space. Left lower lobe atelectasis causes a triangular opacity behind the heart. The lateral border is sharp because of the inferomedial shift of the major fissure. This often produces the appearance of a line that parallels the heart border (Fig 13–7, A). The lateral film confirms a poorly marginated opacity that projects over the lower vertebral bodies and silhouettes the left leaf of the diaphragm (Fig 13–7, B). Complete opacification of a hemithorax with shift of the mediastinum is classic for atelectasis (Fig 13–8, A). In these cases, the shift of the mediastinum toward the opaque side confirms the atelectasis, but the opacification obscures the lung and any underlying abnormalities. A CT scan of the opaque hemithorax will show minimal differences in attenuation and is useful for detecting associated abnormalities such as pleural effusion (Fig 13–8, B).

The diagnostic signs of complete atelectasis of the right lung are not significantly different from those of complete collapse of the left lung. However, since the right lung has three lobes, combinations of atelectasis of two lobes may cause some unique radiologic appearances.[348] The case seen in Figure 13–1 is an example of right middle and upper lobe atelectasis. There is a large opacity involving the right upper thorax, obscuring the right upper lobe vessels and silhouetting the heart border. The diaphragm is pulled up, with the appearance of a pleural peak (juxtaphrenic peak sign).[120] This is probably the result of stretching of the pleura or inferior pulmonary ligament and is often observed as a sign of right upper lobe atelectasis. The lateral view holds the key to the correct diagnosis. The entire major fissure is shifted anteriorly to resemble the left major fissure position in left upper lobe atelectasis. The minor fissure is not visualized because it is surrounded by atelectatic lung. (Answer to question 1 is *e*.) In contrast, right middle and lower lobe atelectasis causes an inferior shift of both the minor fissure and the posterior portion of the major fissure. Compensatory overinflation of the upper lobe displaces the fissure inferiorly and produces a sharp interface with the collapsed lobes that may appear to parallel the diaphragm and thus mimic elevation of the diaphragm or even a subpulmonic effusion. When the opacity silhouettes the pulmonary vessels, atelectasis of the middle and lower lobes should be suspected (Fig 13–9, *A* and *B*).

The several types of atelectasis may be grouped according to their respective causes, as suggested by Fraser et al.[186]: (1) obstructive, (2) compressive, (3) passive, (4) adhesive, and (5) cicatrizing. Furthermore, since airway obstruction is produced by a wide variety of causes (Chart 13–1), this category may be subdivided into large and small airway obstructions, as proposed by Felson.[162] Airway obstruction is by far the most common cause of atelectasis; it can occur as the result of a foreign body, aspiration, endobronchial tumors, or inflammatory reactions such as tuberculosis. Compressive atelectasis is caused by intrapulmonary abnormalities (e.g., a large lung mass) that compress surrounding lung, while lung collapse with passive atelectasis develops from changes in intrapleural pressure (e.g., pneumothorax). Adhesive atelectasis indicates that the lung collapses because the luminal surfaces of the alveolar walls stick together. This occurs in hyaline membrane disease of the newborn, presumably because of a deficiency of surfactant in the alveoli. Finally, cicatrizing atelectasis is the result of scarring by fibrosis, with the loss of volume being a secondary effect. This frequently is a late sequela of tuberculosis.

Large Airway Obstructive Lesions

Bronchogenic carcinoma is one of the most important causes of large airway obstruction. Approximately two-thirds of squamous cell carcinomas of the lung occur in large airways as endobronchial masses. Although carcinoma of the lung is usually expected to present as a mass, the roentgenogram more often shows signs of obstruction, either recurrent atelectasis or pneumonia. When endobronchial masses are small, they are frequently not seen on plain chest films. The abnormalities that do appear while the tumor is small are frequently either segmental or lobar opacities. Other radiologic signs of atelectasis, including displacement of fissures, elevation of the diaphragm, crowding of the ribs, and shift of the mediastinum, should confirm that this radiologic presentation is due to atelectasis.

Patients with bronchogenic carcinoma often have histories that are complex and in some cases difficult to interpret. These histories often include persistent atelectasis, recurrent atelectasis, or recurrent pneumonia. For example, a patient may have a history of a low-grade fever at the time the roentgenogram shows segmental or lobar opacities. This might even appear to suggest the diagnosis of an infectious process. Subsequent treatment with antibiotics may even temporarily reduce the severity of the airway obstruction and also diminish the radiologic signs of atelectasis, thus supporting the original diagnosis. However, most cases of bronchial tumor will not show complete clearing of the radiologic abnormality with such therapy, and these cases then require further evaluation. This is especially important for the middle-aged patient who has a significant history of smoking. In the case of a 45-year-old smoker (Fig 13–10, *A*), the initial film indicated atelectasis of the right upper and middle lobes, a shift of the mediastinum, and an elevation of the right hemidiaphragm. The hilum is partially obscured by the atelectasis, precluding the identification or exclusion of a hilar mass. Although the follow-up film showed marked improvement, the persistent shift of the mediastinum and elevation of the right hemidiaphragm continued to suggest a tumor (Fig 13–10, *B*).

The combination of a hilar mass and lobar atelectasis is strongly suggestive of a primary lung tumor. When the primary tumor is relatively large and obstructs a mainstem bronchus, the plain chest films may reveal a "bronchial cutoff sign," or a "rattail bronchus." Such tumors, however, are not commonly seen, perhaps because they may be very small or are hidden by the superimposition of shadows from other structures. Although primary carcinomas arising in the hilum are not rare, the hilar masses seen on the plain film more often represent metastases to the regional lymph nodes from endobronchial tumors. The obstructing tumor is best diagnosed by CT and bronchoscopy with biopsy.[661]

These central primary carcinomas are frequently lobulated, particularly when multiple nodes are involved. When the nodal metastases are extensive, they may involve hilar and mediastinal nodes. If the patient has no evidence of extrathoracic metastases, chest CT should be used as a staging procedure. Because of the high incidence of liver and adrenal metastases, the examination should be extended into the abdomen.

In current clinical practice, the combination of atelectasis and bronchial obstruction most frequently indicates the presence of a primary malignant tumor, although other lesions can also be responsible. The bronchial carcinoid tumor, frequently found in large bronchi, rarely calcifies[555] and often presents with atelectasis. Although metastatic tumors to the bronchi are not common, they can develop from renal cell carcinoma, breast carcinoma, and occasionally from melanoma,[459] carcinoma of the colon,[42,540] and various sarcomas. Rare benign tumors such as granular cell myoblastoma, amyloid tumor, lipoma, and even fibroepithelial inflammatory polyps all require biopsy for diagnosis. Lymphoma[526] is another tumor that occasionally invades the bronchi with resultant atelectasis; however, this is usually a late stage of the disease and is almost always accompanied by hilar and mediastinal lymphadenopathy. This presentation of lymphoma frequently represents a recurrence of previously treated lymphoma and is not a diagnostic problem.

Today, infectious diseases are seldom the basis of bronchial obstruction, but historically, tuberculosis was an important cause of obstructive atelectasis. In fact, many cases of right middle lobe syndrome (chronic right middle lobe atelectasis) were due to tuberculosis. Bronchial obstruction in tuberculosis most commonly results from peribronchial inflammation. Although there may be associated hilar adenopathy, it is doubtful that the obstruction is simply due to compression by the hilar lymph nodes. In long-term cases of tuberculosis, broncholiths[620]—calcified lymph nodes that erode into the bronchus—may also be a source of bronchial obstruction (see Figs 13–4, *A* and *B*). Occasionally, tuberculosis may even result in endobronchial granulomas that cause obstruction.

In the past, hilar adenopathy was often cited as a cause of atelectasis, but as suggested earlier (see discussions of primary bronchogenic carcinoma, lymphoma, and tuberculosis), the pathologic processes that produce the atelectasis involve more than simple compression of a bronchus by a large lymph node. In fact, it is probably infrequent that enlargement of hilar lymph nodes alone produce obstructive atelectasis. This conclusion is supported by the radiologic presentations of sarcoidosis. Symmetric hilar adenopathy is the most common manifestation of sarcoidosis (see Chapter 11), yet obstructive atelectasis is very rarely associated with sarcoidosis. In those rare cases of sarcoidosis that do develop atelectasis, the atelectasis is often due to endobronchial granulomas rather than to compression of the bronchus by enlarged lymph nodes. All of the entities offered as answers to question 2 may cause atelectasis, but primary bronchogenic carcinoma is, unfortunately, the most common.

Left atrial enlargement from mitral stenosis is an occasional cause of left lower-lobe atelectasis. The diagnosis is easily made when other findings of mitral stenosis, such as a large left atrium and the cephalization of vessels, are present. The lateral radiograph frequently shows the left atrium to be pushing the compressed left main and lower lobe bronchi posteriorly.[343]

The diagnosis of foreign-body obstruction of a bronchus is usually straightforward in adults, since it is commonly associated with the aspiration of food, such as a large piece of meat. The development of atelectasis of the left lung following endotracheal intubation is strongly suggestive of a malpositioned tube. This is the result of advancing the tube too far, so that it enters the bronchus intermedius and occludes the left mainstem bronchus. On the other hand, foreign body aspiration in children may be a difficult problem, since they are unable to give a definite history. In contrast to the adult with a large airway obstruction, a child more commonly presents with overaeration of the lung distal to the obstruction. This is presumably due to collateral air drift that permits air to get into the lung distal to the obstruction. Therefore, an endobronchial foreign body will most likely result in atelectasis in an adult patient, while more frequently causing air trapping in the pediatric patient (see discussion of compressive atelectasis).

Small Airway Obstruction

Mucus plugging is a common cause of both large and small airway obstruction. The bronchial tree branches for approximately seven generations. Bronchi have cartilage in their walls. The airways distal to the seventh generation and without cartilage are defined as bronchioles. Mucus production occurs mainly in the bronchial tree in nonsmokers. Bronchioles in nonsmokers have a ciliated lining and lack mucus-secreting glands, whereas the bronchioles of smokers lose their cilia and have increased numbers of mucus-secreting goblet cells. Although the discussion of large airway obstruction was limited to diseases that occur in the proximal main bronchi, mucus plugging may involve multiple small bronchi and bronchioles. Mucus plugs may form in multiple small bronchi of a patient with an otherwise normal tracheobronchial tree in various clinical settings, such as during general anesthesia, after administration of respiratory-depressant drugs (morphine), or during central nervous system illnesses that produce respiratory depression. Mucus plugging of multiple bronchi is also a frequent complication of abdominal and thoracic surgery. Especially after thoracic surgery, atelectatic opacities are very common in the left lower lobe but may also be more scattered with lobar, segmental, and subsegmental distributions. Subsegmental linear opacities (Fig 13–11, *A* and *B*) most commonly measure from a few millimeters to a centimeter wide, and up to several centimeters long. The exact basis for subsegmental atelectasis has been questioned; some authors believe that collateral air drift should prevent the development of subsegmental atelectasis. However, normal collateral air drift may not be present in patients with impaired bronchial clearance. Rather, when clearance is depressed to the point that mucus obstructs small bronchi and bronchioles, the even smaller passages between sections of lung, such as the canals of Lambert and pores of Kohn, are likely to become obstructed. The transient nature of these subsegmental opacities also further supports the concept that these linear opacities are the result of subsegmental atelectasis.

Atelectasis is not one of the commonly expected presentations of bronchopneumonia, but infections can produce peribronchial inflammation, which may then lead to small airway obstruction followed by atelectasis. This presentation has been occasionally referred to as atelectatic pneumonia. Clinical and laboratory correlations are extremely important in establishing this diagnosis over that of other causes of atelectasis. Patients with bronchopneumonia are usually febrile and have elevated white blood cell counts. Bacteriologic confirmation of the diagnosis is obtained with positive sputum and blood cultures. Atelectasis may also complicate viral and mycoplasma pneumonias, presumably because of the associated bronchial and bronchiolar involvement (see Chapter 14).

Atelectasis from the obstruction of bronchioles may develop during the course of certain chronic obstructive diseases, such as chronic bronchitis, asthma, emphysema, and bronchiolitis obliterans. The atelectasis may develop because many small bronchi and bronchioles can become obstructed as a result of chronic changes in the airway walls that lead to narrowing of the lumen, formation of increased mucus, reduced clearing of secretions, and formation of small intraluminal mucus plugs. Although the radiologic findings in these diseases are frequently minimal, acute exacerbations may result in lobar, segmental, subsegmental atelectasis plus a more diffuse peripheral pattern of atelectasis. The latter appearance sometimes resembles diffuse peripheral air space opacities and may be incorrectly diagnosed as pneumonia without careful clinical and laboratory correlation. A changing appearance with rapid clearing of opacities followed by recurrences should suggest this diagnosis, especially in the intensive care environment.

Compressive Atelectasis

The radiologic appearance of compressive atelectasis is often distinctly different from that of obstructive atelectasis. Compressive atelectasis is a secondary effect of compression of normal lung by a primary, space-occupying abnormality.

The primary abnormality is often a large peripheral lung tumor that collapses adjacent lung.

Extensive air trapping can also compress adjacent normal lung. This type of compression may occur in bullous emphysema, lobar emphysema, and often after an acute bronchial obstruction. The radiologic appearance of bullous emphysema is that of a large area of hyperlucency surrounded by a thin wall. These lucencies are usually in the periphery of the lung. This presentation of bullous emphysema is so characteristic that it is not often a diagnostic problem (see Chapter 22).

In view of the preceding discussion, the finding of distal air trapping with acute bronchial obstruction may appear paradoxical and can be a diagnostic challenge. Presumably, air trapping may result from a ball-valve effect or collateral air drift that allows air to enter the portion of the lung distal to the bronchial obstruction but does not allow air outflow. This unidirectional airflow is a property of the collateral air passages and results in overexpansion of the lung beyond the obstructed bronchus. As the obstructed lung expands, it may compress the normal lung, and it shifts the mediastinum and heart, leading to volume loss in the normal lung (compressive atelectasis). In such cases it is necessary to determine which is the primary abnormality, the lucent lung or the opaque lung. Expiratory films that reveal persistent overexpansion of the lung confirm that the bronchus to that lung is obstructed. Clinical correlation is also important. Obstructive emphysema is most often encountered in a child after an acute bronchial obstruction by a foreign body.

Passive Atelectasis

Although separating atelectasis into passive (relaxation) and compressive categories may seem somewhat artificial, it does focus attention on the source of the primary problem producing collapse. With compressive atelectasis the problem is intrapulmonary, while in the passive form the problem is intrapleural. Two of the most important causes of passive atelectasis are pleural effusion (see Chapter 4) and pneumothorax.

Probably the most important radiologic consideration in the diagnosis of pneumothorax is documentation of the problem and not the specification of its cause. An extensive pneumothorax produces several obvious radiologic abnormalities, including increased opacity of the collapsed lung, the appearance of a pleural line, and a large lucent space between the pleural line and the chest wall. The pleural space lacks normal pulmonary markings. When the pneumothorax is minimal, the pleural line and lack of normal pulmonary markings may be more difficult to identify. In the upright patient, the small pleural line over the apex of the lung frequently appears to parallel the cortex of the ribs. However, close inspection will usually show that the pleural line only partially parallels the rib cortex and crosses the cortex of the ribs laterally. When there is strong clinical suspicion of a pneumothorax but the inspiratory film fails to confirm it, expiratory films may be more useful. Expiration enhances the appearance of the pneumothorax because the increased opacity of the lung during expiration effectively increases the contrast between the trapped air in the pleural cavity and the lung.

When the patient cannot stand up and only supine films are possible, the diagnosis of pneumothorax can be especially difficult.[614,677] Superimposed skinfolds on the supine films may be easily confused with the increased opacity of a pleural line.[173] However, skinfolds can be differentiated from pleural lines, because lines formed by the folds will appear to cross the ribs and thus may be traced off the area of the lungs. A small pneumothorax will collect anteriorly in the supine patient, and the pulmonary markings will extend to the lateral chest wall. In this instance, the best way to confirm a small pneumothorax is to use either an upright film or a lateral decubitus film in which the side with the suspected pneumothorax is up (Fig 13–12, *A* and *B*).

Adhesive Atelectasis

Adhesive atelectasis occurs when the luminal surfaces of the alveolar walls stick together. This type of atelectasis is an important component of two prominent pulmonary diseases: respiratory distress syndrome of the newborn (hyaline membrane disease) and pulmonary embolism. In both diseases, the basis for adhesion is presumed to be a deficiency of surfactant.

HYALINE MEMBRANE DISEASE

The classic radiologic description of respiratory distress syndrome of the newborn does not resemble that of atelectasis (Fig 13–13, *A*). Rather, it has the pattern of a diffuse pulmonary process with a ground-glass appearance that may progress to form coalescent opacities with air bronchograms. It therefore resembles a diffuse airspace disease (see Fig 15–1). Histologic sections of fatal cases of hyaline membrane disease not only demonstrate the pathologically diagnostic hyaline membranes, but also show extensive atelectasis without significant alveolar filling (Fig 13–13, *B*). This is a failure to maintain aeration of the alveoli that results from surfactant deficiency.

PULMONARY EMBOLISM

Pulmonary embolism, on the other hand, may result in radiologic opacities that are typical of atelectasis. An appearance remarkably like that of subsegmental atelectasis is often observed following pulmonary embolism, and lobar opacities may occasionally also be observed in combination with displacement of fissures and elevation of the diaphragm. Such an appearance indicates lobar atelectasis (Fig 13–14, *A* and *B*).

The exact mechanism for atelectasis following pulmonary embolism is not clearly known. Numerous authors have reported that areas of increased opacity following pulmonary embolism often do not represent actual infarction or death of lung tissue. Heitzman[260] emphasized that the radiologic opacities developing after pulmonary embolism are frequently the result of hemorrhagic edema, and as such are pleural-based and larger than the opacities usually attributed to atelectasis.[260] Experimental studies have shown that the parenchymal opacities seen on x-ray films may represent either edema and hemorrhage or atelectasis. In his discussion of the respiratory consequences of pulmonary embolism, Moser[423] described two possible mechanisms leading to atelectasis after pulmonary embolism: (1) When an embolus blocks blood flow to an alveolar area, the volume of alveolar dead space increases; this in turn initiates pneumoconstriction leading to a reduction in total lung volume. Reduced lung volume would also help explain the diaphragmatic elevation that often follows pulmonary embolism. (2) The reduced blood supply may also reduce the availability of surfactant. Surfactant levels may be critically reduced 24 hours after the embolism and may contribute to adhesive atelectasis. There is experimental evidence that a deficiency of surfactant is in fact the major mechanism leading to adhesive atelectasis following pulmonary embolism.

Since atelectasis is a nonspecific finding, careful clinical correlation is essential for this finding to be useful as a diagnostic indicator of pulmonary embolism. This is especially true in the case of postoperative patients, who frequently have atelectasis secondary to mucus plugging but who are also at increased risk for the development of pulmonary embolism. Pleural effusion is an additional radiologic observation that should prompt the radiologist to consider the diagnosis of pulmonary embolism. Certainly mucus plugging is not an adequate explanation for the radiologic combination of atelectasis and pleural effusion. Other conditions, such as thoracic surgical procedures and intra-abdominal processes known to be associated with pleural effusion (e.g., an ovarian tumor and renal and pancreatic surgery), may also produce pleural effusion independent of the presence of atelectasis. When other causes have been eliminated, the combination of pleural effusion and subsegmental atelectasis is highly suggestive of pulmonary embolism. When the clinical history includes pleuritic chest pain, rapid development of pulmonary symptoms with dyspnea, or decrease in arterial oxygen tension, a definitive workup is necessary to rule out pulmonary embolism. This workup should include ventilation/perfusion lung scanning, and in some cases pulmonary arteriography.

Cicatrizing Atelectasis

Cicatrizing atelectasis is primarily the result of fibrosis and scar tissue formation (infiltration) in the interalveolar and interstitial space (interstitial pneumonitis). Because of this fibrosis, the lung loses compliance, and the end result is a reduced lung volume. Although some of the signs of volume loss with cicatrizing atelectasis are similar to those seen in obstructive atelectasis, several important characteristics allow differentiation of the two conditions.

Similar features of cicatrizing and obstructive atelectasis are displacement of the hili and fissures, elevation of the diaphragm, and possibly displacement of the mediastinum. Distinctive of cicatrizing atelectasis are the associated coarse reticular opacities. The classic cause of cicatrizing atelectasis is tuberculosis (see Fig 13–2). Tuberculosis typically involves the development of a reticular pattern in the upper lobe and is also frequently associated with pleural thickening. Elevation of the hilum and distortion of the fissures provide additional clues to volume loss. Entities that can mimic this aspect of tuberculosis are primarily other granulomatous infections such as histoplasmosis. (Answer to question 3 is *c*.) Note the shift of the mediastinum, elevation of the left hemidiaphragm, increased opacity in the left upper lobe, and elevation of the left hilum in Figure 13–2. All of these are indications of volume loss. The thickening and calcification of the pleura and the cavity in the upper lobe confirm the diagnosis of chronic tuberculosis.

Loss of pulmonary volume from cicatrizing atelectasis can also occur with other types of interstitial pneumonitis, such as silicosis, scleroderma, radiation pneumonitis (late stage), idiopathic pulmonary fibrosis, and desquamative inter-stitial pneumonia. However, in contrast to tuberculosis and histoplasmosis, these other diseases do not usually result in segmental or lobar opacities; the volume loss tends to be bilateral and more uniform. Volume loss is manifested simply by an increased opacity, crowding of vessels, and elevation of the diaphragm. Silico-sis, however, may be somewhat different because it tends to be more localized to the upper lobes, which results in the retraction of both hila toward the upper lobes. A history of exposure usually confirms the diagnosis of silicosis. Some of the other types of interstitial pneumonitis, particularly scleroderma, have a ten-dency to involve the lower lobes. The diagnosis of scleroderma is frequently con-firmed by detecting the involvement of other organs, such as the skin and gas-trointestinal tract. The idiopathic forms of interstitial pneumonitis generally result in loss of volume in the lung bases and elevation of the diaphragm. This appear-ance is often mistaken for poor voluntary inspiratory effort and is not usually rec-ognized as atelectasis.

Radiation pneumonitis (Fig 13–15) is another form of interstitial disease that leaves scarring in the lung and a significant volume loss during its later stages. This entity is most often found in patients who have undergone radiation ther-apy. The most distinctive aspect of radiation pneumonitis is the peculiar, nonanatomic distribution of the pathology. It is frequently localized by sharply defined lines that coincide with the portals of the radiation therapy beam to which the patient was exposed. Depending on the specific area irradiated, the re-tracting fibrosis may displace the hilum[249] and interlobar fissures. As with tuber-culosis, the late stage of radiation pneumonitis frequently assumes a reticular pat-tern that is most easily identified around the periphery of the opacity. The diag-nosis can be confirmed by knowledge of previous radiation therapy.

SUMMARY

1. The five major categories of atelectasis are obstructive, compressive, passive, adhesive, and cicatrizing.

2. Obstruction of either large or small airways is the most commonly recog-nized cause of atelectasis.

3. Recurrent atelectasis is a common presentation for bronchogenic carcinoma and may be an indication for further evaluation of the bronchi with bron-choscopy or CT.

4. Compressive and passive atelectasis are rarely considered in the differential diagnosis of lobar or segmental atelectasis.

5. Adhesive atelectasis may follow pulmonary embolism, as a result of a local-ized surfactant deficiency, and may thus produce the radiologic appearance of ei-ther lobar or segmental atelectasis.

6. Cicatrizing atelectasis may occur during the late stages of a number of con-ditions that produce extensive scarring of the lung. In the case of tuberculosis, other associated findings, such as pleural thickening, reticular scarring of the up-per lobes, and cavitation, may be diagnostic.

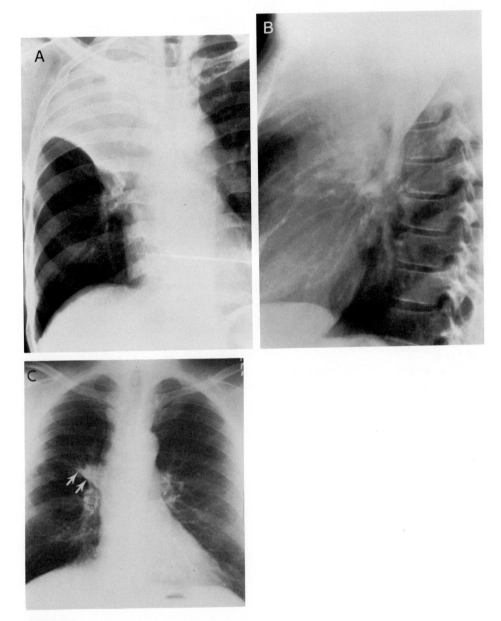

FIG 13–3
A, Complete right upper lobe atelectasis should be recognized by the curved elevation of the minor fissure. This was caused by a bronchogenic carcinoma obstructing the right upper lobe bronchus. **B,** Lateral film shows the right upper lobe opacity to be sharply outlined anteriorly by the minor fissure and posteriorly by the major fissure. **C,** Incomplete right upper lobe atelectasis is less obvious, but this perihilar opacity is sharply marginated inferiorly by the minor fissure *(arrows)*. This confirms the diagnosis of right upper lobe atelectasis.

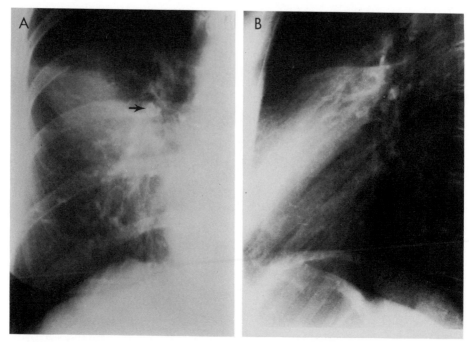

FIG 13–4

A, PA film shows right middle lobe opacity and right hilar calcification *(arrow)*. **B,** Lateral film from same case reveals increased right middle lobe opacity and displacement of major and minor fissures. This is the classic appearance of right middle lobe atelectasis. This is atelectasis secondary to a broncholith. Broncholiths may be secondary to either tuberculosis or histoplasmosis. The diagnosis may be confirmed by CT or bronchoscopy.

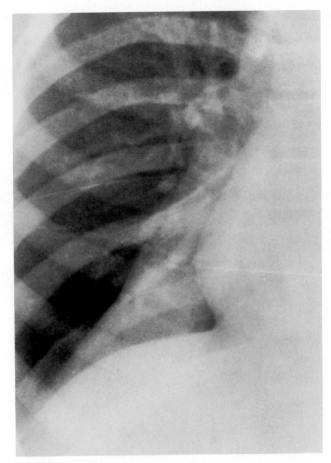

FIG 13–5
Right lower lobe atelectasis causes inferior displacement of the major fissure so that it becomes visible on the PA film. The sharp lateral border of this opaque atelectatic lower lobe is produced by the major fissure. Notice that lower lobe atelectasis does not silhouette the heart border.

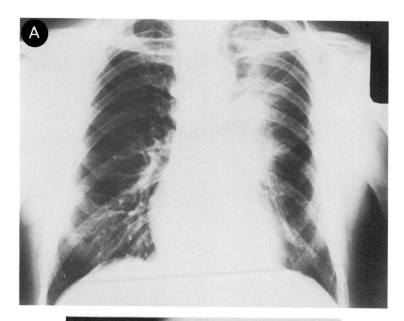

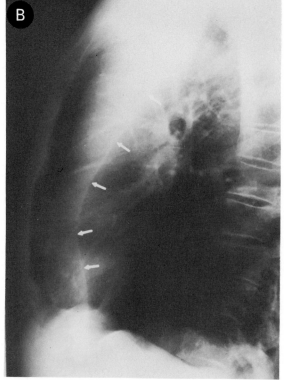

FIG 13–6
A, Left upper lobe atelectasis causes increased opacity medially, elevation of left pulmonary artery, and a decrease in number and caliber of peripheral pulmonary vessels. The volume loss is not easily detected on PA film. **B,** Left upper lobe atelectasis is best recognized by observing displacement of the major fissure *(arrows)* on the lateral film.

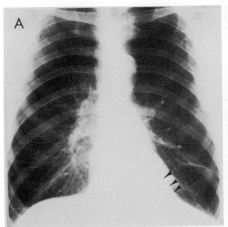
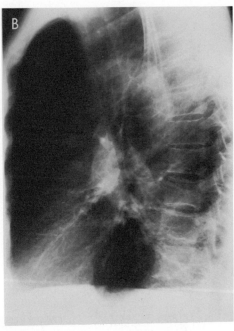

FIG 13–7
A, Increased opacity behind the heart obscures medial half of the left hemidiaphragm. Major fissure forms straight line posterior to the heart *(arrowheads).* This is the classic presentation of left lower lobe atelectasis. **B,** Left lower lobe atelectasis as seen in lateral projection produces increased opacity posteriorly over the vertebral bodies. Fissure displacement is not identifiable on the lateral film.

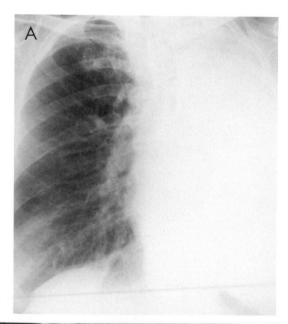

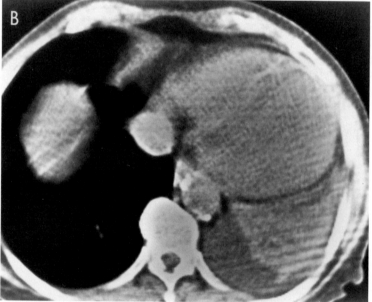

FIG 13–8
A, PA film of patient with carcinoma of the left main bronchus with complete opacification of the left hemithorax. Note that the mediastinum has shifted to the left; this finding excludes the diagnosis of a massive left pleural effusion and confirms atelectasis of the left lung. The opacity obscures the heart and associated abnormalities such as pleural effusion. **B,** CT scan of the patient in Figure 13–8, *A* demonstrates shift of the heart to the left and atelectasis of the left lung. The posterior low-attenuation abnormality confirms the presence of a small pleural effusion, which could not have been suggested on the plain film.

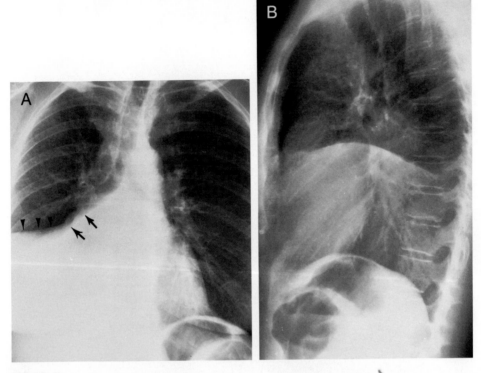

FIG 13–9
A, Right middle and lower lobe atelectasis as a combination may be mistaken for a sub-pulmonic pleural effusion. Note the inferomedial displacement of the major fissure *(arrows)* and the low position of the minor fissure *(arrowheads)*. **B,** The depressed fissures produce a sharp interface with the overaerated upper lobe. This could also be confused with an elevated diaphragm.

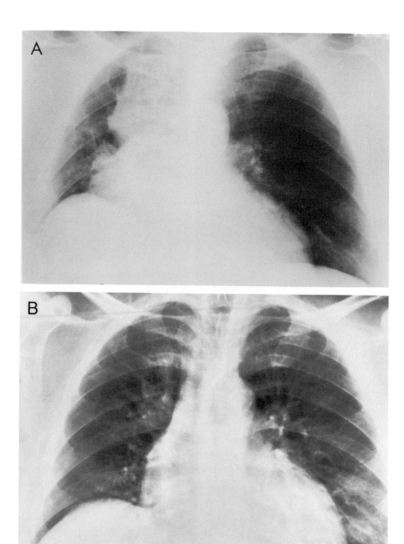

FIG 13–10
A, Note increased opacity in right upper lobe and opacity adjacent to right heart border
(right middle lobe). Right hemidiaphragm is elevated and mediastinum is shifted to the
right. This combination indicates atelectasis of both the right upper and middle lobes.
B, 16 days later, there has been apparent resolution of the atelectasis, but notice the
persistent shift of the mediastinum. This is an important clue to the diagnosis of an
endobronchial tumor (squamous cell carcinoma in this case).

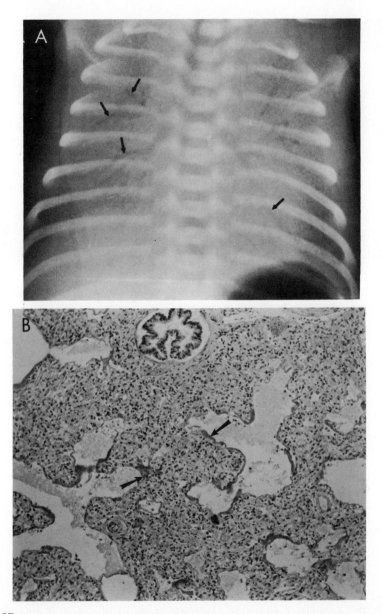

FIG 13–13
A, Diffuse opacities with air bronchograms *(arrows)* are not the radiologic appearance expected of atelectasis. The diagnosis in this newborn is respiratory distress syndrome (hyaline membrane disease). **B,** Histologic section from a similar case reveals extensive collapse of air spaces *(arrows).* This is an example of adhesive atelectasis, since it results from surfactant deficiency. (From Reed JC: Pathologic correlations of the air-bronchogram: a reliable sign in chest radiology. *CRC Crit Rev Diagn Imaging* 1977; 10:235–255. Used by permission. Copyright CRC Press, Boca Raton, Florida.)

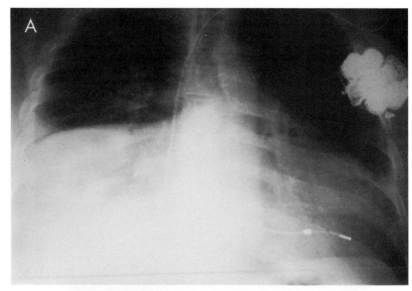

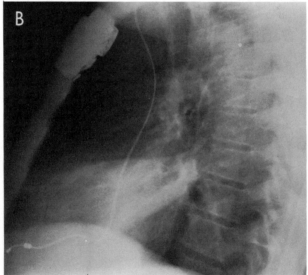

FIG 13–14
A and B, This example of right middle lobe atelectasis was the result of pulmonary embolism with infarction.

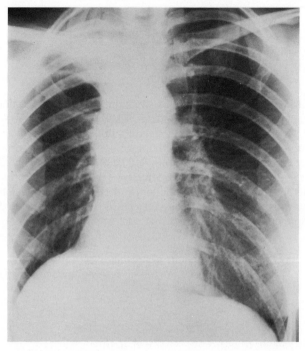

FIG 13–15
Radiation therapy to supraclavicular lymph nodes for carcinoma of the right breast produced increased opacity and volume loss in the right upper lobe. This is another example of atelectasis secondary to parenchymal fibrosis.

ANSWER GUIDE

LEGENDS FOR INTRODUCTORY FIGURES

FIG 13–1
A, Right upper and middle lobe atelectases are an infrequent combination that may have a very characteristic radiologic appearance. Observe that the large area of increased opacity in the right upper thorax obscures the right upper lobe vessels and right heart border. Upper lobe atelectasis alone would not silhouette the heart border. Also, the minor fissure is not visible because it is surrounded by atelectatic lung. In addition, this case illustrates the juxtaphrenic peak sign, which is a reliable indicator of upper lobe atelectasis. **B,** Lateral film demonstrates anterior displacement of the major fissure. This resembles the appearance of left upper lobe atelectasis. The atelectasis in this case resulted from a large endobronchial cancer that obstructed both bronchi.

FIG 13–2
Apical opacity with elevation of left hilum has resulted from tuberculosis. Hilar elevation indicates volume loss. This is the result of chronic scarring, thus the term cicatrizing atelectasis.

ANSWERS

1, e; 2, d; 3, c; 4, b; 5, g, f; 6, e; 7, c, d; 8, a.

CHAPTER 14

Segmental and Lobar Opacities

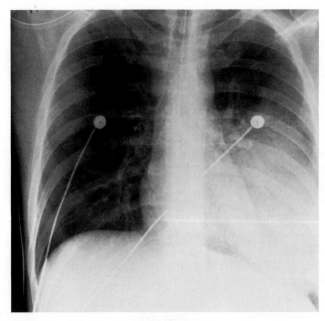

FIG 14–1

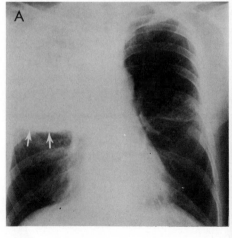

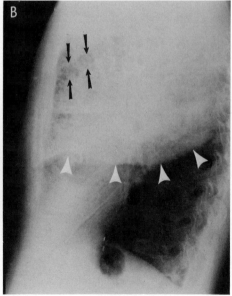

FIG 14–2

QUESTIONS

1. Homogeneous left lower lobe consolidation, as seen in Figure 14–1, is the typical radiologic manifestation of lobar pneumonia. What is the most likely etiologic agent?
   a. *Mycoplasma pneumoniae.*
   b. *Streptococcus pneumoniae.*
   c. *Mycobacterium avium-intracellulare.*
   d. *Legionella pneumophilia.*
   e. *Klebsiella pneumoniae.*
2. Refer to Figure 14–2, *A* and *B.* An expanded lobe with interspersed lucencies *(black arrows)* that are suggestive of multiple cavities is a classic appearance for pneumonias caused by which of the following agents?
   a. *Streptococcus pneumoniae.*
   b. *Klebsiella pneumoniae.*
   c. *Legionella pneumophilia.*
   d. *Mycoplasma pneumoniae.*
   e. Adenovirus.
3. The combination of hilar adenopathy and right middle lobe consolidation in a 15-year-old should suggest which diagnosis?
   a. *Mycoplasma pneumoniae.*
   b. Primary tuberculosis.
   c. *Streptococcus pneumoniae.*
   d. Respiratory syncytial virus.
   e. Gram-negative pneumonia.

CHART 14–1.
Segmental and Lobar Opacities

  I. Lobar pneumonia
      A. *Streptococcus pneumoniae (Diplococcus pneumoniae)*[299,308]
      B. *Klebsiella pneumoniae*[58]
  II. Lobular pneumonia (bronchopneumonia)[676]
      A. *Pseudomonas*[57,58]
      B. *Klebsiella pneumoniae*
      C. *Bacillus proteus*
      D. *Escherichia coli*
      E. Anerobes[31] (*Bacteroides* and clostridia)
      F. *Legionella pneumophila*[151,485]
      G. *Staphylococcus aureus*
      H. Nocardiosis[58,232] and actinomycosis[178]
      I. *Streptococcus pneumoniae*[308]
      J. *Serratia*[25]
  III. Acute interstitial pneumonia
      A. Viruses[383]
      B. Mycoplasma[432]
  IV. Aspiration pneumonia
   V. Tuberculosis[412,550] and atypical mycobacteria
  VI. Pulmonary embolism[295]
      A. Hemorrhage and edema
      B. Infarction

(Continued.)

CHART 14–1. (cont.).

VII. Neoplasms
    A. Obstructive pneumonia (carcinoma of bronchus)
    B. Bronchioloalveolar cell carcinoma[47,146,411]
    C. Lymphoma[270,455]
VIII. Atelectasis (Chapter 13)
 IX. Mitral regurgitation with pulmonary edema localized to the right upper lobe[238]
  X. Lung torsion[163,422]

CHART 14–2.
Lobar Expansion

  I. *Streptococcus pneumoniae*[186]
 II. *Klebsiella pneumoniae*[57,58,186]
III. *Pseudomonas*[57,58]
IV. *Staphylococcus*[57,58]
 V. *Tuberculosis*[550]
VI. Carcinoma with obstructive pneumonia
    (drowned lung)

DISCUSSION

Lobar and Segmental Consolidations

Lobar pneumonia is one of the best examples of classic lobar consolidation. The radiologic appearance of a consolidated lobe is a homogeneous, confluent opacity that obliterates the normal vascular markings throughout the lobe (see Fig 14–1). The opacity is frequently bounded by the fissures, and stretched fissures may even lead to the appearance of an expanded lobe (see Fig 14–2, *A* and *B*). Since the airways are frequently air filled and surrounded by airless lung, air bronchograms are another component of the classic appearance of lobar pneumonia.

From the foregoing description, the distinction of lobar consolidation from atelectasis would appear to be simple. Fraser et al. have emphasized that consolidation of a lobe with fluid is the antithesis of lobar atelectasis. Therefore, bulging fissures that indicate lobar expansion are unequivocal evidence of consolidation.[186] As mentioned in Chapter 13, the displacement of fissures together indicates volume loss in the involved lobe. The problem with applying this approach to the evaluation of a lobar opacity for the purpose of distinguishing atelectasis from consolidation is not in the evaluation of the lobe that is expanded, but rather in the evaluation of the lobe of diminished size. It will become apparent in this discussion that a number of the processes that consolidate the lung also produce small airway obstruction, so that the volume loss produced by the process may be greater than the quantity of fluid that is consolidating the lung. Thus, a consolidating process may also be the cause of atelectasis. For example, bronchopneumonia, which causes airspace consolidations, also leads to small airway obstructions that may result in atelectasis.

Lobar Pneumonia

The distinction between lobar pneumonia and bronchopneumonia has been deemphasized in favor of a bacteriologic classification of pneumonias, which is more relevant in determining appropriate therapy. However, knowledge of the gross morphologic distinctions between the two types of pneumonia is important for understanding the variety of radiologic patterns that may be encountered in acute pneumonias.

The pathogenesis of lobar pneumonia is the key to understanding the spectrum of radiologic patterns of pneumococcal pneumonia. Experimental evidence indicates that the pathogens, in the form of small infected mucus particles, are inhaled to the periphery of the lung, where they set up foci of reaction. Initially, the tissue reaction involves the exudation of watery edema fluid into alveolar spaces. The exudate then spreads into the air passages and their alveoli. As the alveoli fill, the exudate spreads into adjacent lobules and segments. This movement of the exudate occurs via the pores of Kohn, canals of Lambert, and small airways, but it does not appear to spread via the bronchovascular bundle or interstitium of the lung. The watery edema fluid serves as a culture medium for the rapid multiplication of the bacteria. The alveolar walls respond to the organisms by releasing polymorphonuclear leukocytes. The spread of the process through the collateral channels rather than the bronchioles explains why lobar pneumonia often does not follow a segmental distribution. Rather, lobar pneumonia produces opacities that appear to involve multiple segments early in the course of the process. During these early phases, the radiologic appearance is that of a nonsegmental sublobar consolidation (Fig 14–3), which may appear rather sharply circumscribed because of the uniform involvement of contiguous alveoli. This leads to the so-called round pneumonia most commonly seen in children (Fig 14–4, *A* and *B*). Fully developed, classic lobar consolidation is less commonly encountered, since the early diagnosis of bacterial pneumonia followed by appropriate antibiotic therapy frequently arrests the process in its early phases. And since the initial focus of infection is the periphery of the lung, it is not surprising that pleural effusion and empyema are potential complications. However, the occurrence of these complications is also drastically reduced by early antibiotic therapy.

The two most common bacteriologic causes of lobar pneumonia are *Streptococcus pneumoniae,* formally *Diplococcus pneumoniae,* and *Klebsiella pneumoniae.* Which organism is involved can seldom be determined solely from the radiologic appearance. *Streptococcus pneumoniae* is the most common cause of lobar pneumoniae. (Answer to question 1 is *b.*) However, *K. pneumoniae* tends to follow a more aggressive course than *S. pneumoniae,* and it is more likely to expand a lobe and produce necrosis of lung tissue with cavitation (see Chapter 23).

Since the clinical course of lobar pneumonia is characterized primarily by nonspecific symptoms[233] such as productive cough and temperature elevation, additional history should be obtained; for example, is the patient debilitated by alcoholism or immunologic suppression? Considering the combination of the radiologic appearance of an expanding lobar consolidation with cavitation and a history of alcoholism allows the diagnosis of *Klebsiella* pneumonia to be proposed with confidence. (Answer to question 2 is *b.*) However, the definitive diagnosis of a bacterial pneumonia can be made only by analysis of smears and cultures of the sputum, blood, and lung aspirate.

Bronchopneumonia

In comparison with the limited number of radiologic presentations of lobar pneumonia, the spectrum of radiologic patterns associated with bronchopneumonia (lobular pneumonia)[260] is much more diverse.

In bronchopneumonia, the primary sites of injury are the terminal and respiratory bronchioles. The disease starts as an acute bronchitis and bronchiolitis. As it progresses, ulcers are formed in large bronchi by destruction of the epithelial lining, and the bronchial walls become infiltrated with polymorphonuclear leukocytes. These ulcers are covered with a fibrinopurulent membrane that contains large quantities of multiplying organisms. With the more virulent organisms such as *Staphylococcus* and *Pseudomonas,* necrotic bronchitis and bronchiolitis can lead to thrombosis of lobular branches of small pulmonary arteries. This inflammatory reaction also spreads through the walls of the bronchioles to involve the alveolar walls. This is followed by exudation of fluids and inflammatory cells into the acinus to produce lobular consolidations. The alveoli become filled with edematous fluid, blood, polymorphonuclear leukocytes, hyaline membranes, and bacteria.

The foregoing description suggests that the specific radiologic pattern depends on both the virulence of the organism and the host defenses (Fig 14–5). A mild bronchopneumonia in an otherwise healthy individual may lead only to inflammatory peribronchial infiltration and the radiologic appearance of peribronchial thickening with "increased markings." Itoh et al.[293] demonstrated that this peribronchial infiltrate may account for the radiologic appearance of multiple small (5-mm), fluffy, or ill-defined nodules, resembling acinar consolidations. These nodules differ from the expected appearance of miliary nodules mainly in their lack of definition, or fluffy borders. As the inflammatory process spreads, the nodules enlarge. The number of areas involved is highly variable, ranging from a few localized opacities in one area of the lung to diffuse opacities involving both lungs. Lobular pneumonia may therefore present as multifocal, ill-defined opacities, and as such is considered further in Chapter 16.

Although the concomitant appearance of both lobar and segmental opacities may seem paradoxical in the discussion of bronchopneumonia, the combination is consistent with the diagnosis. Recall that bronchopneumonia involves both bronchioles and bronchi. Patients with bronchopneumonia occasionally have both narrowing of the bronchi and mucus plugging; both processes can lead to airway obstruction. Therefore, in contrast to lobar pneumonia, which is characterized by a nonsegmental distribution of opacities and infrequent atelectasis, bronchopneumonia is a common cause of either segmental or lobar opacities accompanied by volume loss. Bronchopneumonia with this presentation has occasionally been referred to as atelectatic pneumonia. If multiple opacities are present in the other lobes, the radiologic appearance is nearly diagnostic. If atelectasis is the only radiologic abnormality, careful clinical and laboratory correlation will be required to distinguish bronchopneumonia from the other causes of atelectasis considered in Chapter 13.

Acute Interstitial Pneumonias

The best-known examples of acute interstitial pneumonia are the viral and mycoplasma pneumonias. The classic radiologic description of these is a diffuse interstitial process.[432] Segmental or lobar opacities are not expected in viral pneumonia, but, as in bronchopneumonia, a viral bronchitis in combination with mucus plugging may lead to atelectasis (Fig 14–6, *A* and *B*). The bronchitis may also produce peribronchial thickening,[260,497] which can be useful in distinguishing viral from bacterial pneumonias (Fig 14–7). Another factor that may contribute to atelectasis in viral pneumonia is injury of the type 2 alveolar cells, which are responsible for surfactant production. Therefore, atelectasis is probably the most significant factor in the development of segmental or lobar opacities as a result of viral pneumonia. Certainly atelectasis will increase the radiologic opacity of an area of lung that is already partially consolidated by hemorrhage or edema. These pneumonias are also frequently distinguished from bacterial pneumonia on clinical grounds. The lack of sputum production may be a significant clue to a nonbacterial pneumonia. The diagnosis is usually confirmed by obtaining complement fixation titers that show at least a fourfold rise between initial and convalescent titers.

Aspiration Pneumonia

Aspiration pneumonia is another important cause of segmental consolidation that may lead to complete consolidation of a lobe. The radiologic feature of aspiration pneumonia that distinguishes it from other causes of segmental consolidation is its distribution. Aspiration pneumonia characteristically occurs in the dependent portions of the lung (see Chapter 15) and is frequently bilateral. However, unilateral involvement can occur, and unilaterality or bilaterality is therefore not a criterion for excluding the diagnosis. In fact, right middle lobe or right lower lobe involvement with sparing of the left side is rather common because of the anatomy of the bronchus intermedius. The diagnosis can often be confirmed on clinical grounds. Occasionally a patient is observed to aspirate either gastric content or food, and subsequent roentgenograms confirm pneumonia. Other cases can be diagnosed on the basis of a radiologic demonstration of segmental consolidation in a dependent portion of the lung and a history of predisposing conditions such as alcoholism, recent anesthesia, head and neck surgery, mental retardation, seizure disorders, and esophageal motility disturbances. In cases of chronic aspiration, segmental consolidation may be a recurring process that never completely clears. On occasion the roentgenogram may document progression from a localized consolidation to interstitial scarring that may even end with the development of an end-stage scar similar to that appearing in honeycomb lung. Pneumonia caused by chronic aspiration is usually distinguished from the other entities that result in honeycomb lung by its localized appearance. A history of mineral oil use is strongly suggestive of chronic aspiration pneumonia (mineral oil or exogenous cholesterol pneumonia). Identification of fat-laden macrophages in the sputum may confirm the diagnosis of mineral oil pneumonia.

Tuberculosis

The initial reaction to the tubercle bacillus (primary tuberculosis) is the exudation of inflammatory cells, including macrophages and polymorphonuclear leukocytes from alveolar capillaries into the alveolar spaces. Initially the alveoli are intact during this exudative phase, but over a period of about a month the exudative reaction is gradually replaced by chronic inflammatory cells as the phase of hypersensitivity reaction begins. After 6 weeks, changes typical of tuberculosis, including caseation necrosis, can be identified in the center of the lesion. This pathogenesis has significant radiologic implications when we contrast the airspace consolidation of the primary exudative phase of tuberculosis with lobar pneumonia. It should be obvious from the preceding description that conventional antibiotic treatment will not clear primary tuberculosis, while adequately treated pneumococcal or *Klebsiella* pneumonia should clear in a few days to 2 weeks. Even with antituberculous therapy, primary tuberculous exudates may require several weeks for complete clearing. Another feature of primary tuberculosis that is extremely important in radiologically differentiating tuberculosis from lobar pneumonia is the presence of hilar or mediastinal adenopathy (see Chapter 11). (Answer to question 3 is *b*.)

Pulmonary Embolism

Pulmonary embolism is an important cause of segmental and lobar consolidations.[295] The consolidations may result from edema and hemorrhage[65] with or without infarction. Jacoby and Mindell[295] emphasized that although these opacities can result from the infarction and necrosis of lung tissue, these opacities more commonly represent incomplete infarction with hemorrhage and edema into the airspaces. Heitzman[260] also indicated that many of the radiologic opacities that appear after pulmonary embolism represent edema and hemorrhage rather than infarction. The radiologic appearance of this type of consolidation is remarkably similar to that of lobar pneumonia. The hemorrhagic edema produces airspace consolidation, with a radiologic appearance of confluent opacities with ill-defined borders, peripheral acinar shadows, and even air bronchograms. Radiologic criteria are frequently inadequate for distinguishing between cases in which the opacities are the result of hemorrhage and edema and those in which they are the result of necrosis with infarction. Air bronchograms are not expected in areas of infarction, but since the infarctions are frequently surrounded by hemorrhagic edema causing airspace consolidation, the presence of air bronchograms is not adequate for excluding the diagnosis of infarction. In cases of angiographically proved pulmonary embolic disease, the radiologic diagnosis of infarction can be made with confidence when the area of consolidation undergoes subsequent cavitation or resolves with a nodular or linear scar.

The combination of segmental or lobar consolidations with pleural effusion might suggest the diagnosis of pulmonary embolism, but this radiologic feature is not useful in distinguishing pulmonary embolism from lobar pneumonia.

Like the radiologic findings, the clinical findings and laboratory tests in pulmonary embolism are frequently nonspecific. Although the classic triad of dyspnea, chest pain, and hemoptysis is seen in only about 20% of cases, the presence of these symptoms in combination with segmental or lobar consolidation and pleural effusion is highly suggestive. Fever, leukocytosis, and sputum production, with the combination of lobar consolidation and pleural effusion, constitute strong evidence for pneumonia, but the diagnosis must be confirmed by laboratory examination of the sputum. A febrile response and leukocytosis do not permit the exclusion of pulmonary embolism, since they may be secondary to severe infarction. This combination probably represents a reaction to the necrosis of lung tissue.

Since the clinical symptoms and radiologic findings are often nonspecific,[227] definitive diagnosis of pulmonary embolism requires either radionuclide studies or pulmonary angiography. In cases with segmental consolidation, the radionu-clide scan requires special care in interpretation. Ventilation and perfusion scans will almost certainly demonstrate that the area of consolidation is neither well perfused nor ventilated, regardless of the cause of the consolidation. In such cases scans are diagnostic of pulmonary embolism only when other areas of abnormal perfusion can be demonstrated. Scans demonstrating abnormalities only in the areas of consolidation should be considered indeterminate, since the consolida-tion could represent infarction, edema and hemorrhage from embolism, or pneu-monia. The most definitive procedure for documenting pulmonary embolism is pulmonary arteriography.

Obstructive Pneumonia

Large airway obstruction was considered in detail in Chapter 13, on atelecta-sis. Atelectasis is the expected result of acute airway obstruction, but with chronic obstruction the collapsed lung re-expands with edema, inflammatory cells, and cholesterol-laden macrophages. This is often described as "drowned" lung, or en-dogenous cholesterol pneumonia (Fig 14–8). When secondary bacterial infection occurs, patients usually experience a febrile response and leukocytosis that is clin-ically typical of pneumonia. The radiologic presentation of an associated hilar mass must be considered as strongly suggestive of obstructive pneumonia. In fact, the combination of a persistent segmental or lobar consolidation with hilar adenopathy in a middle-aged patient strongly suggests an underlying bron-chogenic carcinoma. Radiologic documentation of a lobar opacity that fails to clear completely in response to antibiotic therapy constitutes sufficient clinical grounds for bronchoscopic examination to exclude an underlying tumor. Cavita-tion is another moderately frequent complication of obstructive pneumonia. A persistent abscess following treatment of a pneumonia may also be a clue to an underlying, obstructive bronchial lesion.

Lung Torsion

Torsion[163,422] is a rare cause of either lobar atelectasis or consolidation. It is im-portant because of the risk of complicating infarction and necrosis. Torsion should be suspected when lobar opacities are identified in an unusual position or are as-sociated with unusual hilar displacement. For example, right middle lobe atelec-tasis with elevation of the right hilum should suggest torsion. A major change in position of an opacified lobe on serial films is also evidence to suspect torsion. Torsion has been reported as a complication of thoracic surgery, chest trauma, pneumonia, and both benign and malignant endobronchial tumors.

SUMMARY

1. The classic radiologic appearance of a consolidated lobe is an increased opacity that is homogeneous or confluent, obliterates the normal pulmonary markings, and abuts the fissures. Pure consolidation should not result in volume loss; it frequently even leads to expansion of the lobe.

2. The classic cause of lobar pneumonia is *Streptococcus pneumoniae*, formerly known as *Diplococcus pneumoniae*. Other causes of lobar consolidation include

Klebsiella pneumoniae; primary tuberculosis; aspiration pneumonia; pulmonary embolism with edema, hemorrhage, or infarction; and obstructive pneumonia.

3. Bronchopneumonia and lobular pneumonia are synonyms. The classic appearance of this type of pneumonia is that of multifocal opacities, as described in Chapter 16. There is extensive bronchial involvement, and therefore segmental and lobar opacities with volume loss are not rare. A similar mechanism probably accounts for the segmental and lobar opacities that occur in viral and mycoplasma pneumonias.

4. The bacteriologic diagnosis of pneumonia is not a primary function of the radiologist, since it usually requires laboratory confirmation.

5. Among the radiologic features that occasionally permit the radiologist to suggest a specific etiology for pneumonia are lobar opacities with associated diffuse reticular nodular interstitial disease, which suggest a nonbacterial pneumonia. An expanded lobe with cavitation is strongly suggestive of *Klebsiella* pneumonia.

6. Aspiration pneumonia should be particularly suspected in patients who develop segmental or lobar opacities and who have known predisposing conditions such as alcoholism, recent anesthesia, head and neck tumors, mental retardation, seizure disorders, and disturbances in esophageal motility. Lipid pneumonia should be especially considered in the elderly patient who uses mineral oil.

7. Primary tuberculosis is an important cause of lobar and segmental opacities, which are frequently associated with hilar adenopathy. This combination may also be seen in children with viral pneumonia, and in older patients it may be an important clue to the diagnosis of obstructive pneumonia caused by bronchogenic carcinoma.

8. Obstructive pneumonia is a particularly important cause of segmental and lobar consolidations in middle-aged smokers. The persistence of a lobar or segmental consolidation following antibiotic therapy for a presumed pneumonia is extremely suggestive of obstructive pneumonia. Suspicion of this abnormality warrants further investigation and the collection of sputum samples for cytologic study. Bronchoscopy and biopsy are frequently required for the definitive diagnosis.

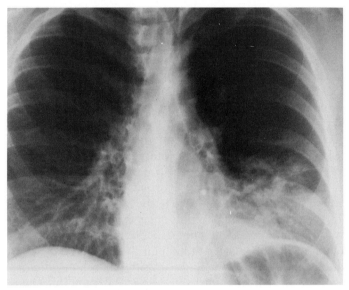

FIG 14–3
Pneumococcal pneumonia has produced a nonsegmental sublobar consolidation of the lingula. Notice loss of the heart border, which indicates that the consolidation is in an anterior location and illustrates the "silhouette sign."[162,369]

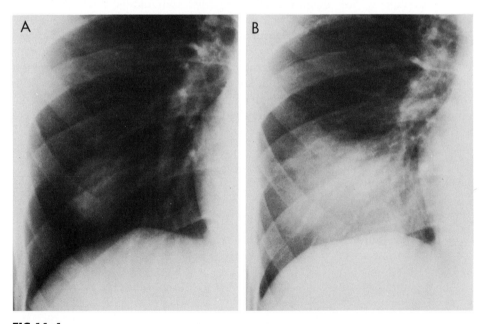

FIG 14–4
A, Localized, rounded opacity with air bronchograms is the result of pneumococcal pneumonia. This has been described as "round pneumonia." **B,** Film obtained 24 hours later shows extensive air space consolidation. Notice nonsegmental distribution, the result of contiguous spread of pneumonia via collateral channels.

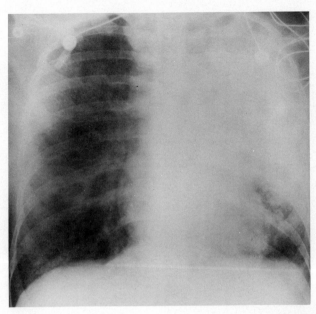

FIG 14–5
Diffuse bronchopneumonia initially involved left upper lobe, but has disseminated via
the airways. Right lung is completely consolidated, resulting in patchy appearance described by Heitzman[260] as "patchwork quilt" appearance. Lobular consolidations separated by aerated lobules give rise to this phenomenon. Disease organism was *Legionella
pneumophila.* (From Reed JC, McLelland R, Nelson P: Legionnaires' disease. *AJR* 1978;
131:892–894. Used by permission.)

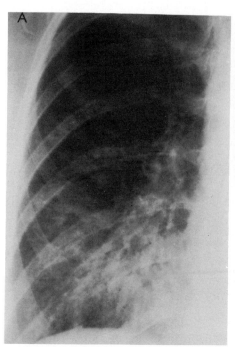 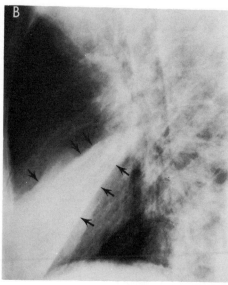

FIG 14–6
A, This case of mycoplasma pneumonia presented with patchy, ill-defined opacities in the right middle and lower lobes, which would not be distinguishable from those in other cases of bronchopneumonia. **B,** Lateral projection film from same case confirms significant atelectasis of right middle lobe. Note displacement of the fissures *(arrows)*. Atelectasis is the result of small airway obstruction caused by a combination of peribronchial inflammation and mucus plugging.

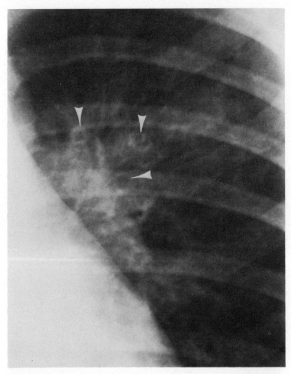

FIG 14–7
Film shows ill-defined opacities in left upper lobe. Additional finding of ring shadows *(arrowheads)* around the hilum confirms presence of peribronchial infiltrates, which are suggestive of associated bronchiolitis. This is mycoplasma pneumonia.

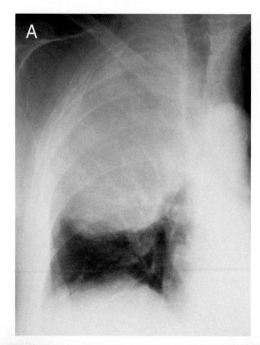

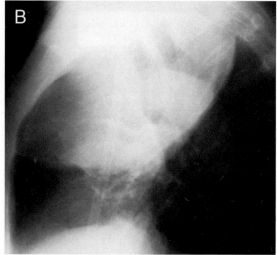

FIG 14–8
A, PA film demonstrates complete consolidation of the right upper lobe with inferior depression of the minor fissure. **B,** Lateral film further confirms the expansion of the right upper lobe by showing displacement of both fissures. This is a "drowned lung" resulting from right upper lobe bronchial obstruction by a bronchogenic carcinoma.

ANSWER GUIDE

LEGENDS FOR INTRODUCTORY FIGURES

FIG 14–1
Homogeneous consolidation of left lower lobe is the result of *Streptococcus pneumoniae.* This organism is the most common cause of lobar pneumonia.

FIG 14–2
A, PA film shows consolidation of right upper lobe with inferior displacement of minor fissure *(arrows).* **B,** Lateral-projection film further confirms consolidation of right upper lobe by revealing posteroinferior displacement of major fissure in addition to depression of minor fissure *(white arrowheads).* Interspersed lucencies *(black arrows)* are due to early cavitation.

ANSWERS

  1, b; 2, b; 3, b.

CHAPTER 15

Diffuse Air-Space Disease

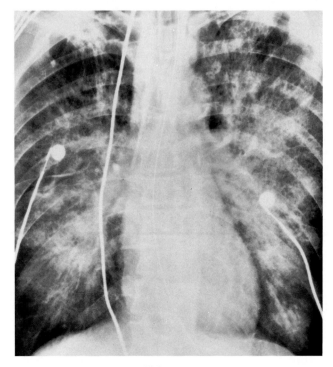

FIG 15–1

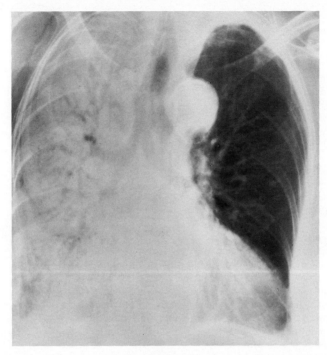

FIG 15–2

QUESTIONS

1. Examine Figure 15–1. Which of the following are signs of air-space disease?
   a. Diffuse coalescent opacities.
   b. Air bronchograms.
   c. Acinar rosettes.
   d. Fine reticular opacities.
   e. Air alveolograms.
2. The asymmetric distribution of the diffuse coalescent opacities in Figure 15–2 is suggestive of which diagnosis?
   a. Bronchopneumonia.
   b. Goodpasture's syndrome.
   c. Chronic renal failure.
   d. Alveolar proteinosis.
   e. Congestive heart failure.
3. A 24- to 48-hour delay in the development of pulmonary edema is commonly observed in which of the following conditions?
   a. Congestive heart failure.
   b. Pulmonary emboli.
   c. Smoke inhalation.
   d. Heroin reaction.
   e. High-altitude pulmonary edema.

CHART 15–1.
Diffuse Air-Space Disease

I. Edema
   A. Cardiac failure
   B. Noncardiac (see Chart 15–2)
II. Exudate (pneumonias)
   A. Bacteria[57,58,126,232,485]
   B. Viruses[260,403]
   C. Mycoplasma[170,279]
   D. Fungi[51,391,474,554]
   E. *Pneumocystis carinii* pneumonia[72,82,103,124]
   F. Parasites (Strongyloidiasis)[664]
   G. Aspiration
   H. Rickettsiae (Rocky Mountain spotted fever)[351,385]
   I. Tuberculosis[433]
III. Hemorrhage
   A. Anticoagulation therapy
   B. Bleeding diathesis (e.g., leukemia)
   C. Disseminated intravascular coagulation (18- to 72-hour delay)[471]
   D. Blunt trauma (usually not diffuse)
   E. Vasculitis
      1. Infections (mucormycosis, aspergillosis, Rocky Mountain spotted fever)
      2. Wegener's granulomatosis[342,377,622] (classic and variant forms)
      3. Goodpasture's syndrome[266,544]
      4. Systemic lupus erythematosus
   F. Idiopathic pulmonary hemosiderosis[176,607]
   G. Infectious mononucleosis[613]
IV. Tumor
   A. Bronchioloalveolar-cell carcinoma[47,411]
   B. Lymphoma and rare lymphocytic disorders including:
      1. Lymphocytic interstitial pneumonitis[56]
      2. Angioblastic lymphadenopathy[314]
      3. Mycosis fungoides[292]
      4. Waldenström's macroglobulinemia
V. Other
   A. Pulmonary alveolar proteinosis[484,509]
   B. Adult respiratory distress syndrome[139,300,301,448,672] or oxygen toxicity
   C. Sarcoidosis (very unusual)[408,481,491]
   D. Desquamative interstitial pneumonitis
   E. Mineral oil aspiration (exogenous cholesterol pneumonia)
   F. Eosinophilic lung disease[95,192]
   G. Chemical pneumonitis from intravenous hydrocarbon
   H. Respiratory distress syndrome of the newborn[481,595]

CHART 15–2.
Noncardiac Pulmonary Edema

  I. Chronic renal failure
 II. Toxic inhalations
   A. Nitrogen dioxide (silo-filler's disease)
   B. Sulfur dioxide[86]
   C. Smoke[307,470]
   D. Beryllium
   E. Cadmium
   F. Silica (very fine particles)   *(Continued.)*

CHART 15–2.   (cont.).

    G. Dinitrogen tetroxide[123]

    H. Carbon monoxide[571]

  III. Anaphylaxis (penicillin, transfusion,[75] radiologic contrast medium[228])

  IV. Narcotics (morphine, heroin)

   V. Drug reaction, (e.g., nitrofurantoin, interleukin-2,[101,535] β-adrenergic drugs[415]

  VI. Acute airway obstruction[449] (e.g., foreign body)

 VII. Near-drowning[472]

VIII. High altitude[285]

  IX. Fluid overload

   X. Cerebral (trauma, stroke, tumor)[491]

  XI. Hypoproteinemia

 XII. Pulmonary embolism

XIII. Adult respiratory distress syndrome (early stages)[135,301]

XIV. Pancreatitis[514]

 XV. Amniotic fluid embolism[557]

XVI. Fat embolism

XVII. Reexpansion following treatment of pneumothorax

XVIII. Organophosphate insecticide ingestion[359]

DISCUSSION

The classic radiologic appearance of diffuse air-space consolidation is shown in Figure 15–1 and consists of diffuse coalescent or confluent opacities with ill-defined borders, a butterfly-shaped perihilar distribution, ill-defined nodular opacities around the periphery of the process ("acinar opacities"),[676] and interspersed small lucencies.[481,484] Air-filled bronchi surrounded by the confluent opacities are seen as dark, branching shadows. These were described by Fleischner[175] as the "visible bronchial tree" and are commonly referred to as "air bronchograms"[162] (see Fig 15–2). The small interspersed lucencies represent groups of air-filled alveoli surrounded by airless consolidated lung. The term "air alveologram" was applied to these lucencies by Felson;[162] they are the alveolar equivalent of the air bronchogram. Other features of air-space consolidation include the lobar or segmental distribution of opacities, discussed in Chapter 14, and a tendency for the process to be labile, changing in severity over a short period. Observation of the changing character of the opacities requires serial roentgenograms. (The only incorrect answer to question 1 is *d*.) Diffuse ground-glass opacity is occasionally used to describe less-opaque diffuse confluent patterns seen on plain film and is more commonly used in reporting high-resolution CT (HRCT). This differs from consolidation in degree of opacity and implies minimal disease. Ground-glass opacities appear on HRCT as gray areas of confluent attenuation that fail to obliterate normal vascular shadows. Ground-glass opacity demonstrated by HRCT results from minimal filling of the alveolar spaces or from thickening of the alveolar walls and septal interstitium.[142]

Pulmonary Edema

CARDIAC PULMONARY EDEMA

Pulmonary alveolar edema is a classic example of a diffuse air-space–filling process. The presence of alveolar edema, however, does not imply the absence of interstitial edema. For example, cardiac pulmonary alveolar edema is always preceded by interstitial edema, but the extensive alveolar consolidation may obscure the fine reticular pattern of the interstitial process. This is in effect a microscopic version of Felson's silhouette sign,[162] since the material in the alveolar space has the same opacity as the edema fluid in the interlobular septa and bronchovascular bundles. Radiologic documentation of the underlying interstitial process entails examination of areas not significantly involved by the alveolar filling process. When alveolar pulmonary edema is secondary to congestive heart failure, the alveolar edema will often have a perihilar distribution, while Kerley's B lines may be present in the costophrenic angles. The latter sign indicates an underlying interstitial process. Other radiologic signs that may be associated with cardiopulmonary edema and can be helpful in suggesting the diagnosis include (1) prominence of the upper-lobe vessels,[479] (2) peribronchial cuffing,[414] (3) increased width of the vascular pedicle,[414] (4) pleural effusion, frequently with fluid in the fissures, and (5) cardiac enlargement with a left ventricular prominence. Correlation of such findings with clinical findings usually confirms the diagnosis. An electrocardiogram (EKG) indicating cardiac enlargement or an old or acute myocardial infarction is also supportive evidence, while an S_3 heart sound, neck vein distention, hepatomegaly, or peripheral edema usually confirms the diagnosis of congestive failure. Also, auscultation over the lungs usually reveals characteristic basilar rales.

Occasionally, the alveolar edema is not distributed uniformly. Owing to gravity, the edema fluid has a predominantly lower lobe distribution when the patient is upright, but when the patient is supine, the fluid tends to have a more posterior distribution. When the patient favors one side, the fluid tends to gravitate to the dependent side. Other causes for atypical or nonuniform distribution of pulmonary edema are usually of pulmonary origin. The best known of these is severe emphysema, which results in patchy distribution of the alveolar edema. Presumably, loss of vasculature in the emphysematous areas of the lung results in the development of edema in the more normal areas. Pulmonary embolism is another complication of pulmonary edema that may result in a nonuniform or patchy distribution of the alveolar edema. Two factors may determine the distribution of the air-space edema following pulmonary embolism: (1) Abrupt interruption of perfusion to an area of lung may prevent the development of typical pulmonary edema. For example, large emboli may occlude the lower lobe vessels so completely that the entire pulmonary blood flow is diverted to the upper lobes. The radiologic result is hyperlucency of the lower lobe and edema in the upper lobe. (2) Ischemia may influence the radiologic appearance of pulmonary edema complicated by pulmonary embolism. Severe ischemia of the lung can give rise to hemorrhagic pulmonary edema, and since pulmonary emboli tend to be scattered, this can lead to the appearance of multifocal ill-defined opacities (see Chapter 16). The significance of this pattern is difficult to determine, because the normal resolution of pulmonary edema is often not uniform; thus clinical correlation is essential. When the plain film reveals patchy air-space consolidation, lung scanning is frequently not diagnostic, and definitive diagnosis of pulmonary embolism may be made only by pulmonary angiography.

Another cause of uneven distribution of pulmonary edema is a concomitant infection. Like the diagnosis of pulmonary embolism, this requires correlation with the clinical history. An elevated temperature, leukocytosis, or purulent sputum should prompt a bacteriologic study to rule out superimposed pneumonia.

Cardiac enlargement in combination with diffuse alveolar opacities that are otherwise characteristic of pulmonary edema is not always a reliable indicator that the patient's primary problem is a cardiac disorder. For instance, chronic renal failure with uremia can cause pulmonary edema (uremic pneumonitis) as well as hypertension and associated heart disease, with the result of cardiac enlargement. Not only does uremia cause true cardiomegaly, which is probably related to chronic hypertension, but it also may cause pericardial effusion. Thus, the pulmonary edema that results from chronic renal failure and uremia is typically associated with enlargement of the cardiac silhouette. Correlation with the clinical history should readily identify uremic pneumonitis.

In contrast to pulmonary alveolar edema and cardiac enlargement, the presence of a normal-sized heart might suggest a noncardiac form of pulmonary edema, but there are situations in which such patients may actually have cardiac pulmonary edema. These include acute cardiac arrhythmias and acute myocardial infarction, which result in pulmonary edema prior to dilation of the heart. Thus, there are at least two mechanisms for cardiac pulmonary edema with a normal-sized heart.

NONCARDIAC PULMONARY EDEMA

The preceding discussion suggests that the radiologic appearance of noncardiac pulmonary edema is similar to that of cardiac pulmonary edema.[568] In general, the most helpful radiologic feature for distinguishing the two is the presence or absence of cardiac enlargement. Accurate assessment of heart size is often difficult. Technical factors—including supine and anterior-posterior positioning, especially when done with portable units—may all contribute to cardiac magnification. Patient condition may also lead to inaccurate cardiac size estimation. Patients with emphysema often have cardiac enlargement, although the plain film is suggestive of a normal or even small heart size. Aggressive intravenous fluid resuscitation may actually enlarge the heart and cause pulmonary edema. The evaluation of serial films is especially useful for distinguishing a number of the causes of noncardiac edema, since the evolution of the edema may be strikingly different. Many of the entities listed in Chart 15–2 may result in acute alveolar edema in the absence of the pulmonary vascular and interstitial changes that precede the edema, owing to either renal failure or cardiac failure. These entities tend to occur in very acute cases of pulmonary edema and are often best diagnosed by clinical correlation,[4] as will be shown in the discussions of acute toxic inhalations, near-drowning, acute airway obstruction, drug reactions, and adult respiratory distress syndrome.

Acute Toxic Inhalations.   Nitrogen dioxide inhalation (silo-filler's disease) is an excellent model for acute toxic pulmonary edema. In the first few days after a grain storage silo is filled, nitrogen dioxide forms. The gas reacts with water in the respiratory tract to produce an irritation of the tracheobronchial tree and alveoli. In the acute phase, this disease has the radiologic appearance of bilateral diffuse alveolar edema. This phase is usually followed within a few days or weeks by complete resolution, although bronchiolitis obliterans may develop weeks to months later as a result of the small airway injury. Roentgenograms from patients with bronchiolitis obliterans often show a fine nodular or reticular pattern. The other chemicals listed in Chart 15–2 produce a similar reaction.

Smoke is a common cause of acute toxic inhalation. Since the most common radiologic presentation of toxic smoke inhalation is a normal chest film, chest roentgenography is not a reliable technique for assessing the acute effects of smoke inhalation. The radiologic appearance of pulmonary edema may be delayed by as much as 24 to 48 hours (answer to question 3 is *c*). Putman et al.[470] suggest that arterial hypoxemia is a more sensitive index of pulmonary injury from smoke inhalation. Another important method for evaluating smoke inhalation is to determine the amount of carboxyhemoglobin in blood. Levels above the normal mean of 2.01% in nonsmokers and 7.22% in smokers reflect carbon monoxide poisoning with potential concomitant lung damage.

Near Drowning.   Near drowning is another important cause of noncardiac pulmonary edema (Fig 15–3). The history should confirm the diagnosis. However, aspiration of water provides only a partial explanation for the diffuse alveolar opacities that may develop in near-drowning victims. Again, there may be a delay of 24 to 48 hours before edema develops. Other mechanisms that may contribute to the development of this type of edema include prolonged hypoxia, respiratory obstruction, and fibrin degradation. Fibrin degradation raises the possibility of a subclinical consumptive coagulopathy with microembolization, which may lead to a diffuse pulmonary capillary leak and thus to pulmonary edema. Severe hypoxia may occur in a near-fatal drowning victim even when the initial chest roentgenogram is normal. Patients should therefore be followed up for 24 to 48 hours to exclude a significant pulmonary injury.

Acute Airway Obstruction.   The diagnosis of acute airway obstruction is usually made on the basis of the clinical history. The obstruction is frequently an aspirated object, such as a large bolus of food or a surgical sponge. The resultant pulmonary edema is most probably related to severe hypoxia. This mechanism may be nearly identical to that described for near drowning. The collection of alveolar fluid is most likely due to a diffuse alveolar leak caused by severe injury to the alveolar capillary membrane.

Drug Reactions.   Acute pulmonary edema may follow the intravenous injection of certain drugs. The drugs best known to produce this type of reaction are morphine, heroin, and other opiates. Although the mechanism for this type of pulmonary edema is unknown, it is generally believed to represent an idiosyncratic reaction. Methadone, a slow-acting narcotic, may cause a slower onset of edema than heroin or morphine.[680] Nonnarcotic drugs, including interleukin-2 and β-adrenergic drugs, have also been reported as causes of acute edema.[101,415,535]

Chronic drug reactions more typically produce a diffuse interstitial pattern, but this is occasionally associated with edema and may thus mimic this pattern.[260]

Adult Respiratory Distress Syndrome.   Adult respiratory distress syndrome (ARDS) is a complex clinical syndrome that may occur after a variety of severe pulmonary injuries,[139] including trauma, shock, sepsis, severe pulmonary infection, transfusion reaction, or cardiopulmonary bypass. These conditions cause an alveolar-capillary injury with leakage of edema fluid into the alveolar spaces. This is so severe that increasing concentrations of inspired oxygen are required to maintain adequate arterial oxygen saturation, while at the same time high ventilator pressures are needed to combat the decreasing lung compliance.

The radiologic appearance is that of diffuse, coalescent opacities similar to those described for alveolar edema, alveolar hemorrhage, or diffuse air-space pneumonia. The sequence of events in patients with ARDS, however, is different from that in patients with typical pulmonary edema. Unlike cardiac pulmonary edema, which clears in response to therapy, the edema and infiltrates in ARDS may persist for days to weeks. As the diffuse coalescent opacities begin to clear, an underlying reticular pattern emerges. Patients who succumb to the illness usually have a complex pulmonary reaction that includes the formation of hyaline membranes, extensive fibrosis, and the development of areas of organizing pneumonia. Grossly, the lungs are stiff and firm. The mechanisms for this catastrophic course are not completely understood. It has been suggested that diffuse intravascular clotting and platelet aggregation within the capillary bed (disseminated intravascular coagulation) probably lead to interstitial edema, altered capillary permeability, atelectasis, and hyaline-membrane formation. Oxygen toxicity may also be a factor in the pathogenesis of many cases of ARDS. In addition, bacterial superinfection is very common. This entity should be suspected on the basis of the clinical presentation and the presence of persistent, diffuse coalescent opacities (Fig 15–4).

Reexpansion pulmonary edema is an infrequent complication of pneumothorax. This is probably the consequence of alveolar capillary injury initiated by ischemia. It develops following the treatment of a large pneumothorax with near-complete collapse of the lung. The history often suggests a delay in treatment of more than 24 hours (Fig 15–5, *A* and *B).*

Other.   Other causes of pulmonary edema that must be diagnosed on the basis of the clinical history include high-altitude pulmonary edema,[285] amniotic fluid embolism,[557] and fat embolism. As indicated in the discussion of smoke inhalation and near-drowning there may be a delay in the development of the diffuse coalescing opacities with fat embolism, but it should not exceed the time of the fracture by more than 24 to 48 hours. Repositioning or orthopedic manipulation of a fracture occasionally accounts for fat emboli occurring days to weeks after the initial fracture. In the absence of a history of manipulation, however, the development of pulmonary opacities from days to weeks after a fracture is more suggestive of other diagnoses, such as venous thromboembolism.

PULMONARY HEMORRHAGE

Hemorrhage is an important cause of diffuse coalescent opacities, since it may lead to extensive air-space consolidation. Some of the causes of pulmonary hemorrhage, such as anticoagulant therapy, Goodpasture's syndrome, and pulmonary contusion, are easily identified from the clinical history. Hemoptysis is a common clinical finding because a large amount of blood fills the lungs.

Some of the bleeding disorders that may lead to pulmonary hemorrhage are hemophilia, anticoagulation therapy, and hematologic malignancy. The differential of diffuse alveolar consolidation in the leukemic patient is that of (1) opportunistic infection, (2) drug reaction, (3) diffuse hemorrhage, (4) leukemic infiltration, and (5) pulmonary edema. Severe hemoptysis confirms the diagnosis of diffuse pulmonary hemorrhage in such a clinical setting, but the absence of hemoptysis does not exclude the diagnosis.

Trauma is not a common cause of diffuse pulmonary hemorrhage, since blunt trauma is usually not sufficiently extensive or crushing to produce it. More frequently, trauma results in a localized area of contusion and therefore in localized opacities on the chest film. Often there are associated fractures and pleural effusion. The history confirms the diagnosis.

Goodpasture's syndrome, although not a common entity, must be seriously considered in a patient with hemoptysis, hematuria, and diffuse air-space consolidations. The diagnosis is usually confirmed by renal biopsy with specific immunofluorescent stains.

Idiopathic pulmonary hemosiderosis is another rare pulmonary disease that causes diffuse pulmonary hemorrhage. The radiologic pattern depends on the stage of the disease. In the acute phases, there are bilateral, diffuse coalescent opacities with air bronchograms. As the disease resolves, the clearing may be patchy, leaving the multifocal, ill-defined opacities described in Chapter 16. This entity tends to be recurrent, with the development of an interstitial pattern that is frequently of a fine reticular nature and occurs as a late complication of the disease. This generally follows many recurrences of the acute alveolar hemorrhage. During the phases of the hemorrhage, the fine reticular pattern is obscured by extensive alveolar consolidation (Fig 15–6).

Wegener's granulomatosis is a diffuse pulmonary vasculitis that may produce either localized or diffuse pulmonary hemorrhage. This diagnosis is easily confirmed when the classic Wegener's triad of pulmonary, nasopharyngeal, and renal involvement is present. The limited form of Wegener's granulomatosis requires lung biopsy for confirmation. Other patterns associated with this entity include multiple ill-defined opacities and multiple lesions that may cavitate (see Chapters 16 and 24).

Inflammation

Acute pulmonary infections are a major consideration in the differential of diffuse coalescent opacities. The entity is commonly distinguished from pulmonary edema on clinical grounds. Patients with diffusely coalescent bilateral pneumonias are usually profoundly ill, with an elevated temperature, elevated white blood cell count, severe dyspnea, and productive sputum.

BRONCHOPNEUMONIA

Bronchopneumonias are the most common infections producing diffuse coalescent opacities. Gram-negative organisms are particularly notorious for producing such fulminant pneumonias.[260] This pattern is frequently preceded by films showing multifocal, ill-defined opacities like those described in Chapter 16. There is a tendency for the patient to have some volume loss because of the bronchial inflammation. The loss of volume may cause one lobe to appear to be predominantly involved during the course of the illness. In some cases the radiologic patterns of bronchopneumonia and pulmonary edema are similar (see the initial description of diffuse air space disease), although an asymmetric, patchy, or even unilateral presentation (see Fig 15–2) is more consistent with the diagnosis of bronchopneumonia. (Answer to question 2 is *a*.) It must be remembered that pulmonary edema may also produce a patchy or asymmetric distribution when there are underlying diseases such as emphysema or pulmonary embolism. Clinical and laboratory data may be useful in distinguishing bronchopneumonia from pulmonary edema. Bronchopneumonia should result in a febrile response, with productive purulent sputum and leukocytosis. Culture of sputum and blood usually confirms the diagnosis and identifies the organisms.

VIRAL PNEUMONIAS

Although viral pneumonias are best known for producing a diffuse interstitial pattern (usually a fine reticular or fine nodular pattern), fulminant cases may also lead to diffuse air-space consolidations. In these cases there is extensive hemorrhagic edema into the alveolar spaces, probably as a result of thrombosis of alveolar capillaries, which leads to necrosis and hemorrhage. Viral pneumonia is especially severe in immunologically compromised patients,[353] in particular those with hematologic malignancies, AIDS, or organ transplants, and especially those who are receiving immunosuppressive therapy. Severe viral pneumonia with air-space consolidation is infrequently encountered in the otherwise normal patient.

ASPIRATION PNEUMONIA

Aspiration pneumonia is another cause of diffuse coalescent opacities that should be diagnosed by correlating the radiologic appearance with the clinical setting. Aspiration pneumonia may produce diffuse bilaterally coalescent opacities, although these tend to be more localized than in pulmonary edema. Since the aspirated material usually goes to the dependent portions of the lung, the distribution of the radiologic abnormality is directly related to the position of the patient at the time of aspiration. Material aspirated while the patient is in the upright position tends to go to the medial basal segments of the lung and to the right middle lobe, while in the supine patient aspirated material tends to collect in the superior segments of the lower lobes and the posterior segments of the upper lobes. Knowledge of the material aspirated and of the patient's position at aspiration usually confirms the diagnosis. In the clinical setting, the postoperative or comatose patient is more susceptible to aspiration. Alcoholic patients are especially prone to aspiration pneumonia.

Chronic aspiration, on the other hand, is more difficult to confirm and requires careful evaluation of the patient's history. For example, air-space consolidation in the right middle lobe in an elderly patient who is otherwise not particularly ill should prompt suspicion of an exogenous lipid pneumonia (mineral oil aspiration). This type of aspiration pneumonia should not result in diffuse confluent opacities. Patients with disturbances of esophageal motility, obstructive lesions of the esophagus, and head or neck tumors are all candidates for chronic aspiration. Aspiration may also be the underlying factor in the tendency for these patients to have gram-negative pneumonias. The gram-negative pneumonias are a much more likely cause of diffuse confluent opacities than is uncomplicated chronic aspiration.

OPPORTUNISTIC PNEUMONIAS

Immunologically compromised patients are susceptible not only to common pyogenic, viral, and fungal pneumonias, but also to a more virulent infection. Viral infections that may cause minimal abnormality in an immune-competent patient may cause a fatal hemorrhagic pneumonia in patients with severe immune suppression. Fungi that are nonpathogenic in patients with normal immunity may cause diffuse coalescent opacities in the immunologically compromised patient. These uncommon pathogenic fungi include *Aspergillus, Candida, Cryptococcus,* and *Phycomycetes.*[391] Infection by *Phycomycetes* is commonly called mucormycosis. Both *Phycomycetes* and *Aspergillus* invade the pulmonary vessels, leading to a diffuse hemorrhagic pneumonia and even pulmonary necrosis or gangrene.

AIDS-RELATED DISEASES

HIV-infected individuals are at risk for a variety of pulmonary infections, neoplasms, and drug reactions. *Pneumocystis carinii* pneumonia (PCP) is one of the most common infections in patients with AIDS, occuring in more than 75% of patients. It is not expected to occur until the CD4 cell count has dropped to less than 200, but it is one of the most common AIDS-defining diseases.[581] The organisms spread through the airways and interstitium with minimal or no visible abnormality on the initial radiograph. During the earliest stages, gallium scans and HRCT are more sensitive for early diagnosis. The earliest plain film appearance is a subtle, fine reticular pattern, but many cases follow a more fulminant course, with rapid development of diffuse coalescent opacities (Fig 15–7, *A* and *B*). This development results from alveolar wall injury followed by filling of the air-spaces with plasma proteins, inflammatory cells, and organisms. The plain film appearance is that of diffuse symmetric coalescent opacities, resembling noncardiac edema (Fig 15–8, *A* and *B*). An atypical upper lobe distribution may result in patients' receiving prophylactic treatment with aerosolized pentamidine (Fig 15–9, *A* and *B*).[82,103] Associated pleural effusions are rare in patients with PCP, occurring as infrequently as in 2% of patients, and should be considered evidence of another diagnosis.

Pyogenic pneumonias are seen in 5% to 30% of HIV-infected individuals, but they typically occur in the earlier stages of infection, before the first AIDS-defining disease. CD4 counts are usually between 200 and 500. Bacterial pneumonias may be severe and cause a pattern of diffuse consolidations in approximately 20% of cases, but lobar consolidations are more common, with a frequency of 50%. The most common organisms are *Haemophilus influenzae* and *Streptococcus pneumoniae.*[112]

Kaposi's sarcoma and lymphoma are common neoplasms in patients with AIDS, but their plain film findings are most often either masses or multiple poorly defined opacities rather than diffuse coalescent opacities (see Chapter 16). Lymphocytic interstitial pneumonia (LIP) is a lymphoproliferative disorder of the lung that is rare in patients with normal immunity but more common in patients with AIDS.[393] LIP in patients without AIDS is a B-cell lymphocytic infiltration of the interstitium and alveolar walls; in patients with AIDS it is a T-cell infiltration. AIDS-related LIP is rare in adults, but it is the second most common disease seen in children with AIDS, occuring in 30% of cases.

Chronic Diffuse Consolidations

Diffuse coalescent opacities usually indicate either an acute process, such as pulmonary edema, or the acute phase of a chronic relapsing disease, such as idiopathic pulmonary hemosiderosis. However, there are a few conditions that, al-

beit rarely, cause persistent chronic diffuse pulmonary consolidations. This somewhat rare radiologic presentation may be seen with chronic granulomatous diseases, neoplasms, and pulmonary alveolar proteinosis.

CHRONIC GRANULOMATOUS DISEASES

Chronic granulomatous diseases rarely cause diffuse coalescent opacities. Fungal infections may produce this pattern in immunologically compromised patients
but rarely in the uncompromised host. Although rarely seen in tuberculosis, this
pattern may occur when there is extensive pulmonary hemorrhage in conjunc-
tion with aspiration of blood to other portions of the lung from a cavitary lesion,
or when patients with miliary tuberculosis develop secondary pulmonary edema
or ARDS.[433] Once this complication develops, the underlying miliary nodules are
obscured by pulmonary edema.

Sarcoidosis is a rare cause of diffuse bilaterally symmetric consolidations that
may resemble pulmonary edema. The mechanism for this pattern is considered in
detail in Chapter 16. Sarcoidosis more often causes multifocal ill-defined opacities, which may have air bronchograms, than a pattern of diffuse confluent opacities. In contrast to all the other entities considered in this chapter, there may be
a striking disparity between the severity of the radiologic appearance of sarcoidosis and the clinical well-being of the patient. Although the abnormalities may
appear to be very extensive, patients with sarcoidosis are often only mildly dysp-
neic and may otherwise be asymptomatic.

NEOPLASMS

Diffuse coalescent opacities are rarely caused by neoplastic processes, but two
categories of tumors do result in this pattern.

Bronchioloalveolar cell carcinoma is a unique airway neoplasm that arises in
either the distal small bronchioles or alveolar walls. In its localized form, bronchioloalveolar cell carcinoma produces an appearance more suggestive of a consolidation than a mass (Fig 15–10). Air bronchograms through the area of tumor
are a common and distinctive feature of this tumor not often encountered in any
other type of primary lung tumor. The air bronchograms may be enhanced by
CT[355]. Bronchioloalveolar cell carcinoma frequently grows along alveolar walls
and produces mucus within the air-spaces. The alveolar walls and bronchi remain
intact. Examination of histologic sections frequently reveals plugs of tumor in the
bronchi, which supports the theory of bronchogenic spread of bronchioloalveolar
cell carcinoma. This theory is consistent with the observation that the carcinoma
may lead to multifocal ill-defined opacities followed by diffuse air-space consolidations. The same mechanism may also account for the occasional lobar consolidations that mimic lobar pneumonia. Because of the large amount of mucus and
tumor tissue in the air-spaces, cytologic examination often provides the diagnosis. Since the radiologic appearance of bronchioloalveolar cell carcinoma is remarkably similar to that of pneumonia, the presence of a chronic, more persistent
air-space consolidation frequently requires biopsy to exclude the diagnosis.

The other major category of neoplastic disease that may lead to diffuse air-space
consolidation consists of lymphoid disorders in the lung (see Chart 15–1). Like
bronchioloalveolar cell carcinoma, lymphoma of the lung tends to be a localized

process. Multifocal areas of air-space consolidation, as discussed in Chapter 16, are much more common than diffuse air-space consolidation, but the latter does occur. In the case of lymphocytic interstitial pneumonia, serial films may reveal an evolution of opacities from a diffuse reticular pattern to a confluent pattern. This once rare disease is now seen with increasing frequency in AIDS patients.[446]

ALVEOLAR PROTEINOSIS

Alveolar proteinosis is an unusual disease that results in diffuse bilateral confluent opacities that often have air bronchograms (Fig 15–11, *A*). It is also a unique disease in comparison with all of the other entities considered in this differential, because it is the model for pure alveolar disease. Occasionally, a fine nodular pattern with ill-defined borders may be seen around the periphery of the confluent opacities, but these are not interstitial nodules like the nodules discussed in Chapter 17. They apparently represent the smallest unit of air-space filling that can be recognized radiologically. Ziskind referred to these fine opacities as "acinar rosettes."[676] Histologic examination demonstrates extensive alveolar filling with proteinaceous material and normal alveolar walls and interlobular septa (Fig 15–11, *B*). These consolidations may appear acutely and resolve spontaneously or may persist, requiring pulmonary lavage. The time required for their spontaneous resolution is highly variable. Alveolar proteinosis is also observed to be a chronic relapsing disease and one of the few diseases that may produce diffuse air-space consolidation while the patient remains relatively asymptomatic. In fact, the radiologic presentation of diffuse bilateral air-space consolidations that are either recurrent or chronic in a patient who complains only of mild dyspnea strongly suggests this diagnosis.

SUMMARY

1. Diffuse coalescent opacities with air bronchograms, air alveolograms, and acinar rosettes constitute the classic radiologic appearance of alveolar disease. Pure alveolar disease is rarely seen, alveolar proteinosis being one of the very few examples. The other entities in Chart 15–1 are all examples of mixed alveolar and interstitial disease.

2. The underlying interstitial component of the disease is obscured by the alveolar disease.

3. The most common cause of this pattern is pulmonary edema. Pulmonary edema may be divided into cardiac and noncardiac categories on the basis of cause. Clinical correlation is extremely important in identifying the cause in pulmonary edema of noncardiac origin.

4. Adult respiratory distress syndrome is a complex clinical syndrome that results in diffuse coalescing opacities. The diagnosis should be suspected when the patient has acute pulmonary edema following severe injury or shock, particularly after drug reactions, gram-negative sepsis, transfusion reactions, snake bite, or the use of pump oxygenators in cardiopulmonary bypass surgery.

5. Diffuse pneumonias are another extremely important cause of diffuse coalescent opacities. They should be easily distinguished from pulmonary edema when seen in an acutely ill and toxic febrile patient. The etiologic agents are fre-

quently gram-negative organisms. The radiologic appearance is of little value in determining the specific organism. Viruses and fungi may also produce this pattern, particularly in the immunologically compromised host. Prompt diagnostic biopsy is essential in the compromised host, since failure to initiate immediate therapy may result in death.

6. Diffuse pulmonary hemorrhage with extensive bilateral confluent opacities is frequently but not invariably associated with hemoptysis. Clinical correlation is essential in determining the cause of diffuse pulmonary hemorrhage (anticoagulation therapy, hemophilia, leukemia, or trauma). Biopsy is required for a diagnosis of the idiopathic sources of such hemorrhage, including Goodpasture's syndrome, pulmonary hemosiderosis, and Wegener's granulomatosis.

7. Bronchioloalveolar cell carcinoma and lymphoid disorders of the lung are the only neoplastic conditions likely to result in this pattern.

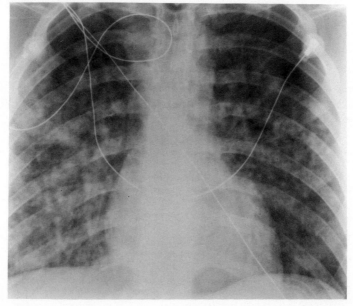

FIG 15–3
Near-drowning produces diffuse bilateral air-space consolidations with a normal heart size. The history is essential to confirm the diagnosis. The radiologic appearance is indistinguishable from that of the other causes of noncardiac pulmonary edema.

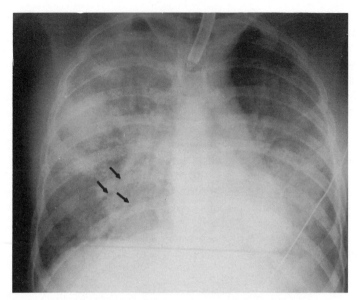

FIG 15–4
Diffuse pulmonary consolidations with air bronchograms *(arrows)* are the result of ARDS following a viral pneumonia. This appearance is radiologically indistinguishable from pulmonary alveolar edema and diffuse pneumonia.

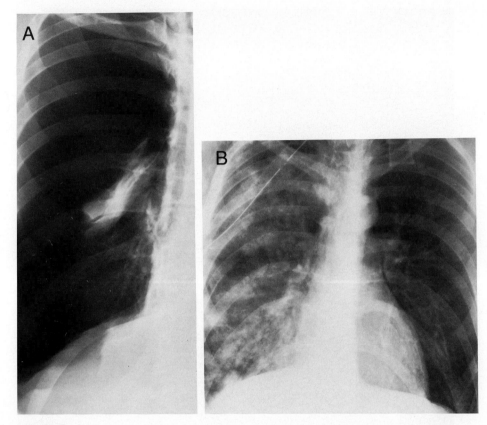

FIG 15–5
A, This large right pneumothorax has caused near-complete collapse of the right lung.
B, Following treatment of the pneumothorax with a thoracostomy tube, the patient developed diffuse confluent opacity throughout the right lung. This has been described as
reexpansion pulmonary edema.

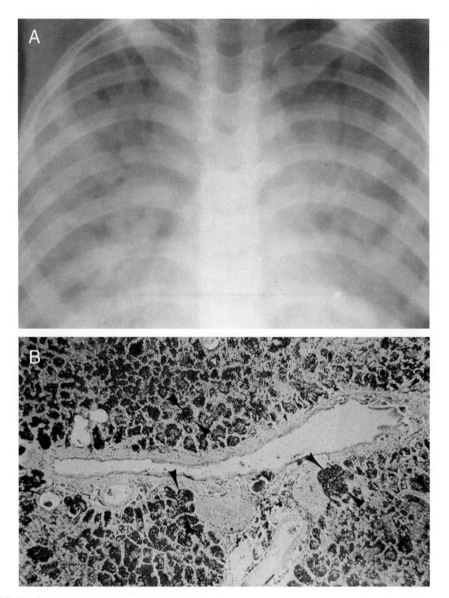

FIG 15–6
A, Pulmonary hemorrhage produces diffuse coalescent air-space opacities that may be indistinguishable from pulmonary edema. Note the air-bronchogram in the left upper lobe. This is a case of idiopathic pulmonary hemosiderosis. **B,** Histologic section from the same case shows diffuse pulmonary hemorrhage filling the air-spaces *(arrowheads)* and surrounding an open airway. (From Reed JC, Madewell JE: The air bronchogram in interstitial disease of the lungs. *Radiology* 1975;116:1–9. Used by permission.)

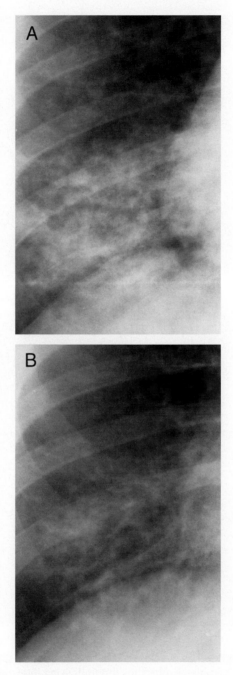

FIG 15–7
A, *Pneumocystis carinii* pneumonia produces a reticular pattern that may be obscured by extensive air-space opacities when the disease is severe. The initial film in this case shows confluent air-space opacities in the right lower lobe. **B,** Film taken 4 weeks later shows a residual reticular interstitial pattern, which may persist for months.

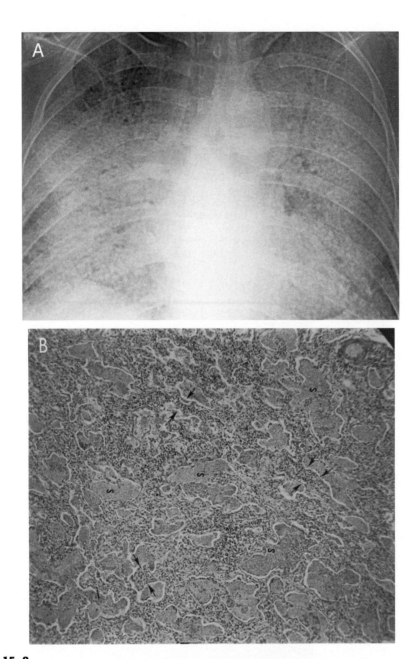

FIG 15–8
A, Another patient with PCP has developed diffuse confluent air-space opacification with air bronchograms. This completely obscures the underlying interstitial disease. **B,** Histologic section from another case of diffuse *Pneumocystis carinii* pneumonia reveals filling of alveolar spaces *(s)* and cellular infiltration of alveolar walls *(arrows)*. (**B** only, From Reed JC, Madewell JE: The air bronchogram in interstitial disease of the lungs. *Radiology* 1975; 116: 1–9. Used by permission.)

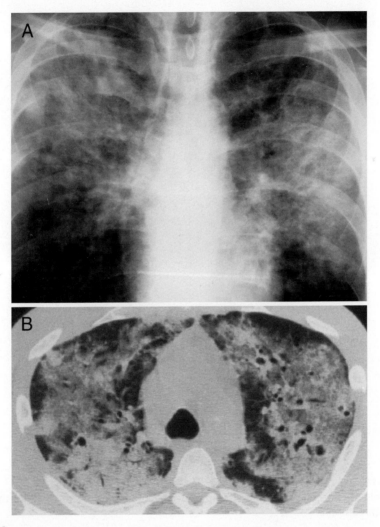

FIG 15–9
A, Prophylactic treatment of patients with AIDS for PCP may cause an atypical upper lobe distribution of the infection. In this case there are confluent opacities in both upper lobes with sparing of the bases. **B,** High-resolution CT section at level of carina shows some consolidation of the posterior segment of the right upper lobes, but extensive ground-glass opacity in both upper lobes. Also note the scattered cystic lesions (see Chapter 24), which are a common complication of PCP in patients with AIDS.

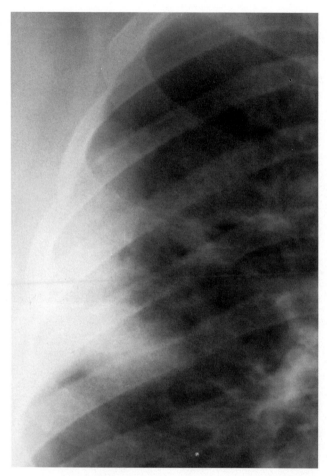

FIG 15–10
Bronchioloalveolar cell carcinoma often produces confluent air-space opacities that resemble pneumonia.

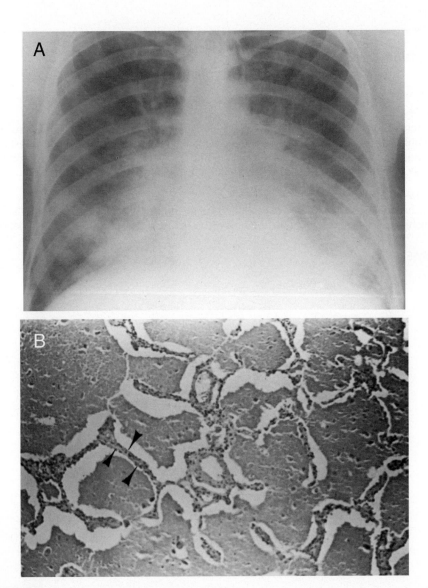

FIG 15–11
A, Diffuse bibasilar confluent opacities are silhouetting the heart. The opacities fade into the more normal-appearing aerated lung with a fine, poorly defined nodular appearance representing acinar opacities. This radiologic appearance is similar to pulmonary edema, hemorrhage, and diffuse pneumonia, but this patient's opacities were chronic, and biopsy revealed pulmonary alveolar proteinosis. **B,** This histologic section is from another case. Pulmonary alveolar proteinosis fills alveolar spaces. In contrast to most diffuse pulmonary diseases, there may be no significant reaction in the alveolar walls *(arrowheads)*. (**B** only, from Reed JC: Pathologic correlations of the air bronchogram: a reliable sign in chest radiology. *CRC Crit Rev Diag Imaging* 1977; 10:235-255. Used by permission. Copyright CRC Press, Boca Raton, Florida.)

ANSWER GUIDE

LEGENDS FOR INTRODUCTORY FIGURES

FIG 15–1
Pulmonary alveolar edema typically causes bilateral symmetric, coalescent opacities with a perihilar distribution. All of the radiologic signs of air-space disease listed in question 1 are present. Fine reticular opacities, which would indicate interstitial edema, are not visible because they are obscured by the confluent alveolar edema.

FIG 15–2
Bronchopneumonia has caused consolidation of the entire right lung. Note the air-filled branching bronchial tree. Air bronchograms are a reliable sign of pulmonary consolidation.

ANSWERS

1, a, b, c, e; 2, a; 3, c.

CHAPTER 16

Multifocal III-Defined Opacities

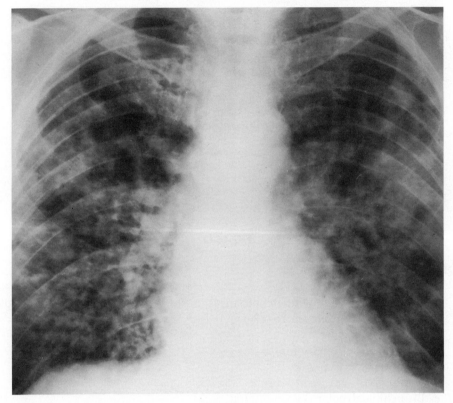

FIG 16–1

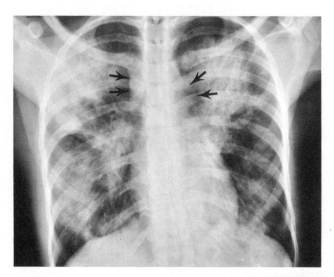

FIG 16–2

QUESTIONS

1. Which one of the following neoplasms is most likely to produce the radiologic appearance seen in Figure 16–1?
   a. Multiple myeloma.
   b. Squamous cell carcinoma.
   c. Melanoma.
   d. Seminoma.
   e. Bronchioloalveolar cell carcinoma.
2. Referring to Figure 16–2, the combination of hilar adenopathy and multifocal ill-defined opacities is most consistent with which one of the following?
   a. Wegener's granulomatosis.
   b. Sarcoidosis.
   c. Farmer's lung.
   d. Eosinophilic granuloma.
   e. Choriocarcinoma.
3. The presence of an air bronchogram throughout a large irregular opacity is inconsistent with which one of the following diagnoses?
   a. Silicosis.
   b. Bronchioloalveolar cell carcinoma.
   c. Lymphoma.
   d. Pseudolymphoma.
   e. Sarcoidosis.

CHART 16–1.
Multifocal Ill-defined Opacities

I. Inflammatory
   A. Bronchopneumonia[131] *(Staphylococcus,*[196] *Streptococcus, Pseudomonas, Legionella,*[517] *Klebsiella, Escherichia coli,* other gram-negative bacteria, *Nocardia*[26,155,260]
   B. Fungal pneumonia (histoplasmosis,[104] blastomycosis,[474] candidiases,[66] actinomycosis,[23,102] coccidioidomycosis, aspergillosis,[51,608] cryptococcosis[252,315,521] mucormycosis,[32] sporotrichosis[100]
   C. Tuberculosis[43,215,412,656]
   D. Sarcoidosis[484]
   E. Eosinophilic granuloma[260] (Langerhans cell histiocytosis[406])
   F. Bronchiolitis obliterans with organizing pneumonia (BOOP)[106,397]
   G. Eosinophilic pneumonitis[95,192,365] (idiopathic and secondary to parasites[370])
   H. Viral[403,615] and mycoplasma pneumonias[183,279]
   I. Rocky Mountain spotted fever[351,370,385]
   J. *Pneumocystis carinii* pneumonia[548]
   K. Paragonimiasis[445]
   L. Q fever[407]
   M. Atypical mycobacteria in AIDS patients[384]
II. Vascular
   A. Thromboemboli[260]
   B. Septic emboli[241]
   C. Vasculitis (Wegener's granulomatosis[342] and variants, including lymphomatoid granulomatosis[363,364,366])
   D. Infectious vasculitis (mucormycosis, aspergillosis, Rocky Mountain spotted fever)
   E. Goodpasture's syndrome[266]
   F. Scleroderma[15]
III. Neoplastic
   A. Bronchioloalveolar cell carcinoma[6,47,411,481]
   B. Lymphoma (Hodgkin's and non-Hodgkin's)[24,502]
   C. Metastasis (vascular tumors, malignant hemangiomas, choriocarcinoma)[361]
   D. Kaposi's sarcoma in AIDS patients[234,434,566]
   E. Waldenström's macroglobulinemia[481]
   F. Angioblastic lymphadenopathy[314]
   G. Mycosis fungoides[292]
   H. Amyloid tumors[271,599]
   I. Post-transplant lymphoproliferative disorder[129]
IV. Idiopathic
   A. Lymphocytic interstitial pneumonia[159]
   B. Desquamative interstitial pneumonia[78,332]
   C. Usual interstitial pneumonia[193]
V. Inhalational
   A. Allergic alveolitis[456,589,592]
   B. Silicosis
VI. Other
   A. Drug reactions[61,260,451,460,518]
   B. Radiation reactions[512]
   C. Metastatic pulmonary calcification (secondary to hypercalcemia)[251]

DISCUSSION

Multifocal ill-defined opacities result from a great variety of diffuse pulmonary diseases. This pattern is sometimes referred to as a patchy alveolar pattern, but it should be contrasted with the bilaterally symmetric diffuse coalescing opacities described as the classic appearance of air-space disease in Chapter 15. Many of the entities that cause multifocal ill-defined opacities do result in air-space filling,[371] but they also may involve the bronchovascular and septal interstitium. Acute diseases may present as patchy, scattered opacities and progress to complete diffuse air-space consolidation. Some of the additional signs of air-space disease are also encountered in this pattern, including air bronchograms, air alveolograms, and a tendency to be labile. Because many of the entities considered in the differential are in fact primarily interstitial diseases, complete examination of the film may reveal an underlying fine nodular or reticular pattern. Distinction of this multifocal pattern from the fine nodular pattern may also become somewhat of a problem, because the definition of the opacities is one of the primary distinguishing characteristics of the two patterns. The description for miliary nodules usually requires that the opacities be sharply defined, in contrast to the less-defined opacities currently under consideration. Also, most entities considered in this differential more typically produce opacities in the range of 1 to 2 or even 3 cm in diameter, in contrast to the fine nodular pattern, in which the opacities tend to be less than 5 mm in diameter. Additionally, this pattern may result from diseases that cause multiple larger nodules and masses. Some tumors may be locally invasive and appear ill-defined because of their growth pattern, whereas others may develop complications such as hemorrhage. Since the differential for multifocal ill-defined opacities is lengthy, its identification obligates the radiologist to review available serial films, carefully evaluate the clinical background of the patient, and recommend additional procedures. When the disease is minimal or the pattern cannot be characterized from the plain film, HRCT (Fig 16–3) may define the pattern, reveal the distribution of the disease and sometimes suggest a specific diagnosis.

Inflammatory Diseases

BACTERIAL BRONCHOPNEUMONIA

The characteristic pattern of a bronchopneumonia is that of lobular consolidations (Fig 16–4). Since this type of infection spreads via the tracheobronchial tree, it almost always produces a multilobular pattern. These lobular opacities[262] tend to be ill-defined because the fluid and inflammatory exudate that produce the opacities spread through the interstitial planes in addition to spilling into the alveolar spaces.[260] In some cases, the lobular pattern may have sharply defined borders where the exudate abuts an interlobular septum. The size of the radiologic opacities depends on the number of contiguous lobules involved. Intervening normal lobules lead to a very heterogeneous appearance, which Heitzman described as a "patchwork quilt." If this pattern of multifocal opacities progresses, the consolidations will begin to coalesce and form a pattern of diffuse air-space consolidation that may be indistinguishable from the pattern commonly associated with alveolar edema.

Knowing the pathogenesis of bronchopneumonia is important for understanding the above pattern. In bronchopneumonia, the primary sites of injury are the terminal and respiratory bronchioles. The disease starts as an acute bronchitis and bronchiolitis. The large bronchi undergo epithelial destruction and infiltration of their walls by polymorphonuclear leukocytes. Epithelial destruction results in ulcerations that are covered with a fibrinopurulent membrane and which contain large quantities of multiplying organisms. With the more aggressive organisms such as *Staphylococcus aureus* and *Pseudomonas,* a necrotic bronchitis and bronchiolitis lead to thrombosis of lobular branches of the small pulmonary arteries. When this becomes extensive, the multifocal opacities may begin to cavitate (see Chapter 24). As the inflammatory reaction spreads through the walls of the bronchioles to involve the alveolar walls, there is an exudation of fluid and inflammatory cells into the acinus. This results in the pattern of multifocal lobular consolidations described in the preceding paragraph. Thus, bronchopneumonia (lobular pneumonia) is in fact a combination of interstitial and alveolar disease. The injury starts in the airways, involves the bronchovascular bundle, and finally spills into the alveoli, which in later stages may contain edema fluid, blood, polymorphonuclear leukocytes, hyaline membranes, and organisms.

This description suggests that the radiologic pattern of bronchopneumonia depends on the virulence of the organism and the host's defenses. A mild bronchopneumonia in a noncompromised host may lead only to peribronchial inflammatory infiltration with the radiologic appearance of peribronchial thickening and increased markings. Itoh and colleagues[293] demonstrated that this peribronchial infiltrate may account for the radiologic appearance of diffuse, small (5 mm), fluffy, or ill-defined nodules that are very similar to the pattern of acinar consolidation. As indicated earlier, these nodules differ from the expected appearance of miliary nodules mainly in their lack of definition, or fluffy borders. In most cases of bronchopneumonia, this small nodular pattern is transient and rapidly replaced by the more characteristic lobular pattern, with opacities measuring 1 to 2 cm in diameter. As noted in Chapter 15, patients with bronchopneumonia occasionally have only one lobe predominantly involved, but there are almost always other areas of involvement. An unusually virulent organism or failure of the patient's immune response will lead to rapid enlargement of the multifocal opacities and finally to diffuse air-space consolidations. This has been observed in patients infected by common organisms[452] and those infected with unusual organisms, including those with legionnaires' and Pittsburgh agent pneumonias.[324,461]

VIRAL PNEUMONIA

The spread of viral infections in the respiratory tract has many similarities to bacterial bronchopneumonia. Most viruses produce their effect in the epithelial cells of the respiratory tract, leading to tracheitis, bronchitis, and bronchiolitis. There is also necrosis of much of the bronchial mucus gland epithelium. The bronchial and bronchiolar walls become very edematous, congested, and infiltrated with lymphocytes. The bronchial infiltrate may extend into the surrounding peribronchial tissues, which become swollen. This infiltrate spreads into the septal tissues of the lung, leading to a diffuse interstitial mononuclear cellular infiltrate. The changes in the airways may extend to the alveolar ducts, but most severe changes occur proximal to the terminal bronchioles. The adjacent alveolar cells, both type 1 and type 2, become swollen and detached. These surfaces then become covered with hyaline membranes. In fulminant cases, there are additional changes in the alveoli. The alveoli are filled with a mixture of blood, edema, fibrin, and macrophages. In the most severely affected areas, there is focal necrosis of the alveolar walls and thrombosis of the alveolar capillaries, leading to necrosis and hemorrhage.

As in bronchopneumonia, the radiologic pattern of a viral pneumonia depends on both the virulence of the organism and the host defenses.[57,58] The mildest cases of viral infection of the airways are confined to the upper airways and manifest no radiologic abnormality. The earliest radiologic abnormalities are the signs of bronchitis and bronchiolitis, which may include peribronchial thickening and signs of air trapping. When the infection spreads into the septal tissues, a reticular pattern with Kerley's lines, as described in Chapter 18, may result. The more serious cases lead to hemorrhagic edema and areas of air-space consolidation. These opacities may be small and appear as a fine nodular pattern similar to that described in Chapter 17, but the nodules tend to be less well defined than the classic miliary pattern. As the process spreads, areas of lobular consolidation develop, as in bacterial bronchopneumonia.[260] In the most severe cases, these areas of lobular consolidation may coalesce into an extensive diffuse consolidation resembling pulmonary edema. In contrast to bacterial pneumonias, viral infections do not result in cavitation. These more fulminating cases of viral pneumonia are rarely encountered in normal patients, but are seen in immunologically suppressed patients, including those receiving high-dose steroid therapy, tumor patients receiving chemotherapy, AIDS patients, organ transplant patients, and even pregnant women.

Confirming a diagnosis of viral pneumonia requires careful correlation with clinical and laboratory findings. In cases of *influenza viral pneumonia,* there are also typical influenza symptoms of fever, dry cough, headache, myalgia, and prostration. As the infection spreads to the lower respiratory tract, the patient notices an increased production of sputum that may be associated with dyspnea, pleuritic chest pain, or both. Physical examination reveals rales that may be accompanied by either diminished or harsh breath sounds. Because of the bronchial involvement, wheezes are occasionally noted. At this time, laboratory examination of the sputum and blood becomes paramount in order to rule out a superimposed bacterial bronchopneumonia. The organisms most likely to present a superimposed bacterial infection are pneumococci, staphylococci, streptococci, and *Haemophilus influenzae.* In this clinical setting, the development of a superimposed cavitary lesion virtually confirms a superimposed infection.

Varicella pneumonia characteristically occurs from 2 to 5 days after the onset of the typical rash. It is most commonly noted in infants, in pregnant women, and in adults with altered immunity. Approximately 10% of adult patients may have some degree of pulmonary involvement. In contrast to the situation in bacterial pneumonias, sputum examination shows a predominance of mononuclear cells and giant cells in which type A intranuclear inclusion bodies may be seen on Giemsa stain. As in the consideration of other viral pneumonias, the possibility of superimposed bacterial infection is best excluded by laboratory examination of sputum and blood. Since the viruses of herpes zoster and varicella are identical, patients with an atypical herpetic syndrome consisting of a rash related to a dermatome and dermatomic distribution of pain are also at an increased risk for development of this type of pneumonia.

Rubeola (measles) *pneumonia* may be more difficult to diagnose by clinical criteria, since the pneumonia occasionally precedes the development of the rash. As with other viral pneumonias, the clinical findings are nonspecific and consist of fever, cough, dyspnea, and minimal sputum production. Increasing sputum production requires exclusion of a superimposed bacterial pneumonia. Timing is important for evaluating a pneumonia associated with measles. The development of primary viral pneumonia in rubeola is synchronous with the first appearance of a rash, while secondary bacterial pneumonias are most likely to occur from 1 to 7 days after the onset of the rash. Bacterial infection is strongly suggested in the patient with a typical measles rash whose condition improves over a period of days before pneumonia develops.

A third type of pneumonia associated with measles pneumonia is histologically referred to as *giant cell pneumonia*. This may follow overt measles in otherwise normal, healthy children, but children with altered immunology may develop subacute or chronic, but often fatal, pneumonias. Pathologically, giant cell pneumonia is characterized by an interstitial mononuclear infiltrate with giant cells containing intranuclear and intracytoplasmic inclusions.

Other viruses, such as cytomegalic inclusion virus,[1] have few distinguishing clinical features. They do, however, have a radiologic presentation suggestive of bronchopneumonia, which is frequently fatal in patients who are immunosuppressed. Histologically, the lung reveals a diffuse mononuclear interstitial pneumonia accompanied by considerable edema in the alveolar walls that may even spill into the alveolar spaces. In addition, the alveolar cells have characteristic intranuclear and intracytoplasmic occlusions. The radiologic opacities are the result of cellular infiltrates in the interstitium, as well as intra-alveolar hemorrhage and edema. Other viruses, including the coxsackieviruses, parainfluenza viruses, adenoviruses, and respiratory syncytial viruses, may result in disseminated multifocal opacities. When the course of the viral infection is mild, confirmation is rarely obtained during the acute phase of the disease, but may be made by viral culture or acute and convalescent serologic studies.

GRANULOMATOUS INFECTIONS

Of the granulomatous infections most likely to produce ill-defined multifocal opacities of varying sizes, histoplasmosis[104] is probably the best known (Fig 16–5). This form of histoplasmosis is usually seen after a massive exposure to *Histoplasma capsulatum*. Since the organism is a soil contaminant found primarily in the Mississippi and Ohio River valleys, the disease should be suspected when this pattern is seen in acutely ill patients from these endemic areas. A history of intense exposure to contaminated soil is frequently obtained and helps confirm the diagnosis. A marked rise in serologic titers is also confirmatory. The radiologic course is characterized by gradual healing of the process, involving contraction of the opacities, resolution of a large number of opacities, and the development of a pattern of scattered, more circumscribed nodules. This may precede the characteristic "snowstorm" appearance of multiple calcifications that develops as a late stage of histoplasmosis.

Blastomycosis[474] and coccidioidomycosis[392] are the two other fungal infections likely to result in this pattern. These fungi are also soil contaminants with a well-defined geographic distribution. Coccidioidomycosis is primarily confined to the desert southwest of the United States, although the fungus may be found as a contaminant of materials such as cotton or wool transported from this area. The geographic distribution of blastomycosis is less distinct than that of either histoplasmosis or coccidioidomycosis, but it is generally confined to the eastern United States, with numerous cases reported from Tennessee and North Carolina. Other fungal diseases, such as cryptococcosis, aspergillosis, and mucormycosis, may produce this pattern but are rarely encountered in immunologically normal patients (Fig 16–6, A–D). These are generally regarded as opportunistic infections and require biopsy confirmation by either transbronchial or open lung biopsy. In the case of mucormycosis and aspergillosis, the densities may actually represent infarction, since the fungus tends to invade the pulmonary vessels.

Tuberculosis[412] less commonly produces multifocal ill-defined opacities but should be strongly considered in the case of an apical cavity followed by the development of this pattern. In such an instance, the opacities most probably are the result of bronchogenic dissemination of the organisms. Usually the diagnosis is easily confirmed by sputum stains for acid-fast bacilli, or by cultures.

Nocardia[26,155,232,522] is another opportunistic organism that may produce multiple, ill-defined opacities. It is probably better known for producing discrete nodules that cavitate, but these nodules are frequently preceded by the less well-defined opacities. As with aspergillosis and mucormycosis, nocardiosis is rarely encountered in the immunologically normal patient but should be strongly suspected in immunocompromised patients. The diagnosis is usually confirmed by either transbronchial or open biopsy.

SARCOIDOSIS

Many authors have emphasized that patients with histologically documented sarcoidosis[260,481,484] may have a radiologic pattern of bilateral nodular foci with ill-defined borders, sometimes becoming confluent and showing air bronchograms (see Fig 16–2). The clinical manifestation of sarcoidosis is in striking contrast to that of the other inflammatory conditions. Patients with sarcoidosis are afebrile and often virtually asymptomatic, although they may complain of mild dyspnea. This marked disparity of the radiologic and clinical findings virtually eliminates all of the entities considered so far in this chapter. When the pattern of multifocal ill-defined opacities is combined with bilaterally symmetric hilar adenopathy and the anomalous clinical presentation of the disease, the diagnosis becomes nearly certain. In this diffuse pulmonary disease, confirmation of the diagnosis is easily obtained by transbronchial biopsy.

The pathologic explanations for this presentation of sarcoidosis have stimulated considerable discussion in the radiologic literature. Some authors describe this pattern as nodular sarcoidosis, while others consider it an alveolar sarcoidosis. The radiologic features supporting the appearance of alveolar sarcoidosis are primarily those of the ill-defined borders and confluent opacities that may contain air bronchograms. It should be pointed out that sarcoidosis rarely causes bilaterally symmetric confluent opacities with a bilateral perihilar (butterfly) distribution, as seen in acute alveolar edema, pulmonary hemorrhage, or alveolar proteinosis. Consequently, sarcoidosis is not a serious consideration in the differential of the pattern considered in Chapter 15. Since pulmonary sarcoidosis is, by histologic definition, a reaction in the interstitium characterized by noncaseating granulomas of unknown origin, there is an apparent conflict between the histologic and radiologic descriptions. In view of the histologic description, sarcoidosis is unlikely to produce confluent opacities with air bronchograms. Such a description, in fact, might suggest intra-alveolar granulomas; however, to date, this concept has not been well documented. Heitzman[260] reported histologic evidence that patients with this "alveolar pattern" may have massive accumulations of interstitial granulomas, which by compression of air-spaces could mimic an alveolar filling process. This would essentially be a form of compressive atelectasis. The histologic observation of a massive accumulation of interstitial granulomas can be easily confirmed by examination of a number of cases with this radiologic pattern (Fig 16–7, A). Therefore, this mechanism almost certainly accounts for some cases with this pattern.

One feature of the alveolar form of sarcoidosis that is not readily explained by the foregoing observations is the very labile character of the infiltrations. Frequently, the opacities accumulate and disappear dramatically, either spontaneously or in response to steroid treatment. It seems unlikely that a massive accumulation of well-organized granulomas could resolve in a matter of days or even a few weeks. Another explanation for this radiologic pattern of fluffy opacities with ill-defined borders and air bronchograms is based on the frequent presence of peribronchial granulomas that cause bronchial obstructions (Fig 16–7, B). Peribronchial granulomas are frequently observed at bronchoscopy and HRCT.[355] Distal to these bronchial obstructions there is, in fact, alveolar filling, not by sarcoid granulomas but by macrophages and proteinaceous material (Fig 16–7, C). Histologically, this pattern is basically an obstructive pneumonia. The clinical variability of alveolar sarcoidosis is probably accounted for by these two major histologic explanations. For instance, the confluent heavy accumulation of sarcoid granulomas with resultant compressive atelectasis would not be expected to resolve in a short time, while the smaller accumulations of granulomas in the peribronchial spaces with distal obstruction could account for cases that follow a much more labile course and respond dramatically to steroid therapy. It should be emphasized that obstructive pneumonia in sarcoidosis is secondary to the obstruction of small distal bronchi and bronchioles. It is very rare for sarcoid granulomas to obstruct large bronchi and produce lobar atelectasis.

EOSINOPHILIC GRANULOMA

Eosinophilic granuloma (Langerhans' cell histiocytosis) is another inflammatory condition of undetermined cause that may produce a pattern of multifocal ill-defined opacities.[260] The nodular phase of the disease is generally believed to represent the earlier radiologic findings, which may precede the development of a reticular pattern and even end with a honeycomb lung. There is typically an upper lobe predominance in both the nodular and reticular phases of the disease. High-resolution CT may confirm this upper lobe distribution and is very sensitive for the detection of small, peripheral cystic spaces[45,419] (Fig 16–8, A–C). Like sarcoidosis, eosinophilic granuloma is an afebrile illness with much milder symptoms than all of the infectious diseases hitherto considered. Pathologically, the lesions consist of a granulomatous infiltrate with histiocytes, eosinophils, plasma cells, lymphocytes, and Langerhans' cells. The earlier nodular lesions are more histologically characteristic than the late honeycomb changes, which basically consist of fibrous replacement of the earlier inflammatory infiltrates. This late appearance may be very similar to that of sarcoidosis. The radiologic identification of associated hilar or paratracheal adenopathy favors the diagnosis of sarcoidosis over eosinophilic granuloma. Eosinophilic granuloma is a biopsy diagnosis.

BRONCHIOLITIS OBLITERANS WITH ORGANIZING PNEUMONIA

Bronchiolitis obliterans with organizing pneumonia (BOOP)[106,397,429] or cryptogenic organizing pneumonia,[347] is assumed to be a subacute or chronic inflammatory process involving the small airways and alveoli. The radiologic presentation resembles that of bronchopneumonia, with multifocal, patchy air-space consolidations. Patients with the disease are often treated with antibiotics, on the basis of a presumed diagnosis of pneumonia, but the process fails to clear. Corticosteroid therapy has been reported to produce clearing of the radiologic abnormalities. However, there is a high relapse rate following steroid withdrawal. The histologic description of bronchiolitis obliterans is similar to that expected with Swyer-James syndrome, but there is much more extensive alveolar exudate and fibrosis that may resemble or overlap the changes of usual interstitial pneumonia (UIP). According to Müller et al., BOOP can be distinguished from UIP. BOOP has multifocal air-space opacities with normal lung volume, while UIP has irregular linear and nodular opacities with reduced lung volume.[429]

EOSINOPHILIC PNEUMONIAS

Pneumonias associated with eosinophilia,[95,192,363] either peripheral eosinophilia or eosinophilic infiltrates of the lung, constitute a category of diseases that may be regarded as either inflammatory or collagen-vascular. Radiologically, these infiltrates appear as patchy areas of air-space consolidation that tend to be in the periphery of the lung (Fig 16–9). When these infiltrates become extensive, the radiologic picture has been compared with a photonegative picture of pulmonary edema, because of the striking peripheral distribution of the opacities. These opacities have very ill-defined borders, tend to be coalescent, and frequently have air bronchogram effects.

There are two important groups of eosinophilic pneumonias. The first group consists of the idiopathic varieties of eosinophilic pneumonia, generally divided into those that are associated with peripheral eosinophilia and are therefore referred to as Löffler's syndrome, and those that comprise primarily eosinophilic infiltrates in the lungs, without peripheral eosinophilia, and are referred to as chronic eosinophilic pneumonia. Besides tending to be peripheral, the infiltrates have the additional characteristic of being recurrent and are frequently described as fleeting.

The second group of pulmonary infiltrates associated with eosinophilia includes those with a known etiologic agent.[370] A variety of parasitic conditions are associated with pulmonary infiltration and are likewise well known for the association of eosinophilia. These include ascariasis, *Strongyloides* infection, hookworm disease (ancylostomiasis), *Dirofilaria immitis* and *Toxocara canis* infections (visceral larva migrans), schistosomiasis, paragonimiasis, and, occasionally, amebiasis.

Correlation of the clinical, laboratory, and radiologic findings often makes a precise diagnosis of parasitic disease a straightforward matter. For example, *Toxocara canis* infection results from infestation by the larva of the dog or cat roundworm and has a worldwide distribution. The disease is most commonly encountered in children. The symptoms are nonspecific, but there is usually the physical finding of hepatosplenomegaly. There is also marked leukocytosis. In addition, liver biopsy usually reveals eosinophilic granulomas containing the larvae. The diagnosis of ascariasis is similarly made by laboratory identification of the organism. Larvae may be detected in either sputum or gastric aspirates, while the adult forms of ova may be found in stool. The disease is usually associated with a marked leukocytosis and eosinophilia. As mentioned earlier, the roentgenographic appearance is that of nonspecific, multifocal areas of homogeneous consolidation that are frequently transient and therefore virtually identical to the opacities described as Löffler's syndrome.[186] Strongyloidiasis, like ascariasis, produces mild clinical symptoms at the same time that the roentgenogram demonstrates peripheral ill-defined areas of homogeneous consolidation. The diagnosis is made by finding larva in the sputum or in the stool. Exceptions to this clinical course occur in the compromised host. A fatal form of strongyloidiasis has been reported in patients who are immunologically compromised, particularly with corticosteroid drugs.

Amebiasis[370] is rather different from the parasitic diseases described above in both its clinical and radiologic presentations. Patients with amebiasis frequently have symptoms of amebic dysentery and complain of right-sided abdominal pain, which is related to the high incidence of liver involvement. There is often elevation of the right hemidiaphragm because of liver involvement and, as in other cases of subphrenic abscess, there is frequently right-sided pleural effusion. Furthermore, the areas of homogeneous consolidation are not evenly distributed throughout the periphery of the lung, as in other cases of eosinophilic infiltration, but tend to be in the bases of the lungs, particularly in the right lower lobe and right middle lobe. Because the roentgenologic opacities correspond to areas of abscess formation, these opacities will occasionally cavitate.

Vascular Diseases

Thromboemboli[260] probably constitute one of the more common causes of multiple ill-defined opacities. These opacities tend to be in the bases of the lungs, are homogeneous, and frequently have either a lobular or a segmental distribution. This segmental distribution has been particularly emphasized by Heitzman et al.[262] Recall that segmental arteries follow the segmental bronchi and that occlusion of a segmental artery therefore results in edema and hemorrhage in the lobule or segment supplied by that vessel. It must be emphasized that not all radiologic opacities resulting from thromboemboli are necessarily areas of infarction. At the time of the acute process, it is usually impossible for the radiologist to distinguish edema and hemorrhage due to ischemia from areas of true infarction. Infarction is the ischemic death of tissue. The radiologist can most accurately diagnose infarction when serial films demonstrate that an area of ill-defined opacities has decreased in size, leaving either a linear or a nodular scar, or when the area of opacities has subsequently cavitated. These opacities are ill defined because of the alveolar filling by the edema and hemorrhage, which spreads between contiguous alveoli.

Septic emboli[241] are another important cause of multifocal peripheral opacities. On occasion, septic emboli may completely mimic the roentgenologic appearance of venous thromboemboli. There is a significantly increased incidence of cavitation following septic embolization. Clinical correlation is essential in the diagnosis of septic embolization. In contrast to cases of venous thromboembolism, there should be a history of a significant febrile illness. Some of the infectious processes known to be associated with septic embolism include osteomyelitis, cellulitis, carbuncles, and right-sided endocarditis. Patients with right-sided endocarditis frequently have a history of drug abuse.

In addition to the embolic obstruction of vessels, inflammatory reactions around the vessels constitute another important category of diseases that may lead to multifocal, ill-defined opacities. Wegener's granulomatosis and its variants are probably the best-known sources of pulmonary vasculitis.[156,342,363,364,366] In such cases, clinical correlation is extremely important, since the classic form of the disease is associated with severe paranasal sinus and kidney involvement. A history of multifocal ill-defined opacities on the chest plain film, hemoptysis, and hematuria strongly suggests Wegener's granulomatosis or a variant. These entities frequently require careful histologic evaluation to differentiate them from other lesions that have been referred to as the pulmonary renal syndromes, including Goodpasture's syndrome and idiopathic pulmonary hemosiderosis. Many opacities appearing on the roentgenogram in Wegener's granulomatosis are areas of edema, hemorrhage, or even lung tissue necrosis (see Fig 16–1). Ischemic necrosis results in cavitary opacities in about 25% of patients with Wegener's granulomatosis.[177] These opacities are therefore more likely to be the result of the vasculitis with ischemia than to be true granulomas. Perivascular granulomas, in fact, may be very small and may contribute minimally to the radiologic opacities. Because of their similar radiologic presentations, there is a tendency for radiologists to combine the variants of Wegener's granulomatosis (limited Wegener's, bronchocentric, and lymphomatoid granulomatosis). Although this is generally appropriate, the entity of lymphomatoid granulomatosis may have a different prognosis, as suggested by Liebow.[364] Liebow described a group of patients who were initially diagnosed as having lymphomatoid granulomatosis and subsequently developed lymphoma. It should be emphasized that associated hilar adenopathy is atypical and unusual in patients with Wegener's granulomatosis. Minimal adenopathy has been shown in a small number of cases and probably represents reactive hyperplasia.[2] The presence of lymphadenopathy should probably be regarded as a warning to question the diagnosis and to suspect the possible development of lymphoma in patients with lymphomatoid granulomatosis.

A small group of acute pulmonary infections tends to invade the pulmonary arteries rather than produce bronchopneumonia. One of the most notorious of these is mucormycosis.[32] Mucormycosis invades the pulmonary vessels and results in distal infarction. The infection is rarely encountered except in the severely compromised host. The invasive form of aspergillosis[608] similarly produces large, multifocal areas of consolidation as a result of pulmonary ischemia. A less well-known cause of pulmonary vasculitis that may lead to the appearance of multiple areas of air-space consolidation, and even an appearance similar to that of pulmonary edema, is Rocky Mountain spotted fever.[351,385] This rickettsial infection results in a diffuse vasculitis. It is best diagnosed by the clinical findings of a rash and central nervous system findings. A history of tick bite and an increase in antibody titers strongly support the diagnosis.

Neoplasms

Neoplasms are not generally regarded as a common cause of multifocal, ill-defined opacities in the lung. However, there are a few neoplasms that do produce this pattern and are somewhat characteristic in their radiologic appearance when compared with other pulmonary tumors.

Bronchioloalveolar cell carcinoma[268,481,605] (Fig 16–10, *A*) is the only primary lung tumor likely to produce multifocal, ill-defined opacities. (Answer to question 1 is *e.*) Air bronchograms may even be seen with this pattern. The biologic behavior of this tumor is significantly different from that of all other primary lung tumors because it tends to spread along the alveolar walls while leaving them intact. At the same time the tumor spreads along the walls, there is a tendency for it to produce significant amounts of mucus, which may contribute to the ill-defined opacities. The preservation of the underlying lung architecture permits the tumor to spread around open bronchi and gives rise to air bronchograms. It must be emphasized that air bronchograms are not readily apparent in all cases of bronchioloalveolar cell carcinoma and that the absence of this sign is not sufficient evidence for excluding the diagnosis. In fact, air bronchograms are frequently enhanced by tomographic sections or CT scanning of the opacity. Because this tumor spreads in the air-spaces, it is frequently postulated that the multifocal appearance of the tumor is the result of bronchogenic dissemination. Histologic sections, such as that shown in Figure 16–10, *B*, tend to support this concept of bronchioloalveolar cell carcinoma.

Lymphoma[481,484,502] is another tumor that may involve multiple areas of the lung and produce the radiologic appearance of ill-defined opacities sometimes accompanied by air bronchograms (Fig 16–11, *A* and *B*). When lymphoma involves the lung parenchyma, either primarily or secondarily, it spreads via the perivascular and peribronchial tissues and even by way of the interlobular septa. Histologically its spread is considered to be an interstitial process. However, it is also well known that lymphomatous involvement of the lung may present with pneumonic opacities that have ill-defined borders, and even with air bronchograms.[357] This type of lymphoma has occasionally been described as alveolar lymphoma. There are at least three feasible explanations for this radiographic appearance of lymphoma: (1) the massive accumulation of tumor cells may destroy the alveolar walls and break into the alveolar spaces, (2) there may essentially be a compressive atelectasis or collapse of the alveolar spaces by the massive accumulation of lymphoma cells in the interstitium, and (3) because of the peribronchial infiltration, there may be an obstructive pneumonitis with secondary filling of the distal air spaces by fluid and inflammatory cells rather than lymphoma cells.

The histologic appearance of the periphery of such a lesion emphasizes the spread through the lung parenchyma via the interlobular septa and peribronchial and perivascular tissues (Fig 16–12, *A*). Thus, the second hypothesis given above is preferable. Histologic sections showing bronchial narrowing by lymphoma cells (Fig 16–12, *B*) provide strong evidence that obstructive pneumonia could also be an important mechanism for the "alveolar" infiltrates in a disease that is, by histologic definition, supposed to be interstitial. It should be emphasized that the histologic entity of pseudolymphoma may present radiologically with multifocal, ill-defined opacities identical to those seen in lymphoma. Other lymphoid disorders of the lung,[159] including Waldenström's macroglobulinemia[481] and angioblastic lymphadenopathy,[314] may result in these patterns.

The occurrence of metastases as multifocal opacities with ill-defined borders is uncommon. It has been suggested in numerous discussions that choriocarcinoma may result in bleeding around the periphery of the tumor, giving the radiologic appearance of ill-defined opacities. However, Libshitz et al.[361] presented over 100 cases showing that this occurrence is exceptional. Superimposition of many nodules probably accounts for the majority of cases in which metastatic nodules appear to have ill-defined borders.

Idiopathic Interstitial Diseases

Two idiopathic conditions that are well known for producing multifocal areas of consolidation are lymphocytic interstitial pneumonia (LIP)[159] and desquamative interstitial pneumonia (DIP).[78, 332] These entities are virtually impossible to diagnosis by clinical and radiologic criteria, instead requiring biopsy diagnosis. Desquamative interstitial pneumonitis produces a true alveolar consolidation because of the large number of polygonal cells that have presumably exfoliated into the alveolar spaces. Like the malignant lymphoid conditions described above, LIP is an interstitial condition that occasionally mimics the appearance of an alveolar process. The histologic appearances of LIP and pseudolymphoma are very similar. In fact, distinction of these entities is based primarily on the gross appearance of the lesion. The more localized forms are referred to as pseudolymphoma, while the more diffuse forms are considered to represent LIP. The association of Sjögren's syndrome, a chronic autoimmune disease, with keratoconjunctivitis sicca, xerostomia, and connective tissue disease is suggestive of LIP.

Usual interstitial pneumonia (fibrosing alveolitis)[193] may present with multifocal opacities that appear to correspond to patches of alveolar fluid. HRCT has shown a peripheral basilar distribution of patchy consolidation and ground-glass opacity. These findings usually precede the development of reticulonodular opacities and are considered to indicate an active phase of alveolitis that may be reversible.[428]

Inhalational Diseases

The inhalational diseases most frequently associated with the pattern of multifocal, ill-defined opacities are those referred to as allergic alveolitis or hypersensitivity pneumonitis.[456,589,592] The prototype for allergic alveolitis is farmer's lung. This is an allergic reaction at the alveolar capillary wall level to the mold that grows in hay. Initially it is an acute reaction consisting of edema with an inflammatory infiltrate in the interstitium. This inflammatory infiltrate may gradually be replaced by a granulomatous reaction with some histologic similarities to sarcoid granulomas. The multiple confluent opacities with air bronchograms tend to represent the acute phase of the disease, while a nodular or even a reticular pattern may be seen in the later stages. Confirmation of the diagnosis is best obtained by establishing a history of exposure followed by skin testing and serologic studies. A large variety of fungal agents in a number of specific environments have been identified as causing similar reactions.

Silicosis is another inhalational disease that frequently results in multiple opacities (Fig 16–13). The border characteristics of these opacities are quite different from those considered in the remainder of this discussion. These borders tend to be more irregular rather than truly ill-defined. The irregularities are the result of strands of fibrotic reaction around the conglomerate masses (Fig 16–14). In addition, the opacities tend to be much more homogeneous, since they represent large masses of fibrotic reaction. There should be no normal intervening alveoli to give a soft heterogeneous appearance. Furthermore, there should be no evidence of air bronchogram effects. (Answer to question 3 is *a*.) These opacities tend to be in the periphery of the lung; however, they are frequently not pleural-based but appear to parallel the chest wall. A history of exposure in mining or sandblasting is usually confirmatory. Comparison with old films is essential to eliminate the possibility of a new superimposed process.

Drug Reactions

Adverse drug reactions,[15,260] such as "chemotherapy lung"[573] constitute another group of pulmonary reactions that may result in multifocal pulmonary opacities. Heitzman[260] states that the most common manifestation of pulmonary drug reaction is an acute alveolar pattern that is often perihilar in distribution and therefore mimics the appearance seen in pulmonary edema of diffuse coalescing disease. In many cases, the patterns are very similar to those encountered in diffuse bronchopneumonia, viral pneumonia, adult respiratory distress syndrome, and even radiation reactions. This leads to a serious diagnostic dilemma in the immunocompromised patient, particularly following treatment for malignant tumor. A number of the examples of acute pulmonary drug reactions cited by Heitzmann[260] did present with patterns that were considerably more patchy or multifocal than the homogeneous appearance expected with pulmonary edema. These opacities frequently change over a relatively short period, particularly in response to steroid therapy, indicating that a significant component of the disease may be alveolar. Pathologic correlations reveal a very nonspecific pneumonitis consisting of an alveolar exudate with an extensive underlying interstitial inflammatory infiltrate. In the acute phases, the alveoli may be filled with proteinaceous fluid, fibrin, and hyaline membranes. The interstitial infiltrate is mainly a round cell infiltrate. As the alveolar component resolves, either in response to discontinuation of the drug or steroid therapy, a reticular pattern may become evident. This is similar to the fine reticular pattern considered in Chapter 18, and may even include the presence of Kerley's B lines. Occasionally these cases progress to a chronic, coarse interstitial pattern resembling the changes seen in honeycomb lung. The exact pathologic mechanism for these drug reactions has been extensively debated. There is considerable clinical and experimental evidence that some drug reactions may represent true allergic responses, while others must be regarded as idiosyncratic.

The diagnosis of drug reaction is best suggested by a history of medication with any of the drugs known to produce pulmonary reactions.[511] In patients who are undergoing chemotherapy for cancer, the differential includes (1) opportunistic infection, (2) diffuse hemorrhage, (3) drug reaction, and (4) spread of the primary tumor.

AIDS-Related Diseases

Although *Pneumocystis carinii* pneumonia is the most common pulmonary infection in patients infected with HIV, it tends to produce a pattern of more uniform reticular or confluent opacities. The appearance of scattered or patchy opacities requires consideration of a greater variety of infections and neoplasms, including bacterial, fungal, and mycobacterial pneumonias, lymphoma, and Kaposi's sarcoma.[558]

Bacterial pneumonias produce the same patterns in patients with HIV infection and in the general population.[112] They occur during the early stages of HIV while immune impairment is mild, with CD4 cell counts between 200 and 500 cells/μl.[387] *Streptococcus pneumoniae* and *Haemophilus influenzae* are the most common organisms, but more virulent organisms such as Staphylococcus should be suspected when the pneumonias are complicated by cavitation.

Tuberculosis in patients with early HIV infection (CD4 counts between 200 and 500) produces the same patterns seen in patients with normal immunity. Postprimary tuberculosis most often causes apical disease with cavitation. Bronchogenic dissemination of organisms from an apical cavity may lead to multifocal opacities that resemble bacterial bronchopneumonia. Following development of AIDS after the CD4 count is below 200, patients are at increased risk for miliary tuberculosis with a fine nodular pattern, as seen in Chapter 17. Additionally, in patients with more severe immune impairment, tuberculosis is likely to cause combinations of segmental, lobar, or multifocal air-space opacities with hilar or mediastinal adenopathy resembling primary infection.[223] Fungal infections are less frequent, but cryptococcosis, histoplasmosis, and coccidioidomycosis have all been reported to produce patterns that are similar to tuberculosis in patients with AIDS.[576]

Mycobacterium avium-intracellulare (MAI) infection most frequently causes a diffuse bilateral reticulonodular pattern in patients with AIDS. In contrast, the patients with normal immunity who are at greatest risk for MAI infection are patients with chronic pulmonary disease. In this latter group of patients, MAI may be radiographically indistinguishable from tuberculosis. The reticular pattern of MAI should be more coarse and disorganized than PCP, but when PCP becomes chronic, it may cause a similar appearance. When MAI causes air-space opacities, it differs from PCP. The air-space opacities of MAI are either segmental or multifocal, and the multifocal opacities are more likely to resemble poorly marginated masses. PCP causes more uniformly diffuse air-space disease. Cases with air-space opacities are also often associated with pleural effusions or adenopathy, which may also be seen in tuberculosis but which are not expected in PCP. Disseminated MAI is a terminal infection that occurs after the CD4 count has declined below 50 cell/μl.

Lymphoma and Kaposi's sarcoma may produce multiple poorly marginated masses and reticular opacities. Lymphoma in HIV-infected patients is usually non-Hodgkin's and differs from patients with normal immunity in that AIDS-related lymphomas are more often extranodal. Lymphoma is probably the most likely diagnosis of lobulated pulmonary masses in patients with AIDS. These masses often show a very aggressive growth pattern and may double in size in 4 to 6 weeks.

Kaposi's sarcoma (Fig 16–15) is the most common AIDS-related neoplasm, but it has decreased in frequency for unexplained reasons. It is a highly vascular tumor that involves any mucocutaneous surface and produces characteristic red plaques. It is most commonly a skin lesion, but it also involves the trachea, bronchi, and lungs. The radiographic appearance of pulmonary opacities may result from atelectasis, hemorrhage, or hemorrhagic masses. Multiple nodules or masses are the most common pattern. More confluent patchy air-space opacities may resemble PCP. Associated adenopathy or pleural effusions are reported to occur in 90% of patients with Kaposi's sarcoma and may help distinguish Kaposi's from PCP, but their occurrence would not permit exclusion of mycobacterial infections. Sequential thallium and gallium scanning has been advocated as a technique for distinguishing PCP, Kaposi's sarcoma, and lymphoma. PCP is thallium negative but gallium positive on 3-hour delayed images. Lymphomas are thallium and gallium positive, and Kaposi's sarcoma is thallium positive but gallium negative. Bronchoscopy may establish the diagnosis of Kaposi's sarcoma. Fine-needle aspiration biopsy has also been advocated for diagnosis of focal and multifocal lesions.[235,547] Lymphoma is an aggressive and often fatal neoplasm, in contrast with Kaposi's, which is an indolent, slow-growing tumor that is rarely fatal.

SUMMARY

1. Small, multifocal, ill-defined opacities are distinguished from miliary nodules by evaluation of their borders. Miliary nodules should be sharply defined.

2. Multifocal ill-defined opacities most commonly result from processes that involve both the interstitium and the air-spaces. Careful evaluation of the roentgenogram frequently reveals the classic signs for both components of the disease.

3. Bronchopneumonias typically present with this pattern.

4. Histoplasmosis is one of the most common fungi to produce the pattern.

5. Unusual pulmonary infections, including aspergillosis, mucormycosis, cryptococcosis, and nocardiosis, may lead to the pattern in the immunologically compromised patient.

6. Sarcoidosis may lead to this pattern when there are extensive accumulations of granulomas or when small granulomas occlude bronchioles with a resultant obstructive pneumonia.

7. Eosinophilic pneumonias should be suspected when the opacities are peripherally located and recurrent or fleeting.

8. Multifocal opacities that develop after pulmonary embolism are usually explained by hemorrhage and edema. True infarction is most accurately diagnosed when serial films demonstrate development of either linear or nodular scars.

9. The large opacities seen in Wegener's granulomatosis frequently represent areas of necrosis or of hemorrhage and edema resulting from ischemia. Remember, Wegener's granulomatosis is a disease of the vessels.

10. Bronchioloalveolar cell carcinoma is the only primary lung tumor that is expected to produce the pattern. Lymphoma and other lymphoid lesions of the lung (pseudolymphoma) may also lead to this pattern.

11. Kaposi's sarcoma in AIDS patients is an increasingly important cause of this pattern. These patients usually have advanced cutaneous Kaposi's sarcoma. The pulmonary involvement must be distinguished from lymphoma and opportunistic infection. For unexplained reasons, the incidence of Kaposi's is declining.

12. Metastases rarely lead to this pattern. Choriocarcinoma has been reported to lead to ill-defined opacities, but this appears to be very rare.

13. Silicosis may lead to large, bilateral, irregular upper lobe masses (con-

glomerate masses). They are fibrotic and should therefore not produce air bronchograms. Peripherally, their margins often parallel the lateral pleura.

14. Drug reactions frequently lead to this pattern. They are best diagnosed by
clinical correlation. Biopsy is frequently required in the immunologically compromised patient to rule out opportunistic infection.

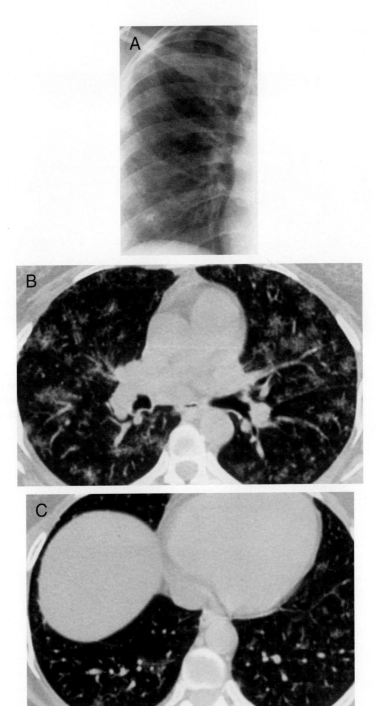

FIG 16–3
A, Patterns are difficult to characterize in patients with minimal diffuse disease. This coned view of the right lung shows poorly defined increased opacity that resembles minimal air-space opacity. **B,** HRCT section of the upper lobes in this patient with sarcoidosis demonstrates multifocal areas of poorly defined ground-glass opacity with associated reticular opacities. **C,** HRCT section through the lung bases confirms relative sparing of the lower lobes, which is a common distribution for sarcoidosis.

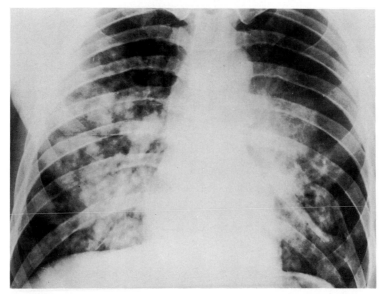

FIG 16–4
This is a common pattern for bronchogenic spread of infection. It is an example of *Kleb-siella* bronchopneumonia. The opacities represent lobular consolidations. The intervening lucencies are normal, aerated lobules. Heitzman has described this as a "patchwork quilt" appearance.

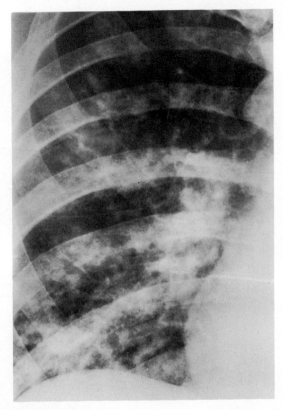

FIG 16–5
Histoplasmosis is caused by a fungus and is well known to produce a radiologic appearance similar to that of lobular pneumonia.

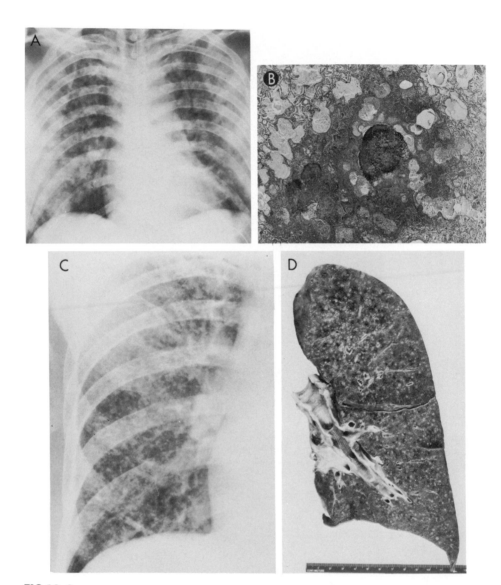

FIG 16–6
A, Invasive aspergillosis with the pattern of lobular pneumonia is rare in the immuno-
competent person but occurs as a frequent manifestation of aspergillosis in immunologically suppressed patients. **B,** Histologic section reveals *Aspergillus* colony with extensive
surrounding hemorrhage, edema, and inflammatory cellular response. Surrounding reaction accounts for lobular opacities seen in **A. C,** Lobular consolidations seen in **A** were
preceded by a fine nodular pattern. **D,** Gross specimen from same case reveals nodular
appearance of fungus colonies *(white)* against background of a lung consolidated by hemorrhagic edema. (From Blum J, Reed JC, Pizzo SV, et al: Miliary aspergillosis associated
with alcoholism. *AJR* 1978; 131:707–709. Used by permission.)

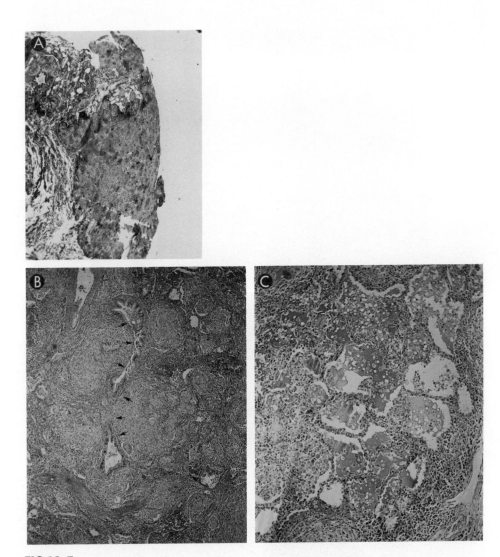

FIG 16–7
A, Large collections of noncaseating granulomas may account for multifocal opacities in cases of sarcoidosis. **B,** Small airway obstruction often occurs as a result of peribronchial granulomas *(arrows)* in sarcoidosis. **C,** Air-space consolidation by proteinaceous material and macrophages may develop distal to a small airway obstruction. This obstructive pneumonia could also account for multifocal opacities in cases of sarcoidosis. (**B** and **C,** from Reed JC, Madewell JE: The air bronchogram in interstitial disease of the lungs. *Radiology* 1975; 116:1–9. Used by permission.)

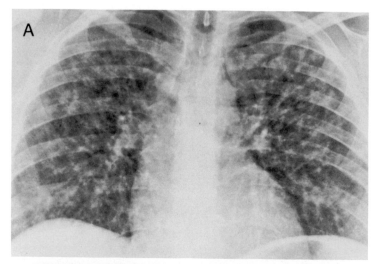

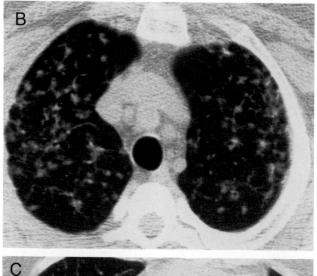

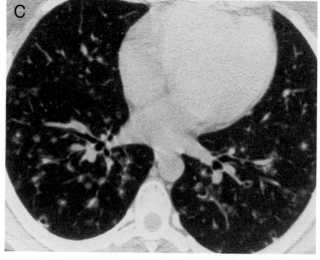

See legend on page 273

FIG 16–8
A, Opacities caused by eosinophilic granuloma are often nonspecific, but there is a tendency toward an upper lobe predominance, as illustrated by this case. **B,** High-resolution CT section through the upper chest reveals multiple poorly marginated nodules with interspersed coarse reticular opacities and peripheral subpleural cystic spaces. **C,** HRCT section through the lower chest confirms that the process is less extensive in the basal portions of the lungs. There are more scattered peripheral cysts. (Case courtesy of Peter Dietrich, M.D.)

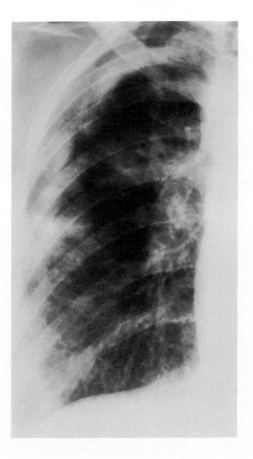

FIG 16–9
Chronic eosinophilic pneumonia typically produces multifocal ill-defined opacities that tend to be in the periphery of the lung. This is often described as the photonegative of pulmonary edema. Note peripheral opacities with a clear area between opacities and the central pulmonary arteries.

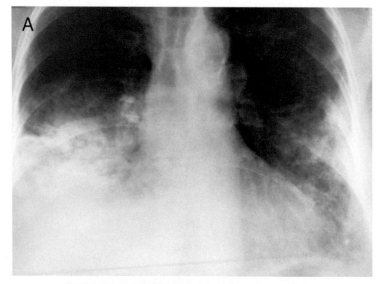

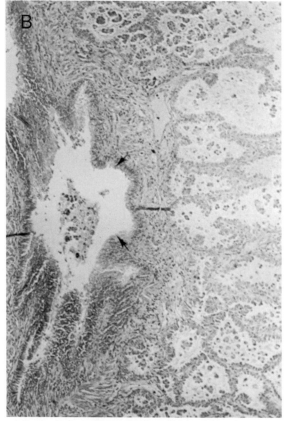

See legend on page 275

FIG 16–10
A, Bronchioloalveolar cell carcinoma fills the air-spaces with mucus and tumor cells. Bronchogenic dissemination accounts for the appearance of multifocal air-space opacities that may progress to cause diffuse consolidation. **B,** This histologic section is from another patient with bronchioloalveolar cell carcinoma. This unique pulmonary neoplasm consolidates lung with mucus and spares the pulmonary architecture. Note the open airway *(arrows)* in the center of this tumor. Plug of tumor in the bronchus supports the hypothesis of bronchial spread, which would account for the pattern of multifocal disease. (**B** only, from Reed JC, Madewell JE: The air bronchogram in interstitial disease of the lungs. *Radiology* 1975; 116:1–9. Used by permission.)

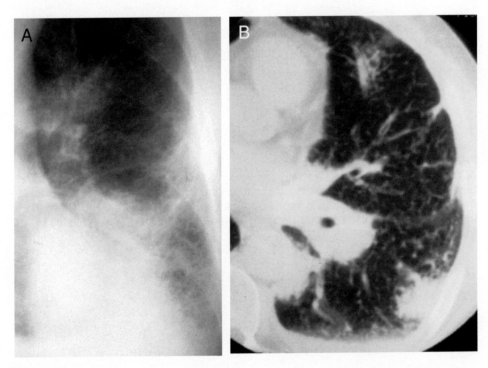

FIG 16–11
A, Pulmonary lymphoma is a cause of poorly marginated masses that may resemble consolidations. This case shows a large opacity in the left lower lobe, a peripheral subpleural opacity, and an opacity above the left hilum. There is also a subtle diffuse fine reticular pattern. **B,** CT section of the same case of lymphoma shows multiple ill-defined opacities. There is an air-bronchogram through the most anterior opacity, which has the appearance of a consolidation. There is also diffuse thickening of the interlobular septae. These findings are all the result of lymphomatous masses and infiltration.

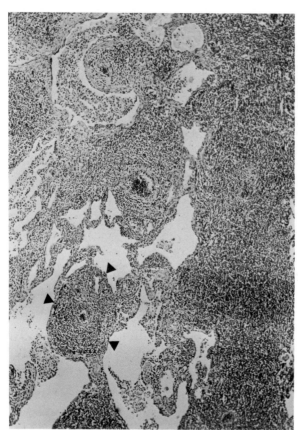

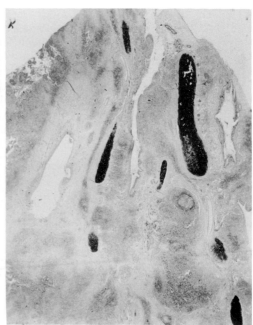

FIG 16–12
A, Cellular infiltration of alveolar walls and perivascular tissues *(arrowheads)* emphasizes how lymphoma may spread through the interstitium. **B,** Separation of bronchial mucosa from cartilage is the result of lymphomatous infiltrate. (From Reed JC, Madewell JE: The air bronchogram in interstitial disease of the lungs. *Radiology* 1975; 116:1-9. Used by permission.)

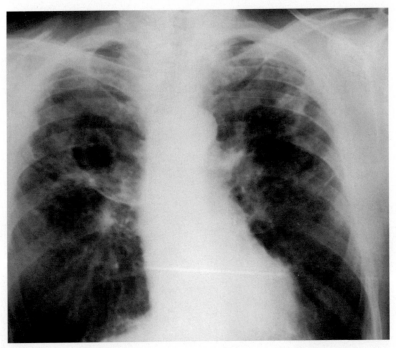

FIG 16–13
Predominantly upper lobe opacities in this case of silicosis are similar to those in other cases in this chapter. Associated coarse reticular opacities are the result of interstitial scars. Latter process often causes the large opacities to have irregular rather than ill-defined borders.

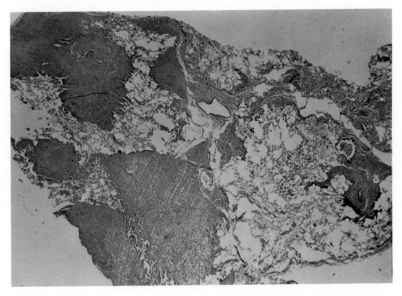

FIG 16–14
Histologic section from a case of silicosis reveals large homogeneous masses of fibrous tissue. Fibrosis accounts for peripheral irregularity.

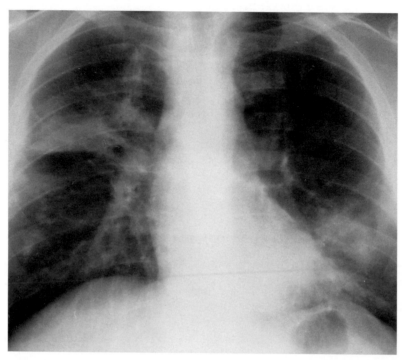

FIG 16–15
Kaposi's sarcoma produces bronchial and pulmonary vascular tumors that are prone to hemorrhage. These opacities are the result of bleeding and often appear more like air-space consolidation than masses.

ANSWER GUIDE

LEGENDS FOR INTRODUCTORY FIGURES

FIG 16–1

This pattern is best described as multifocal ill-defined opacities. The differential is long, but a number of common pulmonary diseases can be eliminated after proper evaluation of the pattern. For example, the only neoplasm listed as an answer to question 1 that is likely to result in this radiologic appearance is bronchioloalveolar-cell carcinoma. This patient had Wegener's granulomatosis.

FIG 16–2

The multifocal ill-defined opacities in this case are very nonspecific, but the observation of enlargement of the nodes in the aortic pulmonary window *(left arrows)* and paratracheal lymph nodes *(right arrows)* combines two patterns and thus narrows the differential. Either sarcoidosis or lymphoma could account for this combination. The fact that the patient is relatively asymptomatic supports the correct diagnosis of sarcoidosis.

ANSWERS

   1, e; 2, b; 3, a.

CHAPTER 17

Diffuse Fine Nodular Disease

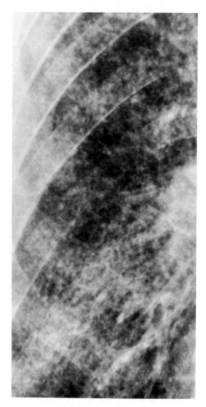

FIG 17–1

QUESTIONS

1. Based on the radiologic appearance of the case illustrated in Figure 17–1, which one of the following diagnoses is *least* likely?
   a. Asbestosis.
   b. Metastatic carcinoma.
   c. Eosinophilic granuloma.
   d. Histoplasmosis.
   e. Sarcoidosis.
2. The patient had chills and a fever. Which of the following is most likely?
   a. Eosinophilic granuloma.
   b. Rheumatoid lung.
   c. Sarcoidosis.
   d. Tuberculosis.
   e. Metastases.

Answer the following questions with True or False:

3. _____ Silicosis and sarcoidosis may present with the pattern seen in Figure 17–1 in combination with hilar adenopathy.

4. _____ Evolution of this pattern to one of multiple, small calcifications is compatible with either healed histoplasmosis or varicella pneumonia.

5. _____ Transbronchial biopsy is contraindicated in the evaluation of patients in whom the pattern is believed to be secondary to tuberculosis.

CHART 17–1.
Diffuse Fine Nodular Diseases

   I. Inhalational diseases (dust)
     A. Silicosis and coal-worker's pneumoconiosis[454]
     B. Berylliosis[186]
     C. Siderosis[186]
     D. Allergic alveolitis (farmer's lung)[516,592]
  II. Eosinophilic granuloma (Langerhans' cell histiocytosis)[603]
 III. Sarcoidosis[435,603]
 IV. Tuberculosis[43,162,260,311]
  V. Fungus infections
     A. Histoplasmosis[104]
     B. Blastomycosis[474,583]
     C. Coccidioidomycosis[186,392]
     D. Aspergillosis (rare)[51]
     E. Cryptococcosis (rare)[217,281]
 VI. Bacterial infections
     A. Nocardiosis[232]
     B. Bronchopneumonias (unusual)[293]
VII. Viral pneumonia (e.g., varicella)[403,476]
VIII. Metastatic tumor[186]
     A. Thyroid carcinoma
     B. Melanoma[88]
     C. Other adenocarcinomas (e.g., pancreas)
 IX. Other
     A. Bronchiolitis obliterans[219]
     B. Alveolar microlithiasis (rare)[491]
     C. Gaucher's disease[657]
     D. Wegener's granulomatosis (rare)[377]

CHART 17–2.
Diffuse Fine Nodular Pattern: Afebrile Patient

   I. Inhalational disease
  II. Eosinophilic granuloma (Langerhans' cell histiocytosis)
 III. Sarcoidosis
 IV. Fungal infection (late stage)
  V. Metastasis
 VI. Miliary tuberculosis (rare)

CHART 17–3.
Diffuse Fine Nodular Pattern: Febrile Patient

   I. Tuberculosis
  II. Fungal infection
 III. Nocardiosis
 IV. Viral pneumonia

DISCUSSION

Compared with some of the other patterns of diffuse pulmonary disease, the evaluation of diffuse fine nodular patterns may appear to be relatively simple. One of the first steps is to confirm the presence of the pattern. This may be difficult, however, because of the small size of the nodules. When they are truly miliary in size (1–2 mm) (see Figs 17–1 and 17–2), they are marginally detectable radiologically and may require HRCT for confirmation. Examination of gross specimens will often reveal many more nodules of a much smaller size than can be resolved as separate shadows on the plain film. Heitzman suggested that miliary nodules are probably seen because of the effect of summation, "a stacked coin effect."[260] These very small nodules are sometimes more easily appreciated on the PA film in the costophrenic angle and on the lateral film in the retrosternal clear space. Furthermore, small nodular opacities may occasionally be confused with very small pulmonary vessels seen on end. This mistake is usually avoided by identifying an associated branching vascular pattern around the nodule. Also, miliary nodules are typically much more diffuse than the fine nodular pattern created by normal vessels.

The sharpness of the borders of the nodules is an important criterion for narrowing the differential. For instance, small opacities may be caused either by small, sharply defined interstitial nodules or by minimal involvement of the distal airspaces (the so-called acinar rosettes), which results in ill-defined opacities.[186,293] This distinction is the key to limiting the differential. If the pattern includes small, fluffy, or ill-defined opacities, then alveolar edema, exudate, or hemorrhage must be considered. Therefore, the presence of ill-defined borders should prompt examination of the films for other signs of air-space–filling disease (see Chapter 15). In contrast, the pattern of very small but sharply defined or discrete opacities should reassure the radiologist that the nodules are more likely interstitial and thus associated with one of the entities listed in Chart 17–1.

Some authors have proposed that miliary nodules should by definition not exceed 1 or 2 mm in diameter.[616] However, this should rarely influence the differential diagnosis, since all of the entities listed in Chart 17–1 may produce larger nodules, up to 3 to 4 mm. It is true, however, that the size of the nodules does occasionally influence the radiologist to favor some members of the differential list over others. For example, the small nodules of eosinophilic granuloma are rarely as small as 1 or 2 mm. Although the very small nodular pattern does not eliminate eosinophilic granuloma from the differential, it makes other diagnoses such as sarcoidosis more likely. Since these small nodules have no distinguishing features, the radiologist must search for associated radiologic and clinical findings to narrow the differential.

Inhalational Diseases

Silicosis and coal-worker's pneumoconiosis[454] are the occupational diseases most commonly associated with the pattern of diffuse, fine interstitial nodules. The predicted distribution of fine nodules based on lung volume would favor a basilar predominance, but this is not the case in silicosis. The fine nodules caused by silicosis are predominantly in the upper lobes (Fig 17–3).[239] Histologically these nodules are localized areas of fibrosis, and the summation of shadows probably contributes to the nodular appearance. In many cases of silicosis the roentgenogram shows a fine reticular and nodular pattern, which suggests that crossing reticulations may contribute to the nodular appearance.

Exposure to free silica occurs in a variety of occupations, including sandblasting, quarrying, and coal mining. There is some controversy as to whether coalworker's pneumoconiosis and silicosis are two separate entities. Radiologic and histologic evidence indicates that the interstitial reaction that results in reticulations, nodules, and conglomerate masses is a reaction to silica rather than to anthracotic pigments. Thus, for the remainder of the text, the term *silicosis* will include the diseases of patients who have worked in coal mines. In most cases, a history of exposure is easily obtained, but the histories must be carefully evaluated. It is also important to compare the current chest x-ray film with old films to confirm the chronicity of the process, as well as to know whether the patient is febrile and to conduct tuberculin skin tests. Remember, patients with a history of coal mining are at increased risk for the development of superimposed tuberculosis or silicotuberculosis. A change in the radiographic pattern, or the rapid development of diffuse, fine interstitial nodules in combination with a febrile response and night sweats, strongly suggests tuberculosis rather than simple pneumoconiosis.

Other occupational exposures known to produce diffuse, fine nodular patterns are berylliosis[186] and allergic alveolitis.[592] Asbestosis, on the other hand, is best known for producing a reticular or linear pattern, as described in Chapter 18, rather than a fine nodular pattern. (Answer to question 1 is *a*.) The diagnosis of berylliosis is usually suggested by a history of exposure. However, the incidence of berylliosis has substantially decreased during the past 20 years, primarily because the number of occupations in which there is potential exposure to beryllium has decreased dramatically. Historically, beryllium was used as a coating for fluorescent light bulbs, and this was one of the most common sources of exposure to the metal. It is still used in the aerospace industry, particularly in aircraft brake linings. Confirming the diagnosis of berylliosis is sometimes difficult because the histologic examination of the nodules reveals a granulomatous reaction that is identical to that seen in sarcoidosis. Chemical analysis of wet tissue is frequently required for confirmation.

Allergic alveolitis is an allergy involving the alveolar wall and may be due to a variety of noninvasive fungi. The fine nodular interstitial opacities frequently represent a subacute or chronic phase of the illness. Histologically they may correspond with the presence of sarcoidlike granulomas in the interstitium. Also, a fine nodular pattern may be encountered around the periphery of the large multifocal parenchymal opacities found in allergic alveolitis. This latter appearance is, in fact, much more common than the fine nodular pattern. More acute phases of the disease produce larger opacities that are considered in detail in Chapter 16.

Eosinophilic Granuloma and Sarcoidosis

Both sarcoidosis and eosinophilic granuloma[603] are inflammatory conditions that may produce a very fine nodular pattern. They may be distinguished from a number of other entities considered in this differential because of their relatively mild symptoms, despite radiologic findings suggesting severe pathology. Patients with these diseases may complain of very mild dyspnea and virtually no other symptoms. The combined presence of hilar adenopathy and a fine nodular pattern is an important feature for distinguishing these illnesses. It must be emphasized that bilaterally symmetric hilar adenopathy in combination with a fine nodular pattern strongly suggests the diagnosis of sarcoidosis (Fig 17–4). Although adenopathy may be an important part of severe histiocytoses seen in children, hilar adenopathy is rarely, if ever, encountered in adult patients who have eosinophilic granuloma of the lung. Examination of previous films is important, since the adenopathy that classically accompanies sarcoidosis may regress as the interstitial disease progresses. Therefore, old films that demonstrate bilaterally symmetric hilar adenopathy are virtually diagnostic of sarcoidosis. Another entity considered in this differential of fine nodules and hilar adenopathy is silicosis, but silicosis rarely leads to symmetric hilar adenopathy, and the adenopathy does not regress. Although eggshell calcification of the hilar lymph nodes is considered a classic sign of silicosis, it has also very rarely been observed in sarcoidosis. (Answer to question 3 is *True*.)

Metastatic Disease

The development of a fine nodular pattern in a patient with a known distant primary tumor, such as a thyroid tumor (Fig 17–5),[491] strongly suggests disseminated metastatic disease. These patients often have signs of severe systemic illness, including weight loss, but careful clinical correlation is required, since many patients with malignant tumors receive chemotherapy with potent immunosuppressing agents. The possibility of opportunistic infection must be ruled out. A febrile response strongly suggests opportunistic infection. Prompt biopsy of the lung, by either transbronchial or open biopsy methods, is advisable for establishing the diagnosis of a treatable infectious disease. Other primary tumors that have been observed to lead to this pattern include melanoma, breast carcinoma, and gastrointestinal tumors, including pancreatic carcinoma (Fig 17–6). These are the same tumors considered in the differential of lymphangitic metastases. CT scanning in patients with lymphangitic spread of tumor often reveals diffuse fine nodules, even when the plain film shows thickened interlobular septae.[46]

Infectious Diseases

The discussion of opportunistic infection in the patient with a known primary tumor leads to the differential diagnosis of infectious diseases that may produce a fine nodular pattern. Eosinophilic granuloma, sarcoidosis, metastases, and most of the inhalational diseases should cause afebrile illnesses. The one exception is allergic alveolitis, which may cause a mild febrile response. The presence of a febrile response requires consideration of tuberculosis, fungal infection, and viral pneumonia.

Miliary tuberculosis implies hematogenous dissemination and almost invariably leads to a dramatic febrile response with night sweats and chills (see Fig 17–1). Exceptions to this clinical presentation are severely debilitated patients, particularly the very elderly. This is probably the result of altered immune response and is most commonly encountered in nursing home populations and patients receiving steroids. It must be emphasized that bacteriologic confirmation of miliary tuberculosis is not always easily obtained. Despite the disseminated disease, the miliary nodules are interstitial. Sputum cultures may continue to be negative in the face of miliary tuberculosis because the organisms are primarily in the interstitium rather than the air-spaces. Therefore, more invasive techniques such as bronchoscopy with transbronchial biopsy may be required to confirm the diagnosis.

Although all of the fungal infections listed in Chart 17–1 may mimic the radiologic appearance of miliary tuberculosis, this pattern is most commonly the result of histoplasmosis, coccidioidomycosis, or, less commonly, North American blastomycosis. The clinical response to these fungal infections may be more varied than in tuberculosis. For instance, some patients have a profound systemic response leading to death, others have a mild influenzalike syndrome, and a few are minimally symptomatic. In the last instance, the radiologic abnormality may be more impressive than the clinical course. A history of exposure to a specific fungus will occasionally be obtained. For example, a history of a trip to the desert virtually confirms the diagnosis of coccidioidomycosis, while exposure to soil contaminated with bird or chicken droppings in the Ohio River Valley area strongly suggests histoplasmosis. Such histories also suggest that the nodules are not always the result of hematogenous dissemination, such as in miliary tuberculosis, but may also be due to an inhaled organism. This difference in etiology helps to explain some of the clinical and radiologic differences in the two conditions. The acute epidemic form of histoplasmosis produces the radiologic appearance of larger ill-defined nodules, like that of bronchopneumonia (see Chapter 16). As the patient recovers, the nodules may regress in size and become more sharply defined. Therefore, the fine nodular pattern may represent either a healing or healed phase of the disease or an acute hematogenous dissemination of the fungus. Some patients with histoplasmosis who develop this diffuse nodular pattern are later observed to develop diffuse small calcified nodules (Fig 17–7). This pattern is virtually specific for histoplasmosis, especially when it is associated with either hilar lymph node or splenic calcifications.

Bacterial infections generally do not produce this fine nodular pattern of pulmonary involvement. However, there are occasional reports of bacterial pneumonias leading to the pattern.[293] For example, salmonella is one organism that can sometimes produce "miliary nodules." *Nocardia,* previously regarded as a fungus, is a gram-positive bacterium. It rarely causes infection in the normal patient; however, in the immunosuppressed patient, *Nocardia* may produce a variety of pulmonary patterns, including miliary nodules.[232]

Viral pneumonia, especially varicella or chickenpox pneumonia, may result in fine nodules (Fig 17–8).[186,403,491] Presumably these nodules represent localized collections of inflammatory cells in the interstitium. If the course of the illness is severe, the pattern may be transient and rapidly followed by larger multifocal ill-defined opacities or even diffuse coalescent opacities and complicated by ARDS. Such a course is frequently encountered in immunologically suppressed patients. As with histoplasmosis, the small nodules caused by varicella pneumonia may heal with the development of multiple calcified nodules. However, confirmation of this etiology of the calcified nodules may be virtually impossible unless the diagnosis is established in the acute phase of illness. Clinical correlation makes diagnosis of the acute illness relatively simple, since most patients have the characteristic skin lesions of chickenpox. Chickenpox pneumonia is much more common in adults than in children. (Answer to question 4 is *True.*)

The Immunologically Compromised Patient

The immunologically compromised patient requires special attention and a more aggressive approach to diagnosis than do other patients.[58] It is important to remember that patients with AIDS or hematologic malignancies, such as lymphoma or leukemia, who develop a fine nodular pattern will most likely have an infectious process such as viral pneumonia, nocardiosis, fungal infection, or tuberculosis. These patients are also subject to many other common infections, such as staphylococcal pneumonia, gram-negative pneumonia, and *Pneumocystis carinii* pneumonia. However, infections of this type are less likely to produce the fine nodular pattern.

Other patients with altered immunity, including transplant patients and those receiving steroids or immunosuppressive agents for such chronic systemic diseases as rheumatoid arthritis and lupus erythematosus, are also susceptible to both common and unusual infections. Because of the suppression of their immunologic response, these patients may not show the dramatic febrile response that is usually seen in the normal host with the same infection. For example, the patient whose roentgenogram is shown in Figure 17–1 was treated for rheumatoid arthritis with steroids and developed a diffuse nodular pattern within 1 month of this treatment. Because of the rapid development of the nodules, chronic diseases such as sarcoidosis and rheumatoid nodules were excluded from the differential. Rheumatoid nodules were also considered unlikely because of the size and distribution of the nodules in the case. Cultures from a transbronchial biopsy confirmed the diagnosis of tuberculosis. (Answer to question 2 is *d*.) Transbronchial biopsy is an excellent method for evaluating diffuse disease. (Answer to question 5 is *False*.)

SUMMARY

1. Miliary tuberculosis is the classic example of a disease producing a fine nodular interstitial pattern on radiographic examination of the chest.

2. The most common fungal infections to produce a fine nodular interstitial pattern are histoplasmosis, coccidioidomycosis, and blastomycosis.

3. Silicosis and coal-worker's pneumoconiosis are the most common inhalational diseases to produce the pattern. Asbestosis, in contrast, produces a reticular interstitial pattern.

4. Sarcoidosis and eosinophilic granuloma may produce a fine nodular interstitial pattern, although the patient may have only minimal symptoms of shortness of breath or easy fatigability. Associated bilateral hilar adenopathy or even previous films revealing hilar adenopathy are virtually diagnostic of sarcoidosis.

5. Immunologically suppressed patients are susceptible to infection by less common organisms (e.g., *Nocardia, Cryptococcus,* and *Aspergillus*), but we must not minimize the frequency of infection by common organisms in these patients (i.e., viral pneumonia, tuberculosis, coccidioidomycosis, histoplasmosis, blastomycosis).

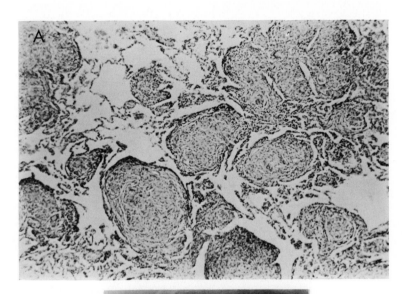

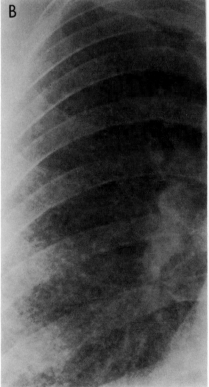

FIG 17-2
A, Histologic section from a case of sarcoidosis reveals microscopic granulomas that would not be expected to be radiologically detectable. **B,** Radiologic detection of such small nodules is probably the result of summation. Heitzman has likened this to a "stacked coin effect." (From Theros EG: RPC of the month from the AFIP. *Radiology* 1969; 92:1557–1561. Used by permission.)

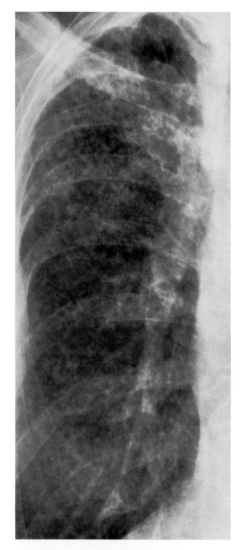

FIG 17–3
The fine nodules in this case are more numerous in the apices, with relative sparing of
the lung bases. This is the typical distribution of silicotic nodules.

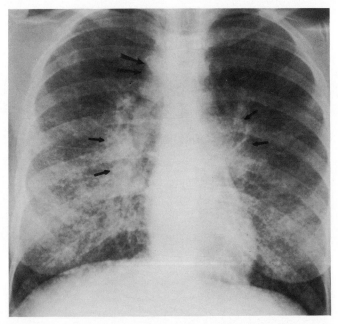

FIG 17–4
Combination of bilateral hilar adenopathy *(small arrows)*, paratracheal adenopathy *(large arrows)*, and diffuse fine nodules is a classic appearance for sarcoidosis. However, the adenopathy may regress prior to radiologic evidence of interstitial disease.

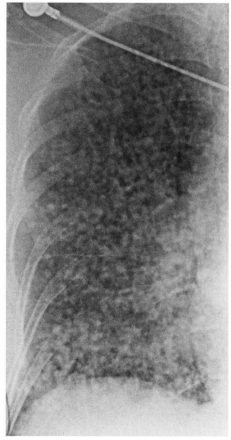

FIG 17–5
Papillary adenothyroid carcinoma is a well-known cause of diffuse small nodular metastases. Since patients with this tumor often have a relatively long survival, the profusion may be great, and the nodules may be larger than the nodules of granulomatous infections.

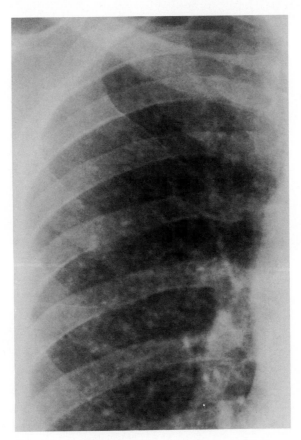

FIG 17–6
Melanoma and adenocarcinomas from breast, lung, and gastrointestinal tract may produce diffuse interstitial nodular metastases. The nodules in this case are the result of
pancreatic carcinoma.

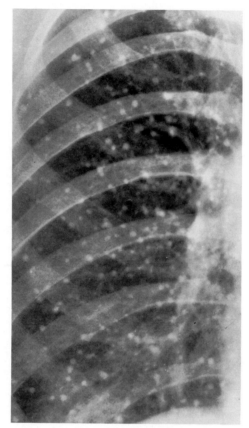

FIG 17–7
Histoplasmosis is the most common cause of disseminated calcified nodules. Chicken-pox pneumonia may also heal and leave residual nodules that may calcify.

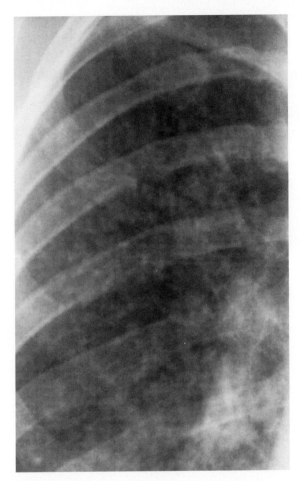

FIG 17–8
Varicella pneumonia is a viral pneumonia that causes diffuse fine nodules. In this case they are very numerous and not well circumscribed. This loss of definition may be the result of superimposition or extension into the airspaces.

ANSWER GUIDE

LEGEND FOR INTRODUCTORY FIGURE

FIG 17–1
Diffuse fine nodular pattern (miliary nodules) is the classic radiologic appearance of miliary tuberculosis.

ANSWERS

1, a; 2, d; 3, T; 4, T; 5, F.

CHAPTER 18

Fine Reticular Opacities

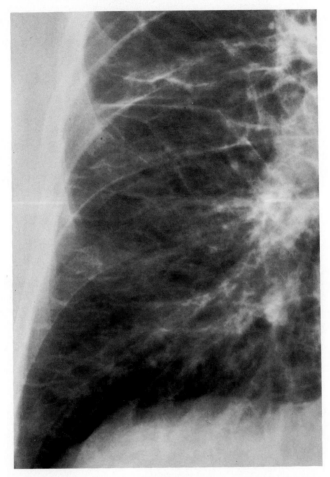

FIG 18–1

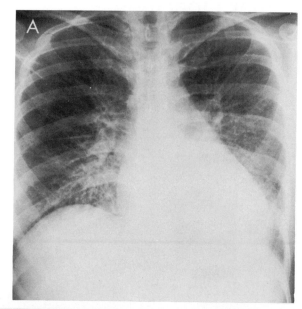

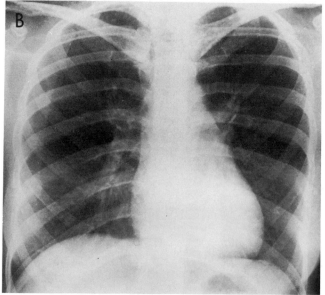

FIG 18–2

QUESTIONS

1. Kerley's B lines (Fig 18–1) represent which one of the following?
   a. Thick interlobular septa.
   b. Dilated lymphatic vessels.
   c. Dilated venules.
   d. Thick alveolar walls.
   e. None of the above.

2. Which of the following diagnoses is most likely in the case illustrated in Figure 18–2, *A* and *B*?
   a. Pulmonary edema.
   b. Lymphangitic metastases.
   c. Lymphoma.
   d. Sarcoidosis.
   e. Lymphangiectasia.
3. Which of the following statements are true?
   a. Kerley's B lines are perpendicular to the pleura.
   b. Kerley's A lines are deep in the lung parenchyma.
   c. Kerley's lines indicate pulmonary edema.
   d. Kerley's lines indicate interstitial disease.
   e. Dilated lymphatics are one cause of Kerley's lines.
4. Which of the following causes of a fine reticular pattern is least likely to be associated with pleural effusion?
   a. Lymphangitic metastases.
   b. Lymphoma.
   c. Scleroderma.
   d. Lymphangiomyomatosis.
   e. Pulmonary edema.

CHART 18–1.
Diffuse Fine Reticular Opacities

I. Acute
  A. Edema
    1. Congestive heart failure[87]
    2. Uremia[186]
    3. Fluid overload
  B. Infection
    1. Viral pneumonia[260,497,569]
    2. Mycoplasma pneumonia[183]
    3. Infectious mononucleosis
    4. Malaria[81] *(Plasmodium falciparum)*
    5. *Pneumocystis carinii* pneumonia
II. Chronic
  A. Chronic edema
    1. Atherosclerotic heart disease
    2. Mitral stenosis[87]
    3. Left atrial tumor (myxoma)
    4. Pulmonary veno-occlusive disease[551]
    5. Sclerosing mediastinitis
  B. Granulomatous disease[260]
    1. Sarcoidosis
    2. Eosinophilic granuloma (Langerhans' cell histiocytosis)[333,406,465]
  C. Collagen vascular disease[189,516,562]
    1. Rheumatoid lung
    2. Scleroderma lung[15]
  D. Lymphangitic spread of tumor[260,288,302]
  E. Lymphocytic disorders
    1. Lymphoma and leukemia
    2. Waldenström's macroglobulinemia[438,655]
    3. Lymphocytic interstitial pneumonia[56,159,263]

(Continued.)

CHART 18–1.   (cont.).

F. Lymphatic obstruction
    1. Mediastinal mass (lymphoma)[260]
    2. Lymphangiectasia (pediatric patient)[161]
G. Inhalational disease[194,454]
    1. Asbestosis[37,203] and talcosis[154]
    2. Silicosis
    3. Hard metals[180]
    4. Allergic alveolitis[69,456,516,589]
H. Drug reactions (see Chart 19–1)[14,61,134,460,584]
I. Idiopathic
    1. Usual interstitial pneumonia[78,109] (Hamman-Rich, fibrosing alveolitis, chronic fibrosing interstitial pneumonia, muscular cirrhosis)[193,465]
    2. Desquamative interstitial pneumonia[332]
    3. Tuberous sclerosis
    4. Lymphangiomyomatosis[326,410,528,563]
    5. Idiopathic pulmonary hemosiderosis[481,484]
    6. Amyloidosis[271]
    7. Interstitial calcification (chronic renal failure)[169]
    8. Alveolar proteinosis (late complication)[283]
    9. Gaucher's disease[657]

CHART 18–2.
Fine Reticular Pattern and Pleural Effusion

I. Acute
    A. Edema
    B. Infection (viral or mycoplasma pneumonia)
    C. Malaria[81] (rare)
II. Chronic
    A. Congestive heart failure
    B. Rheumatoid disease
    C. Lymphangitic spread of tumor
    D. Lymphoma and leukemia
    E. Lymphangiectasis
    F. Lymphangiomyomatosis

CHART 18–3.
Fine Reticular Pattern and Hilar Adenopathy

I. Viral pneumonia (rare combination)
II. Sarcoidosis
III. Lymphoma and leukemia
IV. Primary carcinoma (particularly small cell carcinoma)
V. Metastases (lymphatic dilation or lymphangitic spread)
VI. Silicosis

CHART 18–4.
Differential Diagnosis for the Histologic Changes of Usual Interstitial Pneumonia[*]

  I. Idiopathic
 II. Viral
III. Radiation-induced
 IV. Drug-related (e.g., bleomycin, amiodarone)
  V. Collagen vascular diseases
     A. Scleroderma
     B. Rheumatoid arthritis
     C. Lupus erythematosus
     D. Erythema nodosum
     E. Dermatomyositis
 VI. Pneumoconioses
     A. Asbestosis and talcosis
VII. Noxious gases

[*]Modified from Gaensler EA, Carrington CB, Coutu RE: Chronic interstitial pneumonias. *Clinical Notes on Respiratory Diseases*, vol 10. New York, American Thoracic Society, 1972, pp 1–16.

DISCUSSION

The diffuse, fine reticular pattern (see Fig 18–1) is one of the most reliable patterns for identifying diffuse interstitial disease.[260] Since this pattern is linear, the lines must be distinguished from the normal pattern of blood vessels. In the early stages of an interstitial disease, this may be impossible.[144] The most reliable radiologic observation for making this distinction is the identification of Kerley's lines.[162,186,260] Kerley's B lines are short lines that are perpendicular to the pleura and continuous with it. The latter feature distinguishes the Kerley B lines from small vessels. Kerley's B lines are most commonly observed in the costophrenic angles on PA films and occasionally on lateral films in the retrosternal clear space. They were first thought to represent only enlarged lymphatics, but, based on pathologic correlations, Heitzman[260] has shown that these lines represent more generalized enlarged interlobular septa. (Answer to question 1 is *a*.) Although it is true that the engorgement of septal lymphatic vessels contributes to Kerley's B lines, this has probably been overemphasized. Lymphangiectasia and lymphangitic spread of a malignant tumor are examples of a reticular pattern that is secondary to dilation of lymphatics, but in the other entities listed in Chart 18–1, dilation of lymphatics is not a sufficient explanation for the presence of Kerley's B lines. Furthermore, in congestive heart failure, edema of the loose connective tissue of the interlobular septum accounts for Kerley's lines, rather than the engorged lymphatics.[260]

Kerley's A lines are also important and reliable signs of interstitial disease. These lines are linear opacities that appear to cross the normal vascular markings. Heitzman[260] has shown that they correspond anatomically to thick interlobular septa. They differ from Kerley's B lines only by their location, representing thick interlobular septa that are deep in the lung parenchyma. Kerley's C lines have not been well defined anatomically and continue to be a topic of considerable controversy.[186,260] (Answers to question 3 are *a, b, d,* and *e*. The only incorrect answer is *c*; pulmonary edema is only one cause of Kerley's lines.)

Pulmonary Edema

The most common cause of a fine reticular pattern is pulmonary interstitial edema.[186,260] The next step in the evaluation of this pattern is to check for other signs that might suggest congestive heart failure. These include a large heart with left ventricular or left atrial enlargement, prominence of upper lobe vessels, constriction of lower lobe vessels (cephalization of flow), peribronchial cuffing,[414] increased width of vascular pedicle,[414] and signs of pleural effusion, including thickening of the interlobar fissures[87] (see Fig 18–2, A). Prominence of the left atrium without left ventricular enlargement, in combination with a fine reticular pattern and prominence of upper lobe vessels, strongly suggests mitral stenosis. A clinical history of rheumatic fever and a murmur indicating mitral stenosis should be sufficient to confirm the diagnosis. Cardiac ultrasound examination is a reliable, noninvasive method for confirming such a diagnosis and for excluding the rare atrial myxoma, which may also produce the classic plain film findings of mitral stenosis.

Fluid overload is another common cause of interstitial edema. Fluid overload may be iatrogenic, but it is also commonly encountered in patients suffering from chronic renal failure.[186] Correlation with the clinical setting is particularly important in renal transplant patients, since they are susceptible to interstitial edema and to infections. Therefore, a febrile response should suggest an interstitial pneumonia rather than interstitial edema. In addition, any cause of severe hypoproteinemia, including cirrhosis and nephrosis, may lead to interstitial edema.

All of these causes of interstitial edema, except mitral stenosis, are acute processes; the pattern tends to be transient and changes rapidly. A changing course can be ascertained by examining old films and obtaining serial films (see Fig 18–2, B).

Acute Interstitial Pneumonias

After pulmonary edema has been eliminated, viral, *Pneumocystis carinii*, and mycoplasma pneumonias are the major causes of an acute fine reticular pattern (Fig 18–3). The acuteness of the interstitial pattern is best documented with serial films. These patterns will usually change over a few days. Both viral and mycoplasma pneumonias characteristically produce a febrile response and a nonproductive cough. They are commonly associated with a flulike syndrome. The reticular pattern may appear coarse on occasion, but this is the result of a heavy accumulation of inflammatory cells in the interstitium and should not be confused with honeycombing (see Chapter 19 for a discussion of honeycomb lung).

Chronic Interstitial Inflammatory Disease

Distinguishing acute from chronic interstitial patterns requires careful clinical correlation and serial films; a single film is rarely adequate. Serial films not only document the chronicity of the disease but may also reveal information about changing patterns. This is particularly important in the diagnosis of diseases that may change from a nodular to a fine reticular pattern. Eosinophilic granuloma and sarcoidosis are two diseases well known for this type of radiologic evolution (nodules to lines).[260,486] Both diseases may be very similar in their radiologic appearances except for the presence of hilar adenopathy, which is not seen in eosinophilic granuloma and is therefore diagnostic of sarcoidosis. The first manifestations in the classic pattern of the progression of sarcoidosis are bilaterally symmetric hilar adenopathy and paratracheal adenopathy.[186] A small percentage of patients have radiologically detectable fine nodules (described in Chapter 17) at the time of their initial visit. The nodules are small, noncaseating granulomas. If the nodules become very extensive, they appear to line up along the bronchovascular bundles and interlobular septa. This arrangement of the nodules produces a fine reticular pattern and may occur at the time of the adenopathy, but it more typically occurs in the later stages of the disease, after the adenopathy has regressed. The granulomas may regress spontaneously or in response to steroids. In some cases, the diffuse reticular pattern will resolve, but in a small number of patients the granulomas will gradually be replaced by fibrosis. This replacement may not be radiologically detectable. In other cases the fine reticular pattern will increase. This fibrotic reaction may eventually lead to a coarse reticular or honeycomb pattern.[260]

In eosinophilic granuloma the change from a nodular to a fine reticular pattern suggests that histiocytes and eosinophils, which give rise to the nodular pattern, are being replaced by fibrosis.[486] As in sarcoidosis, if the fibrotic reaction continues, the fine reticular pattern will progress to a honeycomb pattern. In eosinophilic granuloma an upper lobe distribution of the reticular interstitial disease is frequently observed, in contrast to the entities listed in Chart 18–2 that characteristically have a lower lobe distribution. Hilar adenopathy is not typically seen in any stage of eosinophilic granuloma,[186,260] although slightly enlarged hilar and mediastinal nodes have been reported in histiocytosis X.[35,386,634]

Of the collagen vascular diseases, rheumatoid arthritis and scleroderma most commonly produce a fine reticular interstitial pattern.[189] The clinical presentation of these entities is usually distinctive, and the pulmonary changes are almost always seen in a late stage of the disease. However, Fraser[186] et al. have emphasized that patients may occasionally be seen with rheumatoid involvement of the lung prior to the development of joint disease. Rheumatoid lung disease may be associated with pleural effusions or pleural thickening (Fig 18–4), either of which helps to distinguish it from sarcoidosis. Pleural reactions secondary to sarcoidosis are rare. Rheumatoid lung disease has a tendency to involve the bases in the early stages of the process but will be diffuse if the interstitial disease becomes extensive. This is in contrast to scleroderma, which is usually but not necessarily confined to the bases even after it has progressed from a fine reticular to a coarse honeycomb pattern. In addition to the fine reticular pattern, multiple areas of airspace consolidation may be observed in patients with scleroderma. These areas of consolidation are also in the bases and frequently represent localized areas of edema. Gaensler et al.[193] postulated that the alveolar edema is organized and incorporated into the interstitium. This would suggest that the consolidations represent acute or early phases of the disease and might therefore precede the fine reticular pattern. Another possible factor contributing to the development of the air-space pattern in scleroderma is aspiration. Many patients with significant pulmonary involvement from scleroderma have a serious esophageal motility disturbance with a dilated, atonic esophagus. It is necessary to document any acute changes in the patterns of pulmonary disease in patients with either scleroderma or rheumatoid arthritis in order to detect an acute pneumonia. This is most important in patients with rheumatoid arthritis who are being treated with steroids and are thus susceptible to opportunistic infections or reactivations of previous granulomatous infections, particularly tuberculosis.

Neoplasms

A fine reticular pattern with Kerley's A and B lines is the classic radiologic appearance of lymphangitic spread of a tumor.[186,260] This is most commonly a bilateral process with a predominantly basilar distribution. In the early stages, lymphangitic carcinomatosis may be very subtle. High-resolution CT is very sensitive for the detection of early spread of tumor through the bronchovascular and septal interstitium (Fig 18–5, *A–C*). The procedure has also been reported to be useful for distinguishing carcinomatosis from benign diseases such as sarcoidosis, UIP, and drug reactions.[45,319,582] The radiologic appearance of a reticular pattern correlates well with the typical histologic appearance of tumor that has spread through the bronchovascular bundles and interlobular septa (Fig 18–6, *A*). As the tumor becomes more extensive, the radiologic pattern may change from a reticular to a reticulonodular or even a fine nodular pattern (see Chapter 17). However, this nodular pattern does not correlate well with the histologic appearance. Heitzman[260] suggests that these nodular and reticular nodular patterns do not in fact represent structural nodules, but are a summation of shadows produced by the crossing-line shadows. As the tumor becomes more extensive, it may even give the appearance of basilar consolidation and thus mimic the appearance of an airspace consolidation (see Chapter 15). The most common primary tumors to spread through the lymphatic vessels are adenocarcinomas from the breast, colon, stomach, pancreas, and lung. A primary lung tumor is the most common tumor to undergo unilateral lymphangitic spread. It sometimes produces a characteristic pattern of either parenchymal or hilar mass in combination with a unilateral, fine reticular pattern. This is not to say that the combination of a pulmonary or hilar mass with a bilateral fine reticular pattern is not also very suggestive of a primary lung tumor. Another finding commonly associated with lymphangitic spread of any of the above tumors is pleural effusion. Pleural effusion is usually the result of extensive infiltration of the pleural lymphatic vessels by tumor that appears to be continuous with the pulmonary lymphatic vessels. The combination of a fine reticular pattern and pleural effusion is not specific for lymphangitic spread of a malignant tumor (see Chart 18–2), but thoracentesis with pleural biopsy is a good means of confirming the diagnosis.

Hilar adenopathy (Chart 18–3) is occasionally observed in patients with lymphangitic metastases,[297] but it may be more suggestive of lymphoma,[260,263] which commonly produces hilar or mediastinal adenopathy and occasionally spreads through the interstitium of the lung (Fig 18–6, *B*), producing a fine reticular pattern. This is a late stage of the disease, and the diagnosis of lymphoma is usually known from previous lymph node biopsies. It may be more common for patients with lymphoma to have been seen earlier, with adenopathy, and to have been treated, with resolution of the adenopathy prior to the development of the fine reticular pattern. In the latter situation the development of the pulmonary disease raises the differential of (1) opportunistic infection, (2) drug reaction, and (3) diffuse spread of the lymphoma. Since the treatment of these three entities is quite different, a precise diagnosis is essential. Early biopsy is an essential procedure, since delay in treatment of the opportunistic infections may be fatal. In addition to lymphoma, leukemia is another malignant disorder that may disseminate through the lung and produce a fine interstitial pattern. Like lymphoma, the diagnosis of leukemia is usually known by the time the interstitial pattern develops, and the differential problem is to exclude opportunistic infections and drug reactions.

Lymphocytic interstitial pneumonia is an infrequent cause of a fine reticular pattern. It involves an infiltration of the pulmonary interstitium with mature lymphocytes and may closely resemble a lymphocytic lymphoma histologically. It is imperative that patients with LIP be carefully evaluated, perhaps even by CT scanning. Associated adenopathy is strong evidence against the diagnosis of LIP and would therefore influence the histologist to favor the diagnosis of a well-differentiated lymphocytic lymphoma.[159,263] Recently, LIP has been observed as an additional complication of AIDS (see Chapter 15).[446]

Inhalational Diseases

A fine reticular pattern may occur with any inhalational disease that produces a significant interstitial fibrotic reaction. Silicon and asbestos dusts are the most common causes of interstitial fibrosis.[37,186,194] Silicosis is a reaction to free silica, which may be encountered in a number of occupations, including mining (particularly of coal), stone quarrying, and sandblasting. The patterns seen in silicosis may vary considerably. The interstitial disease may be extensive and is frequently progressive. The fine reticular pattern is generally considered to be a simple form of pneumoconiosis, which may precede the appearance of extensive honeycombing fibrosis and the development of large conglomerate masses. The combination of small nodules and reticulations is more common than a pure reticular pattern (see Chapter 17).

The radiologic pattern of asbestosis is strikingly different from that of silicosis.[186] The classic description of asbestosis is of a fine reticular pattern localized predominantly in the bases and which may be associated with pleural thickening and pleural calcification, as described in Chapter 5. In some cases, the reticulations may be very subtle and require HRCT for confirmation.[197] Magnesium silicate, a salt of silicic acid, is believed to be the component of asbestos that produces the pulmonary disease. It is believed to form silicic acid when it contacts moisture in the lung. The very dilute acid may then diffuse through the alveolar walls and interlobular septa and produce a fibrotic response that initially follows the normal anatomic planes. Histologically, asbestosis entails extensive reactions in the alveolar walls, involving fibrosis and inflammatory cells, including foreign body giant cells that may even contain asbestos bodies. Talc is another compound that contains magnesium silicate and produces a radiologic picture identical to that in asbestosis.[154]

Idiopathic Diseases

Usual interstitial pneumonia is one of the most common diffuse chronic interstitial diseases, but it does not have a universally accepted name. In 1944 Hamman and Rich described a group of patients with diffuse pulmonary fibrosis that experienced a short, fulminant, fatal course.[243] Since their report many patients have been diagnosed as having Hamman-Rich syndrome, but many cases in which the radiologic and histologic findings are compatible with diffuse chronic fibrosing interstitial pneumonia do not have such a short course. The acute course is currently believed to represent a variant of UIP that is often labeled acute interstitial pneumonia. Other terms that are used to describe UIP include fibrosing alveolitis, cryptogenic fibrosing alveolitis, diffuse chronic fibrosing intersitital pneumonia, and idiopathic pulmonary fibrosis (IPF).

Serial radiographs of patients with UIP often document a slowly progressive course that presents with a basilar reticular or reticulonodular pattern. There may be intermittent episodes that appear as minimal basilar confluent opacities, but as the disease progresses it appears more reticular, and there is progressive volume loss. The final stages produce end-stage scarring with honeycombing fibrosis (see Chapter 19). Plain films provide an excellent chronologic record of disease progression, but precise characterization of the pattern and distribution of the disease is limited by plain film assessment (Fig 18–7, *A* and *B*). HRCT is the most effective technique for confirming the presence of minimal disease and evaluating distribution of disease. Small reticular opacities and cystic changes that are predominantly in the periphery of the lung are reported to be characteristic of UIP.[427,428,465] HRCT (Fig 18–8, *A* and *B*) has also been advocated as a technique to assess the stage and activity of UIP. During the active alveolitis stages of the disease, HRCT shows patchy areas of ground-glass opacity, which are the result of alveolar wall inflammation, intra-alveolar edema with cellular infiltration, and fibrosis.[142,428] Because similar radiologic and histologic changes are seen in scleroderma, systemic lupus erythematosus, dermatomyositis, and rheumatoid arthritis, this is a diagnosis of exclusion requiring clinical correlation (Chart 18–4).

Desquamative interstitial pneumonia[332] more commonly involves areas of consolidation and is discussed in Chapter 16, but the air-space–filling component of the process may resolve and leave a fine reticular interstitial pattern.

Tuberous sclerosis may result in a smooth muscle proliferation in the lung and therefore in a diffuse, fine reticular pattern.[327] It is best diagnosed on clinical grounds, since patients with the disease usually have other associated signs.

Lymphangiomyomatosis[326] is a rare cause of a fine reticular pattern, but the clinical setting may be very specific (Fig 18–9, *A* and *B*). It typically occurs in young women and is accompanied by recurrent pleural effusions and pneumothoraces. Examination of pleural fluid reveals a chylous effusion. This complex of radiologic and clinical findings may be so specific that biopsy may be unnecessary. In addition, HRCT has been reported to show extensive small cystic changes with very thin walls that may not be visible on the plain film.[45]

Idiopathic pulmonary hemosiderosis most commonly produces diffuse air-space consolidations (see Chapter 15); however, after multiple episodes of bleeding, a fine reticular pattern may develop.[481] This is most prominent in the bases and is the result of an accumulation of iron-laden macrophages in the interstitium, which may gradually be replaced by fibrosis. The pattern can be observed only between episodes of acute bleeding and occurs as a late complication of the disease.[403,607]

Amyloidosis[271] is a rare cause of a diffuse fine reticular pattern. In fact, this is possibly the most rare of the pulmonary manifestations of amyloidosis.[618] Amyloidosis should be suspected in patients with multiple myeloma and a slowly progressive interstitial pattern, but care must be taken in this setting to rule out both opportunistic infections and drug reactions.

Drug reactions, particularly to cytotoxic agents such as bleomycin and busulfan, should be suspected when a patient receiving one of these agents develops a diffuse fine reticular pattern.

SUMMARY

1. A fine reticular or linear pattern with Kerley's A and B lines is specific for interstitial disease.

2. One of the earliest steps in evaluating a fine reticular pattern is to determine whether the process is acute or chronic.

3. The most common acute cause of the pattern is interstitial edema, which should be divided into cardiac and noncardiac edema on the basis of cause.

4. Other radiologic signs of cardiac pulmonary edema include cardiomegaly, prominence of upper lobe vessels, constriction of lower lobe vessels, loss of definition of vessels, pleural effusion, perihilar haze, and air-space consolidations.

5. Viral, mycoplasma, and *Pneumocystis carinii* pneumonias are the other major causes of an acute interstitial pattern.

6. Chronic pulmonary edema is most commonly associated with mitral stenosis and, rarely, with left atrial myxoma. These may be distinguished by cardiac ultrasound examination.

7. Clinical correlation is essential for evaluating chronic causes of a fine reticular pattern. Biopsy is usually not necessary in rheumatoid arthritis, scleroderma, silicosis, asbestosis, tuberous sclerosis, and lymphangiomyomatosis.

8. The most important reason for lung biopsy in patients with a known primary malignancy or lymphoma and who exhibit a fine reticular pattern is to exclude an opportunistic pneumonia.

9. It is important not to assume that a chronic, fine reticular pattern is due to fibrosis. Even when biopsy confirms the diagnosis of a disease that may ultimately lead to fibrosis, such as sarcoidosis, the pattern may be due to an extensive inflammatory reaction rather than fibrosis.

10. Some of the diagnoses considered in Chart 18–1 must be confirmed by biopsy. These are UIP, DIP, LIP, lymphangiectasis, eosinophilic granuloma, and sarcoidosis.

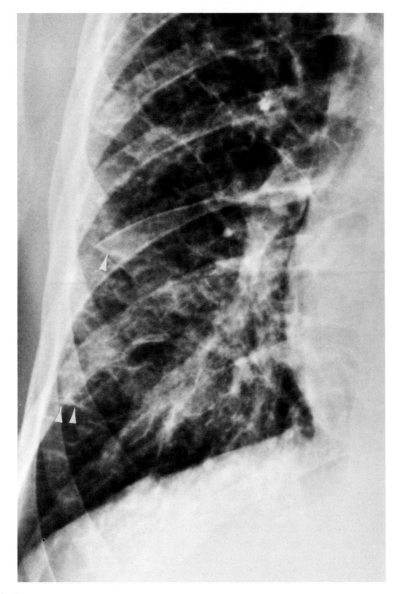

FIG 18-3

Case of mycoplasma pneumonia illustrates Kerley's B lines *(arrowheads)*. These lines are typically in the costophrenic angles and perpendicular to the pleura. (Case courtesy of Peter Dempsey, M.D.)

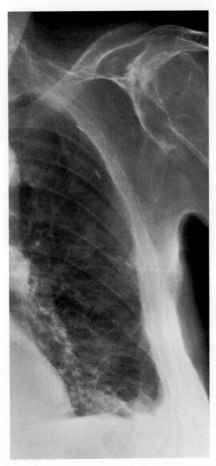

FIG 18–4
The combination of a fine reticular pattern that is most severe in the bases with pleural thickening and advanced destructive arthritis of the shoulder is diagnostic of rheumatoid disease.

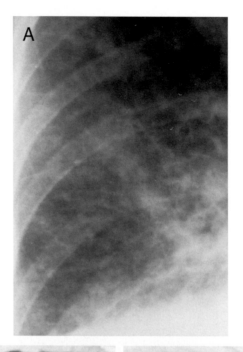

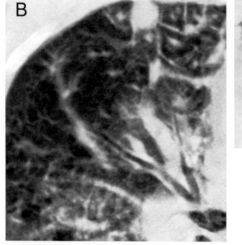

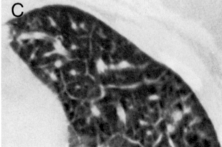

FIG 18–5

A, Coned view of the right lower thorax of a patient with prior breast cancer shows a peripheral reticular pattern that appears more confluent centrally. The left lower chest was partially obscured by the heart but had a similar appearance. **B,** HRCT section of the right middle lobe shows peribronchial thickening, peripheral reticular opacities, and an anterior subpleural nodule. **C,** HRCT section coned to the anterior portion of the left upper lobe shows thickening of the interlobular septae. This is the typical appearance of interstitial spread of metastatic cancer. HRCT often shows a combination of reticular opacities with thickening of the septal tissues and nodules.

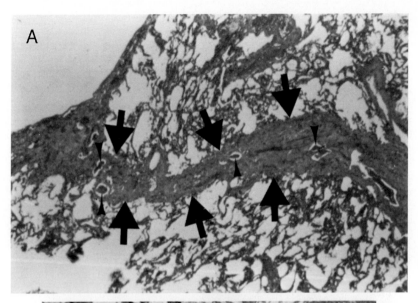

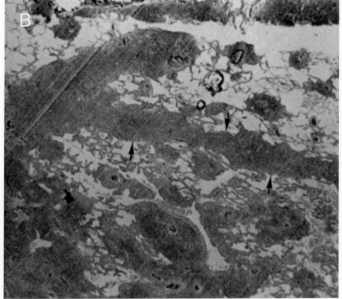

FIG 18–6
A, Lymphangitic metastases *(small arrowheads)* often lead to extensive thickening of interlobular septa *(large arrows).* Some thickening is the result of a desmoplastic reaction (fibrosis). Tumor appears to fill the lymphatic channels. **B,** Lymphoma has thickened the interlobular septum *(arrows)* and spread through the perivascular interstitium. This would account for the radiologic appearance of a fine reticular pattern with Kerley's lines. (**B** only, from Reed JC, Madewell JE: The air bronchogram in interstitial disease of the lungs. *Radiology* 1975; 116:1–9. Used by permission.)

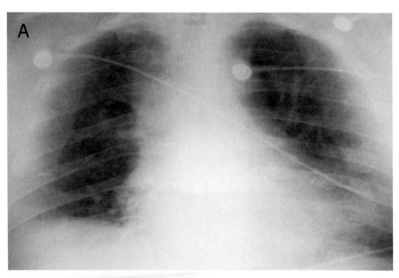

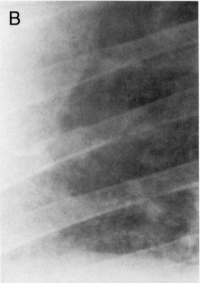

FIG 18–7
A, UIP causes peripheral basilar fine reticular opacities with volume loss. **B,** Coned view of the right lower lobe better shows the diffuse disease, but characterization of the pattern is difficult when there is volume loss and crowding of the abnormal opacities.

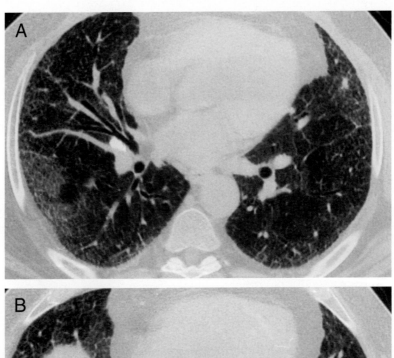

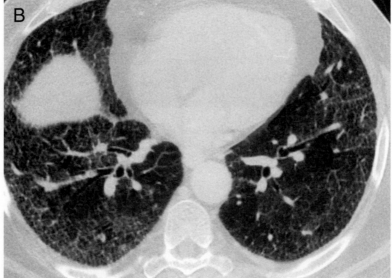

FIG 18–8
A, HRCT image taken above the diaphragm in the patient discussed in Figure 18–7 shows a peripheral distribution of a diffuse fine reticular pattern with an area of ground-glass opacity in the periphery of the right lower lobe. **B,** Another HRCT image taken at the level of the diaphragm shows more-extensive peripheral fine reticular opacities. This is a characteristic appearance of UIP on HRCT.

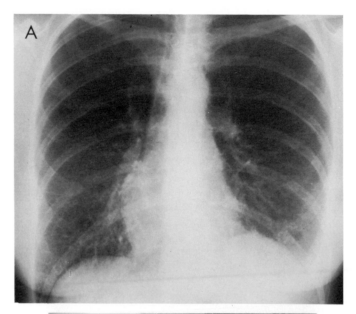

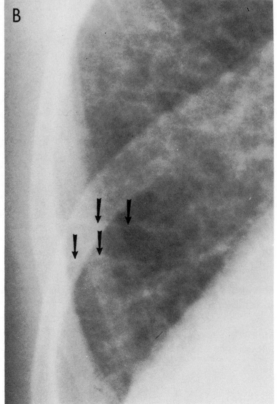

FIG 18–9
A, Lymphangiomyomatosis is a rare cause of a reticular pattern, which is typically associated with pleural disease including either recurrent pleural effusion or pneumothorax. **B,** Interstitial character of disease is confirmed by identification of Kerley's B lines *(arrows).*

ANSWER GUIDE

LEGENDS FOR INTRODUCTORY FIGURES

FIG 18–1
A fine reticular pattern is confirmed by identifying Kerley's B lines, which appear as thin linear opacities in the periphery of the lung, extending to the pleura. These lines result from thick interlobular septa. This patient had interstitial edema caused by congestive heart failure.

FIG 18–2
A, Combination of fine reticular pattern in the bases, cardiac enlargement, fluid in the minor fissure, and congestion of upper lobe vessels is the classic appearance of interstitial pulmonary edema secondary to congestive heart failure. **B,** Follow-up examination of case illustrated in **A,** after therapy, reveals complete resolution. Comparison with previous normal or follow-up films is often helpful in perceiving abnormalities and further confirms the transient character of the process.

ANSWERS

1, a; 2, a; 3, a, b, d, e; 4, c.

CHAPTER 19

Coarse Reticular Opacities (Honeycomb Lung)

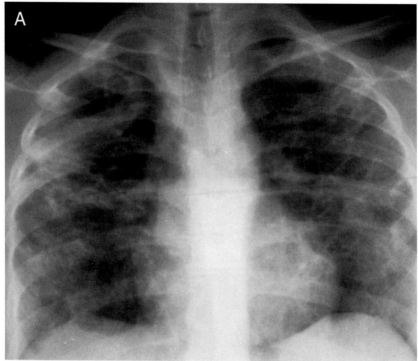

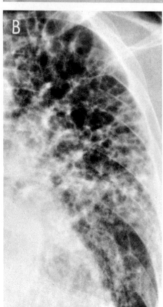

FIG 19–1

QUESTIONS

1. Refer to Figure 19–1, *A* and *B*. The term *honeycomb lung* indicates which one of these processes?
   a. Emphysema.
   b. Cystic bronchiectasis.
   c. Interstitial emphysema.
   d. End-stage interstitial fibrosis.
   e. None of the above.

2. Which one of the following diagnoses is least likely in the cases shown in Figure 19–1, *A* and *B*?
   a. Lymphangitic metastases.
   b. Sarcoidosis.
   c. Asbestosis.
   d. Usual interstitial pneumonia.
   e. Rheumatoid lung.

3. Basilar distribution of the interstitial disease is commonly expected in which of the following entities?
   a. Asbestosis.
   b. Usual interstitial pneumonia.
   c. Scleroderma.
   d. Silicosis.
   e. Eosinophilic granuloma.

CHART 19–1.
Coarse Reticular Opacities (Honeycomb Lung)

I. Collagen vascular diseases
   A. Rheumatoid lung[553]
   B. Scleroderma
   C. Dermatomyositis[546]
   D. Ankylosing spondylitis (upper lobe)[54,658]
II. Inhalation
   A. Pneumoconiosis[194]
      1. Silicosis
      2. Asbestosis[37]
      3. Berylliosis
   B. Chemical inhalation (late)[193]
      1. Silo-filler's disease
      2. Sulfur dioxide
      3. Other noxious gases
   C. Allergic alveolitis (e.g., farmer's lung)[456,516,592]
   D. Oxygen toxicity
   E. Chronic aspiration (e.g., lipid pneumonia) (usually localized)[486]
III. Inflammation
   A. Sarcoidosis[260]
   B. Eosinophilic granuloma[486]
IV. Drug reaction[14]
   A. Nitrofurantoin
   B. Methotrexate
   C. Hexamethonium
   D. Busulfan

(Continued.)

CHART 19–1.   (cont.).

  E. Cyclophosphamide (Cytoxan)
  F. Bleomycin
  G. Amiodarone
 V. Idiopathic
  A. Usual interstitial pneumonia[78,109,193]
  B. Desquamative interstitial pneumonia[78]
  C. Tuberous sclerosis
  D. Lymphangiomyomatosis[326]
  E. Neurofibromatosis (very rare)[486]

DISCUSSION

 Honeycomb lung is characterized by coarse reticular interstitial opacities with intervening lucencies that appear as cystic spaces.[196] The feature of cystic spaces distinguishes honeycomb lung from the fine reticular opacities described in Chapter 18. The typical appearance of a honeycomb lung is shown in Figure 19–1, *A* and *B*. Diseases that produce honeycomb lung tend to be diffuse, although the degree of involvement is frequently not uniform. The cystic spaces of honeycombing are pathologically different from true cavitary lesions in that they do not result from necrosis (Fig 19–2). They are radiologically recognizable by their large number and the associated reticular opacities. Furthermore, these lucencies should not be confused with those seen in emphysema (see Chapter 22), which have a different pathogenesis. Emphysema involves tissue destruction without fibrosis, while honeycombing involves tissue destruction by retracting fibrosis. Honeycombing has also been called paracicatricial emphysema because the cystic spaces develop from retracting fibrosis, but honeycombing is not an obstructive airway disease. HRCT (Fig 19–2, *A*) of honeycombing fibrosis shows thick-walled cystic spaces that correlate with the appearance of gross pathologic specimens or low-power microscopic sections (Fig 19–2, *B*). HRCT should reliably differentiate the thick-walled spaces caused by honeycombing from emphysema, which causes spaces that lack walls. HRCT also provides a map of the distribution of the honeycombing and often permits the radiologist to determine a specific etiology.[465]

 Recognizing the honeycomb pattern is helpful in narrowing the differential diagnosis for fine reticular interstitial opacities. As previously suggested, the honeycomb appearance indicates end-stage scarring of the lung with revision of the pulmonary architecture by fibrosis. (Answer to question 1 is *d*.) Therefore, serial films may reveal progression from a fine interstitial pattern to honeycombing. This is often the case in the pneumoconioses. Additionally, identification of the cystic spaces of honeycomb lung permits exclusion of other causes of reticular opacities such as acute pulmonary edema, viral pneumonia, mycoplasma pneumonia, lymphangitic spread of carcinoma, lymphoma, and LIP. (Answer to question 2 is *a*.) Honeycomb lung also has grave prognostic implications, since the cystic spaces are due to end-stage, irreversible scarring.

 Cystic bronchiectasis (Fig 19–3) sometimes produces a radiologic appearance of coarse irregular opacities with intervening cystic spaces that resemble honeycombing fibrosis.[491] Bacterial, viral, and tuberculous pneumonias may all cause bronchial wall necrosis with late scarring and bronchiectasis, but this necrosis rarely causes diffuse bronchiectasis that would be confused with honeycombing fibrosis. The late stages of cystic fibrosis do, however, produce diffuse disease with extensive scarring.[543] The scarring of cystic fibrosis is caused by recurrent pneumonias that complicate the chronic problems of thick mucus and impaired bronchial clearance. The radiologic appearance differs from the primary interstitial diseases that cause lung fibrosis by the presence of perihilar bronchial thickening. Additionally, since cystic fibrosis is an obstructive bronchial disease, there is often increased lung volume, in contrast with restrictive scarring from the fibrotic interstitial diseases that reduce lung volume.

Collagen Vascular Diseases

Rheumatoid arthritis and scleroderma are the collagen vascular diseases that are most likely to result in end-stage scarring of the lung.

The characteristic radiologic appearance of rheumatoid interstitial disease changes with the stage of the disease. In the earliest stages there is congestion of the alveolar capillaries, edema of the alveolar walls, and lymphocytic infiltration. There may even be an alveolar fibrinous exudate. This leads to the radiologic appearance of patchy areas of air-space consolidation (multifocal ill-defined opacities). The patchy alveolar opacities usually resolve and are followed by the development of a fine interstitial pattern that histologically consists mainly of histiocytes and lymphocytes. At this intermediate stage, the radiologic appearance is that of a fine reticular pattern or reticulonodular pattern. As the disease progresses, the cellular infiltrate is gradually replaced by fibrosis that tends to destroy the alveolar walls and distal bronchioles, leading to the cystic spaces of honeycomb lung. There is a definite tendency for this interstitial reaction to be localized in the bases of the lungs. Since rheumatoid interstitial disease is a restrictive lung disease, there may be evidence of pulmonary volume loss with elevation of both leaves of the diaphragm; this may occur even when the patient attempts to inspire deeply. Clinically the patient usually has the characteristic joint involvement of rheumatoid arthritis. However, rheumatoid lung disease rarely occurs before the development of the characteristic joint disease. The pulmonary symptoms may be nonspecific and include cough, dyspnea, and even cyanosis. The dyspnea often exceeds what might be expected from the physical signs and radiologic findings.

Scleroderma (progressive systemic sclerosis) is another collagen vascular disease that frequently produces interstitial fibrosis and honeycomb lung. As in rheumatoid arthritis, there is a tendency for the interstitial fibrosis to have a basal distribution (one answer to question 3 is *c*); also, the early phases of scleroderma may produce patchy air-space consolidations, which may be recurrent, followed by the development of a fine reticular interstitial pattern. Histologically there may be prominent alveolar capillaries and thickened cellular alveolar walls. This process is gradually replaced by fibrosis, which progresses from a fine reticular to a honeycomb pattern. The air-filled cystic spaces left by retracting fibrosis tend to be in the bases of the lung. This peripheral distribution helps to distinguish honeycomb lung from bronchiectasis, which is more severe in the central portions of the lung.

Other clinical signs of progressive systemic sclerosis are often present and confirm the diagnosis. These include skin changes, soft tissue calcifications, disturbances of esophageal motility, and dilation of the esophagus. Radiologically, an upper gastrointestinal tract series may demonstrate both esophageal dilation and decreased motility, as well as the characteristic small bowel dilation.

In general, symptoms of progressive systemic sclerosis include weight loss, slight productive cough, progressive dyspnea, and low-grade fever. However, dyspnea is rarely found at first admission and usually occurs late in the disease. Half of patients with pulmonary symptoms also have dysphagia accompanied by substernal and epigastric pain related to the esophageal involvement.

The other collagen vascular diseases, including systemic lupus erythematosus and dermatomyositis, less frequently involve the lungs and rarely progress to the degree of interstitial fibrosis required for development of the honeycomb appearance.

A coarse reticular interstitial pattern may also occur as a result of hypersensitivity to such drugs as nitrofurantoin, methotrexate,[575] hexamethonium, methysergide (Sansert), cyclophosphamide (Cytoxan), busulfan, amiodarone,[451] and bleomycin.[260] Reaction to these agents usually produces interstitial cellular infiltrates and is reversible. The common radiologic manifestation of this type of reaction consists either of fine reticular opacities or multifocal consolidations. When the reaction is progressive and chronic, it may lead to fibrosis and true honeycombing. Clinical correlation is obviously necessary for a diagnosis of drug reaction. Nitrofurantoin is an antibiotic used for urinary tract infections and may be easily overlooked as an etiologic agent in progressive interstitial disease. Since the cancer chemotherapeutic agents, including methotrexate, busulfan, cyclophosphamide, and bleomycin, are immunologic suppressants, it is necessary to distinguish drug reactions from opportunistic infection. Opportunistic infections would be unlikely to result in the pattern of honeycombing.

Inhalational Diseases

The confirmation of pneumoconiosis as a cause of honeycomb lung is best achieved by clinical correlation, but the radiologic appearances of this condition, particularly when serial films are examined, may be quite distinctive. Asbestosis, for example, produces a basilar distribution that may progress from a fine reticular interstitial pattern to a coarse interstitial pattern with honeycombing. The basilar distribution has been emphasized by the classic description of a "shaggy heart." (One correct answer to question 3 is *a*.) The basilar reticular or honeycomb pattern is also frequently associated with pleural thickening and may even be associated with pleural calcification. Therefore, a combination of basilar interstitial disease, pleural thickening, and calcification is virtually diagnostic of asbestosis.

Most cases of asbestosis are easily confirmed by a clinical history of asbestos exposure; however, some patients may have been subjected to significant asbestos exposure from unrecognized sources. The most common sources of asbestos exposure include asbestos mills, shipyards, and plumbing, pipe fitting, insulation, and automobile brake lining work. Exposure is not limited to the industrial worker; asbestosis can also occur in members of the asbestos worker's family. In particular, spouses are exposed to asbestos in the worker's dust-contaminated clothing.

Silica is another inorganic compound that may result in extensive interstitial disease. The radiologic manifestations of silicosis are more varied than those of asbestosis. The diagnosis of silicosis is also reviewed in the chapters on fine nodular patterns, fine reticular patterns, hilar adenopathy, and large mass lesions.

The largest population of patients with exposure to silica comes from coal-mining areas. There has been considerable controversy about the classification of pneumoconiosis and silicosis in coal workers. Histologic evidence suggests that the progressive interstitial fibrosis that leads to extensive scarring and revision of the pulmonary architecture (honeycomb lung) is due primarily to silica exposure. Other components of coal dust, such as anthracotic carbon pigments, excite very little histologic reaction and are therefore not the source of the severe reactions seen in honeycombing fibrosis. Other sources of silica exposure include quarry working, sandblasting, and gem polishing. Since honeycomb lung is a late stage of silicosis, serial roentgenograms are particularly important in documenting its progression. A fine interstitial nodular pattern or a fine reticular interstitial pattern may precede the appearance of the honeycomb lung. Furthermore, hilar and mediastinal lymphadenopathy may also be associated with silicosis. Although there may be associated pleural thickening, pleural calcification does not occur in silicosis; this is an important difference from asbestosis. Another radiologic feature helpful in distinguishing silicosis from asbestosis is the predominant upper lobe distribution of silicosis,[239] whereas asbestosis has a basilar distribution.

Chemical inhalation does not rapidly lead to end-stage scarring of the lung, but patients who have had either massive or recurrent exposures to nitrogen dioxide (silo-filler's disease), sulfur dioxide, chlorine, phosgene, cadmium, or other noxious gases may experience extensive parenchymal scarring with revision of the architecture and resultant honeycombing fibrosis.

Allergic alveolitis is another inhalational disease that may lead to honeycombing fibrosis.[516,592] The pathogenesis of allergic alveolitis is in marked contrast to the diseases caused by exposure to metal and more closely resembles that of the collagen vascular diseases. Injury first occurs at the alveolar capillary level and results in localized alveolar edema, which may resolve with no significant residual effect. However, as exposure to the offending allergen continues, the patient may develop chronic changes, the ultimate effect being honeycombing fibrosis. A model for allergic alveolitis is farmer's lung disease, an allergy to a fungus that grows in hay. A large variety of fungi have been identified that may provoke a similar allergic reaction. Other sources of this type of reaction include saw mills (maple bark disease), sugar mills (bagassosis), bird excrement (bird-fanciers' disease), and cork (suberosis). Air-conditioning systems may also be a source of these offending but noninvasive fungi. The diagnosis of allergic alveolitis as a cause of chronic lung disease frequently requires considerable detective work on the part of the clinician.

Oxygen toxicity is another form of inhalational disease that may lead to extensive interstitial scarring. This is probably best known for its occurrence in the pediatric age group; however, it may also occur as a complication of oxygen therapy in any age group and as a complication of any severe pulmonary illness requiring prolonged concentrated oxygen therapy. Many patients who are clinically diagnosed as having ARDS ultimately have extensive interstitial fibrosis with revision of pulmonary architecture that is in large part due to oxygen toxicity. Oxygen toxicity does occasionally differ significantly from the other causes of interstitial fibrosis in that the fibrosis appears to improve slowly over a period of months.

Chronic aspiration, particularly of mineral oil, may also lead to interstitial fibrosis. This fibrosis tends to be a localized rather than a diffuse process. It most commonly involves the dependent portions of the lung. The right middle lobe is not a rare location. A history of mineral oil use should suggest the diagnosis.

Inflammatory Diseases

Sarcoidosis[260] and eosinophilic granuloma[486] are the most common inflammatory diseases to produce true honeycomb lung. As mentioned earlier, honeycombing as a complication of tuberculosis, rather than true honeycombing, is most often the result of tuberculous bronchiectasis.

In the case of sarcoidosis, a small percentage of patients who develop pulmonary disease with interstitial nodules or fine reticular interstitial disease will have progression of their interstitial disease with replacement of the granulomas by fibrosis (Fig 19–4). This has the effect of revising the pulmonary architecture through retracting fibrosis, in a manner similar to that seen in the collagen vascular diseases, inhalational diseases, and the idiopathic group of diseases to be discussed later in this chapter. Some of the cystic spaces resulting from sarcoidosis may be quite extensive, and may even suggest the presence of cavities. However, pathologic documentation of necrotic cavities in sarcoidosis is extremely rare. Most patients who develop large cystic spaces in the end stage of sarcoidosis have retracting fibrosis with exaggerated revision of the normal pulmonary architecture. Serial roentgenograms are particularly helpful in evaluating these patients. Such late end-stage findings are usually preceded by some classic findings, including hilar adenopathy and an interstitial nodular or fine reticular interstitial pattern (see Chapters 11, 17, and 18). The classic description of sarcoid involvement of the lung involves regression of the hilar adenopathy as the interstitial disease progresses. However, the coexistence of hilar adenopathy and extensive interstitial disease still favors the diagnosis of sarcoidosis. In fact, associated hilar adenopathy is particularly helpful in the radiologic distinction of sarcoidosis from eosinophilic granuloma.

Eosinophilic granuloma, like sarcoidosis, is an idiopathic inflammatory process. Initially there is extensive infiltration of the lung with histiocytes and eosinophils; the radiologic result is a coarse, ill-defined nodular pattern. In the early phases of this disease, the pattern may gradually resolve as the size of the nodules decreases. As the disease progresses, the nodular appearance may be completely replaced by a fine reticular pattern. As the histiocytic and eosinophilic cellular response is replaced by fibrosis, the fibrosis retracts, producing thick, coarse reticular opacities and cystic spaces, and therefore qualifying as a cause of honeycomb lung. As mentioned in the discussion of sarcoidosis, these spaces are rarely true cavities; they are typically due to destruction of lung parenchyma by the retracting fibrosis (paracicatricial emphysema). The presence of hilar adenopathy at any time during the course of the interstitial disease is strong evidence against the diagnosis of eosinophilic granuloma. Additionally, there is a tendency toward an upper lobe distribution, which may help distinguish eosinophilic granuloma from a number of other entities considered in this differential. In fact, the costophrenic angles are the last parts of the lung to be involved in eosinophilic granuloma.[337]

In 1953 Lichtenstein suggested that "histiocytosis X should include Letterer-Siwe disease, Hand-Schüller-Christian disease, and eosinophilic granuloma."[486] Although these three conditions are histologically related, because histiocytes are the dominant cell type in each, they are clinically quite different. Letterer-Siwe and Hand-Schüller-Christian disease occur in infants and children and follow a more severe, often fatal course. In contrast, eosinophilic granuloma tends to occur most frequently in people between the ages of 15 and 40 years and has a comparatively mild course. In about 25% of patients, the honeycomb lung of eosinophilic granuloma is accompanied by pneumothorax, presumably owing to rupture of some of the cystic spaces.

Idiopathic Diseases

Usual interstitial pneumonia is possibly the most common cause of honeycomb lung, but the radiographic and even the histologic findings are not always specific (see Chart 18–4 for histologic differential diagnosis). The initial injury is at the alveolar capillary wall, with episodes of active alveolitis that may cause a pattern of basilar ground-glass or air-space opacities, followed by a progressive development of a peripheral basilar reticular pattern. (One correct answer to question 3 is *b.*) The disease ends in severe scarring with revision of the pulmonary architecture. The radiologic appearance is a pattern of coarse, disorganized reticular opacities with cystic spaces. Honeycombing occurs in about 50% of cases of UIP. This extensive fibrosis also leads to severe volume loss that is radiographically apparent in as many as 45% of cases. Because UIP is a slowly progressive disease, it must be emphasized that the histologist may appreciate revision of the pulmonary architecture and report honeycombing by biopsy at a time when the radiograph appears to have only minimal abnormality. Carrington et al.[78] reported that 7.6% of patients with UIP may have a normal radiograph. HRCT permits earlier diagnosis of fibrosis and may detect active alveolitis even after development of honeycombing (Fig 19–5). HRCT often shows a nonuniform patchy peripheral distribution that is diagnostic and correlates with the histologic hallmarks of UIP.[428] Mediastinal adenopathy is not an expected plain film finding in patients with UIP and should be considered evidence to consider other causes such as sarcoidosis, but it has been reported as an infrequent CT observation.[44]

Desquamative interstitial pneumonia is another idiopathic interstitial disease that occasionally ends with honeycombing fibrosis.[78,193] However, severe honeycombing fibrosis is a less-frequent complication of DIP than of UIP, occurring in only 12.5% of cases. Likewise, severe lung volume loss is less frequent in DIP (23%) than in UIP (45%). On the other hand, areas of patchy air-space consolidation (see Chapter 16) are more common in DIP. These opacities are frequently basilar. Histologically, DIP is characterized by a massive filling of air-spaces by polygonal mononuclear cells. The exact relationship of DIP and UIP has not been determined, but some authors believe that DIP is one manifestation of the early phases of UIP. Perhaps more important, however, are the prognostic differences between the two diseases. The 10-year mortality is 30% in DIP and 71% in UIP. Also, DIP responds to steroid therapy much more frequently than does UIP.

Tuberous sclerosis is another idiopathic disease that may lead to extensive interstitial scarring with the appearance of honeycombing.[326] This entity is best suggested in the presence of other signs of tuberous sclerosis, particularly when there is involvement of the brain, kidney, skin, and bones. Pulmonary manifestations of tuberous sclerosis are relatively rare, but when present they tend to dominate the clinical picture. Tuberous sclerosis is another interstitial disease that is associated with pneumothorax, which is presumably due to rupture of the cystic spaces.

Lymphangiomyomatosis is a rare cause of a honeycomb appearance that may have a distinctive clinical presentation.[326] As with many other entities in this differential, the honeycombing may be preceded by a fine reticular interstitial pattern identified by the presence of Kerley's B lines. The associated findings include recurrent pleural effusion and pneumothorax. In addition, lymphangiomyomatosis has been reported only in young and middle-aged women who have respiratory symptoms of gradually progressive dyspnea. This disease is frequently aggravated by hormone therapy, and particularly birth control pills. It is postulated that lymphangiomyomatosis may represent a forme fruste of tuberous sclerosis. In fact, rather than fibrosis, there is extensive smooth muscle proliferation in the interstitium that contributes to the revision of the pulmonary architecture.

In contrast to UIP and DIP, lymphangiomyomatosis is not a typical restrictive disease. The cystic lesions may lead to air trapping, resulting in normal or even increased lung volume. High-resolution CT is reported to yield a characteristic appearance in lymphangiomyomatosis when compared with the other causes of honeycomb lung. It is a cystic process with thin walls, in contrast to the thick fibrotic walls of the cystic spaces seen in UIP.[45]

Neurofibromatosis is another rare cause of honeycombing fibrosis. However, this diagnosis should be considered only in the presence of other signs of neurofibromatosis.[486,491]

SUMMARY

1. The term *honeycomb lung* indicates interstitial fibrosis.

2. The radiologic appearance of honeycombing fibrosis may be mimicked by severe cystic bronchiectasis, particularly in patients with cystic fibrosis or tuberculous bronchiectasis.

3. Honeycombing fibrosis results in revision of the pulmonary architecture, with cystic spaces that are not consistent with the diagnosis of pulmonary interstitial edema, lymphangitic metastases, or acute viral pneumonia. Therefore, such common causes of interstitial disease can essentially be ruled out by correct identification of the pattern.

4. Distribution of the disease is extremely important in considering the differential. For example, an exclusively peripheral location of the cystic spaces in honeycombing fibrosis makes exclusion of cystic bronchiectasis more simple.

5. A basilar distribution is suggestive of asbestosis, scleroderma, rheumatoid lung, UIP, or DIP.

6. An upper lobe distribution is suggestive of silicosis, eosinophilic granuloma, or tuberculous bronchiectasis.

7. Clinical correlation frequently confirms the diagnosis of a collagen vascular disease such as rheumatoid arthritis, scleroderma, or drug sensitivity.

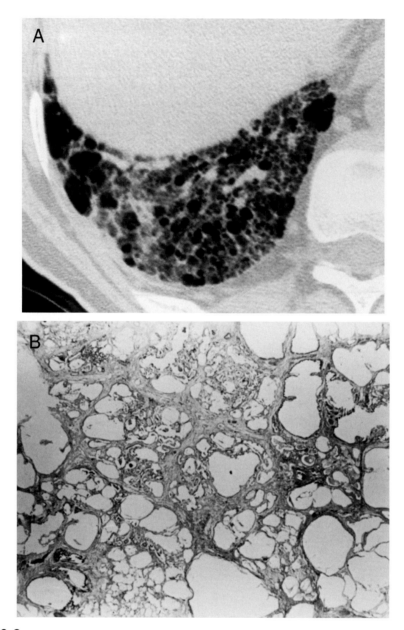

FIG 19–2
A, High-resolution CT of this patient with UIP shows coarse reticular opacities with a disorganized pattern and cystic spaces. This appearance of thick-walled spaces is the result of retracting fibrosis. The thick fibrotic walls distinguish this from emphysema. **B,** This low-power microscopic section from another case shows how idiopathic fibrosis can extensively revise the pulmonary architecture. Thick septations between spaces produce a radiologic appearance of coarse reticular opacities. Spaces have formed as the result of destruction of normal alveolar walls by retracting fibrosis. These spaces may become very large and may be radiologically confused with cavities. HRCT reliably correlates with this appearance.

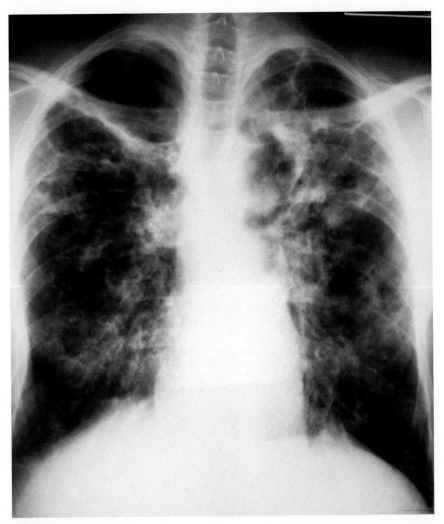

FIG 19–3
Severe diffuse cystic bronchiectasis, as seen in adults with cystic fibrosis, causes coarse reticular scarring with multiple cystic spaces. Associated bronchial thickening around the hilum and increased lung volume distinguish this appearance from honeycombing fibrosis.

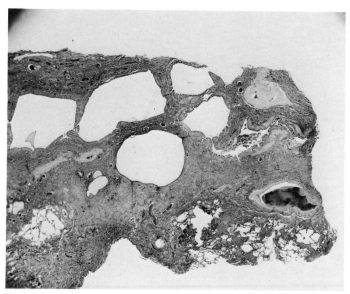

FIG 19–4
In late stages of sarcoidosis, interstitial granulomas may be replaced by fibrosis. Cystic spaces must not be confused with cavities. Even very large spaces are the result of destruction of lung by retracting fibrosis and are therefore a manifestation of honeycombing.

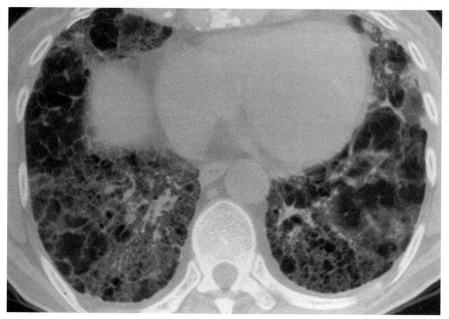

FIG 19–5
The HRCT of a case of UIP shows advanced revision of the pulmonary architecture with coarse reticular opacities and thick-walled cystic spaces. The peripheral ground-glass opacities in the posterior peripheral areas of both lungs suggest continued active alveolitis.

ANSWER GUIDE

LEGEND FOR INTRODUCTORY FIGURES

FIG 19–1
A, Sarcoidosis is illustrated by a diffuse bilateral coarse reticular pattern. **B,** Another case of advanced sarcoidosis illustrates a combination of coarse reticular opacities and intervening lucencies known as honeycomb lung. The lucencies accentuate the coarse reticular pattern.

ANSWERS

1, d; 2, a; 3, a, b, c.

CHAPTER 20

Solitary Pulmonary Nodule

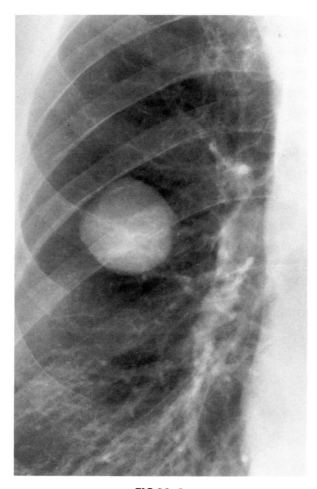

FIG 20–1

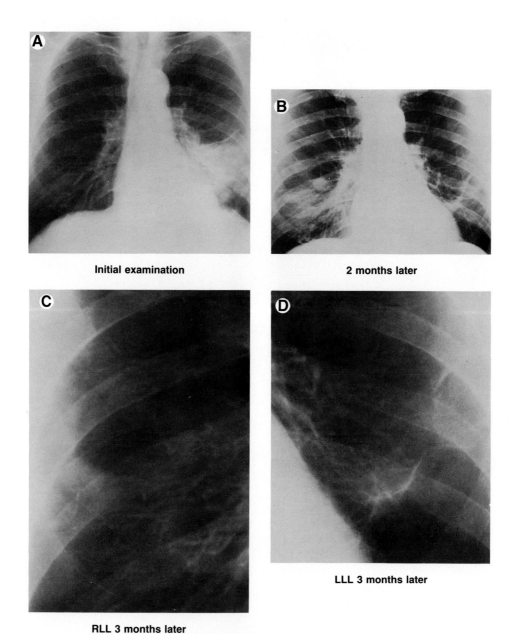

Initial examination

2 months later

RLL 3 months later

LLL 3 months later

FIG 20–2

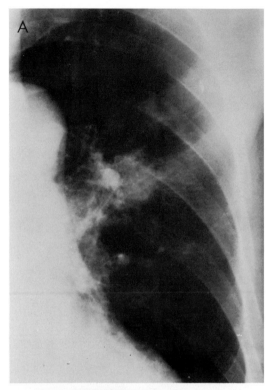

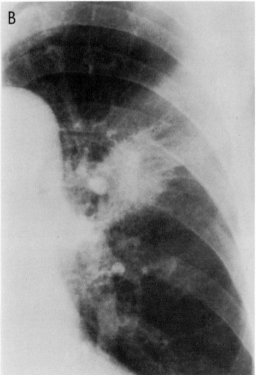

FIG 20–3

QUESTIONS

1. Refer to Figure 20–1. Which of the following is the least likely diagnosis?
   a. Bronchial carcinoid.
   b. Metastasis.
   c. Hamartoma.
   d. Lymphoma.
   e. Granuloma.
2. Serial films (Fig 20–2, *A–D*) revealing the development of a sharply defined nodule (Fig 20–2, *C*) are consistent with which of the following diagnoses?
   a. Nocardiosis.
   b. Epidermoid carcinoma.
   c. Infarct.
   d. Cryptococcosis.
   e. Bronchioloalveolar cell carcinoma.
3. The changing pattern illustrated by the films in Figure 20–3, *A* and *B,* is virtually diagnostic of which of the following?
   a. Tuberculoma.
   b. Infarct.
   c. Hamartoma.
   d. Primary carcinoma.
   e. Metastatic carcinoma.
4. Which one of the following features of a peripheral nodule would be most diagnostic?
   a. Spiculated borders.
   b. Air bronchograms.
   c. Central calcification.
   d. Central cavitation.
   e. Eccentric calcification.

CHART 20–1.
Most Likely Causes of Solitary Nodule

  I. Mimicking opacities
    A. Artifacts (e.g., button, snap)[491]
    B. Nipple shadow
    C. Skin and subcutaneous lesions (e.g., mole, neurofibroma, lipoma)
    D. Pleural lesions (loculated effusion or pleural mass)
  II. Infections
    A. Histoplasmosis[104,216]
    B. Tuberculosis
    C. Coccidioidomycosis
    D. Organizing pneumonia
 III. Neoplasms
    A. Malignant
       1. Primary lung tumor (Chart 20–2)[47,98,200,257]
       2. Metastasis[213,344]
    B. Benign (less common)[375]
       1. Hamartoma
       2. Arteriovenous malformation[137]
 IV. Vascular
    A. Infarct

(Continued.)

CHART 20–2.
Solitary Pulmonary Nodule or Mass

I. Neoplastic
   A. Malignant
      1. Primary carcinoma of the lung (see Chart 20–2)[47,98,195,200,257,499,501,564]
      2. Metastasis (e.g., kidney, colon, ovary, testis, Wilms' tumor, sarcoma)[213,344]
      3. Lymphoma[502]
      4. Primary sarcoma of lung
      5. Plasmacytoma (primary or secondary)
   B. Benign[375,493]
      1. Hamartoma
      2. Chondroma
      3. Arteriovenous malformation
      4. Lipoma (usually pleural lesion)
      5. Amyloidosis[271]
      6. Leiomyoma
      7. Hemangioma
      8. Intrapulmonary lymph node
      9. Endometrioma
      10. Fibroma
      11. Neural tumor (schwannoma and neurofibroma)
      12. Paraganglioma (chemodectoma)
      13. Inflammatory pseudotumor (fibroxanthoma, histiocytoma, plasma cell granuloma, sclerosing hemangioma)
II. Inflammatory
   A. Granuloma
      1. Tuberculosis[412]
      2. Histoplasmosis[104,216]
      3. Coccidioidomycosis
      4. Cryptococcosis (torulosis)[217,252,400]
      5. Nocardiosis[522]
      6. Talc
      7. *Dirofilaria immitis* (dog heartworm)
      8. Gumma
      9. Atypical measles infection
      10. Sarcoidosis[458]
      11. Q fever[407]
   B. Abscess
   C. Hydatid cyst (fluid-filled)
   D. Bronchiectatic cyst (fluid-filled)
   E. Fungus ball
   F. Organizing pneumonia (atypical measles pneumonia,[669] cytomegalic inclusion virus)[480]
   G. Inflammatory pseudotumor[143,375]
   H. Bronchocele[354] and mucoid impaction[417]
   I. Intrapulmonary lymph node[323]
III. Vascular
   A. Infarct (organizing)[21,244,276]
   B. Pulmonary vein varix or anomaly[40]
   C. Rheumatoid nodule
   D. Wegener's granulomatosis
   E. Arteriovenous malformation
   F. Pulmonary artery aneurysm (Behcet disease)[7,441]
IV. Developmental
   A. Broznchogenic cyst (fluid-filled)[487]
   B. Pulmonary sequestration[610]

(Continued.)

CHART 20–2 (cont.)
Solitary Pulmonary Nodule or Mass

 V. Inhalation
    A. Silicosis (conglomerate mass)[648]
    B. Mucoid impaction (allergic aspergillosis)
    C. Paraffinoma (lipoid granuloma)
    D. Aspirated foreign body
 VI. Other
    A. Hematoma
    B. Extramedullary hematopoiesis
    C. Emphysematous bulla (fluid-filled)
    D. Thrombolytic therapy[76]
    E. Mimicking opacities[491]
      1. Fluid in interlobar fissure
      2. Mediastinal mass
      3. Pleural mass (mesothelioma)
      4. Chest wall opacities (nipple, rib lesion, skin tumor)
      5. Artifacts
    F. Post-transplant lymphoproliferative disorder[129,248]

CHART 20–3.
Solitary Pulmonary Nodule in Childhood*

 I. Neoplasms
    A. Malignant
      1. Metastasis (neuroblastoma, Wilms' tumor, Ewing's sarcoma, osteosarcoma)
      2. Primary carcinoma (exceedingly rare)
      3. Blastoma[245]
    B. Benign
      1. Arteriovenous malformation
      2. Hamartoma
      3. Hemangioma
 II. Inflammatory
    A. Granuloma
    B. Organizing pneumonia (especially atypical measles pneumonia)
 III. Developmental
    A. Bronchopulmonary sequestration
    B. Bronchogenic cyst

*Modified from Young LW, Smith DI, Glasgow LA: Pneumonia of atypical measles, *AJR* 1970; 110:439–448.

CHART 20–4.

Classification of Primary Carcinoma of the Lung*
  I. Squamous cell carcinoma (30%–40%)
     A. Well differentiated
     B. Moderately differentiated
     C. Poorly differentiated
 II. Adenocarcinoma (25%–30%)
     A. Well differentiated
     B. Moderately differentiated
     C. Poorly differentiated
III. Bronchioloalveolar cell carcinoma (subtype of adenocarcinoma)
 IV. Large cell undifferentiated carcinoma (10–15%)
  V. Small cell undifferentiated carcinoma (20%)
 VI. Typical carcinoid (low grade malignant tumor 5% metastasize to lymph nodes)
VII. Atypical carcinoid tumor (malignant tumor with prognosis similar to other non-small cell tumors)
VIII. Adenoid cystic carcinoma (uncommon malignant tumor)
 IX. Mucoepidermoid carcinoma (uncommon malignant tumor)
  X. Multicomponent tumors (adenosquamous or small cell adenocarcinoma)

---

*Modified from Haque AK: Pathology of carcinoma of lung: an update on current concepts, *J Thorac Imaging* 1991;7(1):9–20.

CHART 20–5.
TNM Definitions of Primary Tumor*

TX   Tumor proven by the presence of malignant cells in bronchopulmonary secretions but not visualized radiographically, or any tumor that cannot be assessed, as in a retreatment staging.
TIS Carcinoma in situ.
T1   A tumor that is 3 cm or less in greatest dimension, surrounded by lung or visceral pleura, and without evidence of invasion proximal to a lobar bronchus at bronchoscopy.
T2   A tumor more than 3 cm in greatest dimension, or a tumor of any size that either invades the visceral pleura or has associated atelectasis or obstructive pneumonitis extending to the hilar region. At bronchoscopy, the proximal extent of demonstrable tumor must be within a lobar bronchus or at least 2 cm distal to the carina. Any associated atelectasis or obstructive pneumonitis must involve less than an entire lung.
T3   A tumor of any size with direct extension into the chest wall (including superior sulcus tumors), diaphragm, or the mediastinal pleura or pericardium without involving the heart, great vessels, trachea, esophagus, or vertebral body, or a tumor in the main bronchus within 2 cm of the carina without involving the carina.
T4   A tumor of any size with invasion of the mediastinum or involving heart, great vessels, trachea or carina, esophagus, vertebral body, or presence of malignant pleural effusion.

---

*Modified from Mountain CF: A new international staging system for lung cancer, *Chest* 1986; 89 (4 Suppl): 225S–233S.

CHART 20–6.
TNM Definitions: Nodal Involvement*

N0   No demonstrable metastasis to regional lymph nodes.
N1   Metastasis to lymph nodes in the peribronchial or the ipsilateral hilar region, or both, includ-
     ing direct extension.
N2   Metastasis to ipsilateral mediastinal lymph nodes and subcarinal lymph nodes.
N3   Metastasis to contralateral mediastinal lymph nodes, contralateral hilar lymph nodes, or ipsi-
     lateral or contralateral scalene or supraclavicular lymph nodes.

*Reprinted from Mountain CF: A new international staging system for lung cancer, *Chest* 1986; 89 (4 Suppl):
225S–233S.

CHART 20–7.
TNM Definitions: Distant Metastasis*

M0   No (known) distant metastasis.
M1   Distant metastasis present—specify site(s).

*Reprinted from Mountain CF: A new international staging system for lung cancer, *Chest* 1986; 89 (4 Suppl):
225S–233S.

CHART 20–8.
Stage Grouping of TNM Subsets*

Occult Carcinoma	TX	N0	M0
Stage 0	TIS	N0	M0
Stage I	T1	N0	M0
	T2	N0	M0
Stage II	T1	N1	M0
	T2	N1	M0
Stage IIIa	T3	N0	M0
	T3	N1	M0
	T1–3	N2	M0
Stage IIIb	Any T	N3	M0
	T4	Any N	M0
Stage IV	Any T	Any N	M1

*Reprinted from Mountain CF: A new international staging system for lung cancer, *Chest* 1986; 89 (4 Suppl):
225S–233S.

DISCUSSION

   Perception is the first challenge confronting the radiologist in the evaluation of
the solitary pulmonary nodule.[17,62,221,254,312,335,426,525,662] Good radiographic technique is required for detection of a pulmonary nodule. The standard chest exam
includes a frontal film, taken with the patient facing the film and the x-ray beam
passing posterior to anterior, and a lateral film, which is taken with the patient's
left side against the film (left lateral). Both films should be taken at maximum inspiration. There is no perfect technique for all cases. The ideal frontal film pro-

vides good detail of the central structures (e.g., the trachea, carina, thoracic spine, and intervertebral disk). This permits visualization of the normal vasculature posterior to the heart and thus makes possible detection of nodules posterior to the heart and posterior to the domes of the diaphragm. Adequate penetration of these dense areas must be done while preserving good visualization of the peripheral vascular markings. This cannot be accomplished with low peak kilovoltage (kVp) techniques. For example, a PA chest film taken at 60 kVp will be too light for adequate evaluation of the mediastinum if the lungs are properly penetrated. With the low-kVp technique, the lungs will be black if the mediastinum and the left lower lobe are adequately penetrated. Low-kVp chest film technique would therefore require two films so that the radiologist can detect both peripheral and central tumors. This has led to the development of higher kVp techniques for standard chest radiography. It is generally agreed that the optimal kVp is in the range of 120 kVp to 150 kVp. This is a major limiting feature of portable chest radiography, which makes it inadequate for exclusion of pulmonary nodules. The only major disadvantage of the high-kVp techniques is the reduced visibility of calcium.

A major problem affecting radiologic visualization of a peripheral lesion is superimposition of the normal structures, including ribs, costal cartilage calcifications, clavicles, scapula, heart, pulmonary vessels, aorta, and great vessels (Fig 20–4, *A* and *B*). Even the dome of the diaphragm may obscure posterior lower lobe nodules. Variations in position of the nodule caused by differences in respiratory effort also account for some of the variations in visibility of small nodules. For example, a small difference in inspiratory effort may result in a 5 mm nodule projecting over a rib or an interspace. Other characteristics of the nodule that affect detectability include shape and borders. A well-circumscribed nodule has better contrast with the surrounding lung and is therefore more visible than a poorly marginated tumor, which has borders that imperceptibly fade into the surrounding lung. Lung cancers are frequently ill-defined because they are locally invasive and may also incite a desmoplastic reaction. This may further reduce the radiologic detectability of early lung cancers, particularly those that are less than 1 cm.

Many of the special techniques in chest radiology are in fact used in an attempt to overcome the problem of superimposed shadows and render the nodule more conspicuous. Special procedures that may be used in the evaluation of a nodule include oblique films, fluoroscopy, apical lordotic films, stereoscopic films, and CT. Ordinarily a suspicious opacity must be detected on the plain film before a special procedure can be used successfully. Detection of less-visible lesions is improved by knowing in which anatomical areas lesions are likely to be obscured.[586] Comparisons are vital. For example, crossing ribs are seen many times on a single film and therefore provide an opportunity for comparison. A slight increase in the opacity of one pair of crossing ribs should be carefully evaluated to rule out a superimposed nodule. The right and left pulmonary arteries should be symmetrically opaque. Asymmetric opacity at the junction of the costal cartilage and the rib must be carefully scrutinized. Lesions in the medial portions of the lung may be obscured by large vessels or the heart and may for this reason be more easily detected on the lateral film than on the PA film (Fig 20–5, *A* and *B*). Obvious abnormalities that may even be insignificant sometimes capture the viewer's attention and interfere with the detection of a subtle pulmonary nodule. Observers should make a conscious effort to complete the review of the film and avoid the phenomenon of satisfaction of search as a cause of missed abnormalities.[525] Comparisons with prior examinations enhance the visual search and may also make subtle or minimal opacities more detectable.

Even with optimal film techniques, careful review of films, and application of a thorough knowledge of the anatomic structures that may obscure small pulmonary nodules, radiologic detection of the solitary nodule continues to be a difficult challenge for the radiologist.[462] The reported error rate for the detection of early lung cancer has been reported to vary between 20% and 50%.[662] Studies that were specifically designed for screening patients who were at high risk for lung cancer suggest that the error rate may be even higher. Muhm et al.[426] designed a study for screening cigarette smokers who were over age 45 with chest radiographs taken at 4-month intervals. The examinations were double read. The study included more than 4,000 patients and detected 92 lung cancers. Of these 92, 50 cancers presented as peripheral pulmonary nodules. The researchers reported that, in retrospect, 90% of the peripheral cancers were detectable on earlier films. Although 27 of the tumors had been visible for a year or less, 14 were identified between 12 and 24 months and 4 had been visible for more than 2 years. Woodring's review[662] of the pitfalls in the diagnosis of lung cancer reminds us that detectability of small pulmonary nodules requires good technique and careful review of the film and still depends on the size of the nodule. Kundel[335] reported that nodules less than 1 cm in size are not usually detected by plain film. Heelan et al.[254] suggested that the threshold nodule size for detectability of peripheral lung cancer is larger; they reported prospective detection from screening plain film to range from 0.7 cm to 9.4 cm nodule size, with an average size of 2.4 cm. Even with optimal radiographic technique and knowledge of the pitfalls in viewing a film, the radiologist faces the problem of calling insignificant opacities suspicious for cancer and at the same time continues to detect lung cancers that should have been detected on earlier film. When an abnormal nodular opacity is suspected, it is essential to select, from all of the available procedures, the least invasive and costly procedures required to confirm the presence of an early lung cancer.

When a nodule is suspected on a plain film, radiologic confirmation is the next step. Fluoroscopy is an underutilized but useful procedure for verifying the location of opacities that are identified on the plain film. This should easily permit recognition of superimposed structures such as artifacts and healed rib fractures. Repeat film with nipple markers should be obtained to evaluate nodules that project over the lower chest. Fluoroscopic spot films are also valuable for the detection of calcification. Since the routine plain film is obtained with a technique in the 120 kVp–140 kVp range, calcification of small nodules may not be obvious on the plain film. The optimal kVp for detection of calcium is approximately 68 kVp. When oblique films are used in the evaluation of peripheral nodules, the patient should be placed in a minimally oblique position (for example, 5°). Steep oblique positions, which are routinely used for cardiac fluoroscopy, are usually too steeply angled and result in a suspected nodule moving so far that it may be superimposed over the heart or spine, thus being imperceptible. For this reason, fluoroscopic spot films are the best technique for obtaining the optimal oblique position. Lordotic or reverse lordotic projections similarly may separate a questionable pulmonary nodule from overlying opacities. The use of the apical lordotic film for verifying suspected tuberculosis is excellent. However, apical tuberculous disease is usually in the posterior apical portions of the lung, which are well demonstrated on the apical lordotic film. Use of apical lordotic films in evaluation of possible apical nodule has received considerable criticism, primarily because the anterior portion of the lung is not completely visible on the apical lordotic film. If this modality is selected, an abnormal apical lordotic film may be acceptable proof of an apical mass, but a normal apical lordotic film must be accepted with reservations. The diagnostic value of the apical lordotic film is probably enhanced if the apical reverse lordotic film is performed at the same time. This has the effect of giving a more complete look at both the anterior and posterior portions of the lung, but CT is the most direct and valuable method of assessing a suspected apical lesion.

CT is currently the procedure of choice for confirmation and evaluation of a suspected pulmonary nodule[216] (Fig 20–6, *A* and *B*). It provides precise localization of the nodule and is reliable for detection of other radiologic features of the nodule, including calcification, cavitation, and spiculated borders.[543,679] CT should be done without intravenous contrast when the scan is performed for the detection of calcification. Tumors have been shown to take up iodinated contrast, whereas granulomas do not enhance.[593]

CT is also useful for detecting additional abnormalities (e.g., other nodules and hilar or mediastinal adenopathy). Identification of multiple nodules substantially alters the differential considerations, suggesting either metastases or multiple granulomas. Detection of enlarged hilar or mediastinal nodes in a patient with a solitary nodule would change the approach to both diagnosis and treatment, especially when a primary carcinoma is suspected. The presentation of a primary lung cancer as a solitary pulmonary nodule with adenopathy would indicate an advanced stage of the disease,[193] and fine-needle aspiration biopsy or mediastinoscopy and biopsy of nodes might be considered rather than biopsy and resection of the nodule.

Calcification is the most diagnostic feature of a pulmonary nodule. Central, laminated, or complete calcification is virtually diagnostic of a granuloma[580] (Fig 20–7, *A* and *B*). (Answer to question 4 is *c*.) Thin-section, HRCT is the procedure of choice for confirmation of benign calcification. Although concentric swirls of calcification in the center of the mass are virtually diagnostic of a granuloma, eccentric calcification in the periphery of a lesion should not be regarded as an indication of a benign process. Tumors occasionally arise around preexistent calcific scars, at times engulfing a previous granuloma. In such cases the calcification is most likely to be eccentric. Another explanation for eccentric calcification is reactivation of an old granulomatous process. In either case, the presence of a mass with eccentric calcification warrants further diagnostic evaluation. In the case of multiple pulmonary nodules, it must be emphasized that patients may have calcified granulomas and also develop carcinomas. Therefore, the presence of calcium in one nodule is meaningless with regard to the evaluation of a second nodule. The detection of minimal calcification in a mass must be cautiously interpreted. Microscopic calcifications in primary lung tumors and metastatic tumors, particularly from mucin-producing adenocarcinomas (Fig 20–8, *A* and *B*) and certainly from primary bone tumors, are not rare.[379] Calcification from metastases of osteosarcoma may be readily detected by conventional x-rays, but the microscopic calcifications seen in primary lung tumors are very rarely detectable by conventional radiography. Detection of minimal calcification by thin-section CT or CT with a reference phantom may lead to an incorrect diagnosis of a benign process.[313,594,629,678]

The following criteria are recommended for avoiding the potential pitfalls of thin-section CT: (1) Benign calcifications should extend over 10% of the cross-section area of the nodule. (2) The calcification must have a symmetric pattern of deposition (e.g., diffuse, laminated, or central nidus). (3) Benign nodules have smooth margins. (4) Benign nodules should not be larger than 3 cm in diameter. (5) Nodules meeting the preceding criteria should show no change in 24 months of follow-up.

Once the presence of a noncalcified nodule has been confirmed, such radiologic features as the borders and texture of the lesion should be characterized. The borders may be smooth, lobulated, ill-defined, or spiculated. Although the border characteristics are valuable, they are rarely reliable in making a definitive diagnosis. Nordenström[440] described the characteristic irregular, spiculated borders of a primary carcinoma of the lung as a "corona maligna"; however, he later modified this view and used the term "corona radiata" (Fig 20–9). Heitzman's[257] pathologic correlations of the irregular, spiculated border indicate that some of the spiculations are related to the spread of the tumor into the pulmonary parenchyma, whereas others represent fibrotic strands that presumably are part of the desmoplastic reaction to the tumor. He also observed that similar border characteristics may be seen in organizing processes, including organizing infections and infarcts. The corona radiata sign is therefore no longer regarded as pathognomonic of malignancy,[269] but it is nevertheless strongly suggestive of malignancy. The value of this sign is greatly enhanced by serial roentgenograms, since the organizing processes tend to become smaller and less spiculated as the inflammatory reaction around the resolving infection or infarct fades. This is in marked contrast to the changing border characteristics that are anticipated in a primary carcinoma of the lung. As the primary carcinoma of the lung grows, it continues to invade the surrounding parenchyma. The mass not only enlarges but becomes more irregular (more spiculated) and possibly even ill-defined (see Fig 20–4, A and B). Therefore, while the border characteristics may not be diagnostic on a single film, on serial films they may be virtually diagnostic.[501] The answer to question 3 is primary carcinoma, because of the increasing size and loss of definition of the border.

As indicated in the discussion of irregular, spiculated masses, a very smooth border is not typical of primary lung carcinoma, but this appearance should not be used to exclude the diagnosis. Well-differentiated adenocarcinomas and squamous cell tumors may present as well-circumscribed solitary nodules (Fig 20–10). In contrast, a sharply circumscribed nodule is the expected appearance for a solitary metastasis. Metastases are usually hematogenous implants. They are not locally invasive and maintain a sharply defined margin as they enlarge. Knowledge of a distant primary lesion requires consideration of metastasis. In such a case a sharply marginated nodule favors the diagnosis of metastasis, while an irregular border indicates a probable primary lung tumor. Bronchial carcinoids, which most frequently occur in the proximal bronchi, may also arise from more peripheral bronchi and present as solitary nodules. They are noninvasive tumors that have sharply defined borders. Benign tumors[375] such as hamartomas (see Fig 20–1) also have a sharp interface with surrounding lung, and granulomas become more sharply defined as the surrounding inflammatory reactions are replaced by fibrosis. In answer to question 1, lymphoma is a primary interstitial process that spreads through the lung, following the bronchovascular bundles and septal planes. Lymphoma is therefore not an expected cause of a well-circumscribed solitary pulmonary nodule. (Answer to question 1 is *d*.)

The texture of a nodule is most frequently described as homogeneous. It should be obvious that any of the causes of a solitary pulmonary nodule may present with a homogeneous nodule, but deviations from this homogeneous character do add diagnostic information to the radiologic appearance of the nodule. Intervening lucencies suggest either that the process is spreading through the lung in an infiltrative manner, leaving some aerated alveoli, or that central necrosis and cavitation may have occurred. This distinction may require CT for verification. Multiple small lucencies throughout the opacity are more in keeping with an infiltrative process such as a resolving pneumonia. However, caution is warranted in these cases since lymphomas and bronchioloalveolar cell carcinomas may spread in a very infiltrative manner, mimicking organizing pneumonias.

Demonstration of air bronchograms through the opacity might be considered to be a diagnostic feature in favor of an organizing process. However, it must be emphasized that bronchioloalveolar cell carcinoma and lymphoma[481,484] occasionally spread around the bronchi, leaving open, air-containing bronchi throughout the tumor. The air-bronchogram is therefore not a reliable feature for distinguishing tumor from organizing pneumonia. If the air bronchogram persists over a period of weeks, particularly after antibiotic therapy, the possibility of neoplasm must be ruled out by sputum cytology or biopsy.

As suggested in the discussion of border characteristics, the second most valuable step in the evaluation of the pulmonary nodule, after verification of the presence of the nodule, is the comparison of serial films.[98] It is absolutely imperative that any previous chest x-ray film be obtained for all patients with pulmonary nodules. A report of a previously normal chest x-ray is not adequate, since minimally perceptible nodules are frequently identifiable when films are reviewed in retrospect. Such a review makes is possible for the radiologist to document change in size of the nodule over time. In the case of a nodule that has decreased in size, it is possible to radiologically confirm the presence of a benign process, even in the absence of calcification. The radiologist's level of confidence should be particularly high when the nodule not only decreases in size but becomes more sharply defined (see Fig 20–2, *A–D*). Growth of a nodule is a more difficult problem.[200,201] Nathan[436] and Nathan et al.[437] emphasized the importance of evaluating the growth characteristics of a nodule. Growth rates are usually described in terms of doubling time. Collins et al.[98] indicated that a nodule must go through approximately 30 doublings to reach 1 cm in diameter and therefore become radiologically detectable. It has been estimated that bronchogenic carcinomas are present for 8 to 10 years in most patients before becoming radiologically detectable. Rate of growth is probably most useful in those cases in which an extremely rapid growth rate is observed. For example, the appearance of a sharply defined nodule measuring 1 to 2 cm in diameter after 1 month provokes the following considerations.

Very rapid growth would be atypical for a bronchogenic carcinoma and might even seem unlikely to result from metastases. Some very aggressive anaplastic metastatic tumors do grow rapidly, such as osteosarcomas and choriocarcinomas.

History of a known primary tumor usually confirms these possibilities. Other considerations in the diagnosis of rapidly appearing nodules include infectious processes[138] and infarcts. Very rapid growth of a pulmonary nodule has been observed with so-called "round" pneumonias caused by pneumococcal infection, and with unusual organisms, such as the Pittsburgh pneumonia agent.[138] The diagnosis of infarction implies the diagnosis of pulmonary embolism, but pulmonary vasculitis (Wegener's granulomatosis) may also result in necrosis of lung and therefore in the rapid appearance of a pulmonary nodule. When old films reveal that the nodule was preceded by a larger, ill-defined opacity, the diagnosis of an organizing process is confirmed. The radiologic combination of bilateral basilar subsegmental opacities and pleural effusion prior to the development of a sharply defined nodule is strong evidence in favor of an infarct. (Answer to question 2 is *c*.) Clinical and laboratory correlation is necessary to distinguish an organizing pneumonia from an infarct.

Nodules that enlarge very slowly are more likely to be benign.[375] For example, a nodule that doubles its diameter every 18 months suggests a benign tumor such as hamartoma. Additional diagnostic considerations for slow-growing nodules include bronchial carcinoids, inflammatory pseudotumors, and even granulomas.[216] It may be surprising to list granulomas as nodules that may grow, but granulomas form as an immunologic response to an organism. If this immunologic response continues to be active, there will be continued accumulation of inflammatory cells and even fibrosis around the periphery of the nodule. Therefore, granulomas are occasionally observed to increase slowly in size. Unfortunately, slow growth makes absolute exclusion of a malignant tumor difficult, since low-grade adenocarcinomas and metastases such as renal cell carcinoma may enlarge very slowly. Despite the lack of specificity in growth rate, some authors[437] have advocated following solitary nodules with serial films. These authors have emphasized that distant metastases from slowly growing tumors are slow to develop, while if the development of a metastatic tumor is fast, the patient will not benefit from immediate resection of the primary tumor. Nathan[436] cited a series of patients in whom there was a 6- to 12-month delay in surgery for peripheral nodular bronchogenic carcinoma, and indicated that their survival was longer than that of patients who underwent surgery with less than 6 months delay. On the basis of the studies cited, Nathan[436] suggested that a nodule can be safely followed for 2 weeks and, if no growth is demonstrated, a subsequent examination can be performed after 4 weeks. He further suggested that if no change is detected at that time, progressive x-ray films can be obtained at increasing intervals for up to 2 years. When no change is detected after 2 years, it is generally recommended that the lesion be considered benign. On the basis of these and similar studies, a nodule that is documented to be stable for 2 years is usually labeled benign, while growth is a generally accepted indication for biopsy.

Rarely, pulmonary nodules may assume a characteristic shape. Extremely lobulated masses are not expected with either metastases or primary carcinomas, since both tend to grow concentrically. An extremely lobulated opacity is much more in keeping with the diagnosis of an organizing mass, which may have bands of fibrosis that have the effect of pinching off lobulations. A very lobulated mass may also result when a tumor contains multiple cell types growing at different rates. An example of the latter is the hamartoma, but the presence of a lobulated mass is not adequately specific to confirm the diagnosis. Calcification is an additional radiologic finding that may be present in as many as 20% of hamartomas. In contrast to typical granulomatous calcifications, hamartomatous calcifications consist of rings and dots that may be scattered through the bulk of the tumor. This calcification resembles the calcified cartilaginous matrix seen in cartilaginous bone tumors and is, in fact, ossification of the cartilage contained within the tumor. As with granulomas, hamartomatous calcification may be confirmed with CT scan.

Arteriovenous malformation (AVM) is another lesion that may assume a characteristic shape. The presence of large vessels entering a nodule should strongly suggest the diagnosis of AVM. The definitive diagnostic procedure is a contrast-enhanced CT scan (Fig 20–11). It is imperative to rule out the possibility of AVM prior to either transbronchial or percutaneous biopsy.

Pulmonary vein varix[40] is another vascular abnormality that may present as a solitary opacity. The lesions occur in the medial portion of the lung just before the veins enter the left atrium. Fluoroscopy is a valuable procedure for their identification, since Valsalva maneuver will demonstrate a change in size, indicating a vascular mass. Pulmonary arteriography distinguishes pulmonary vein varix from AVM.

Clinical Correlations

The value of clinical correlation for evaluating the solitary pulmonary nodule is obviously limited, since many of the entities listed in Chart 20–3 have no characteristic clinical presentation and therefore require biopsy for diagnosis. Specific clinical backgrounds, however, are strongly suggestive and even diagnostic of some of these entities. For example, a primary carcinoma elsewhere suggests metastatic disease.

Of the benign neoplasms, pulmonary AVMs may have either strongly suggestive or diagnostic clinical associations. Patients with pulmonary AVMs may have dyspnea, hemoptysis, cyanosis, clubbing of the fingers, and polycythemia, which may be followed by congestive heart failure. Physical findings may include extracardiac humming sounds or bruits over the chest, particularly when the fistulas are large. Arteriovenous fistulas most commonly occur spontaneously, but they have also been reported to occur as sequelae to trauma. In addition, there are hereditary associations. The clinical syndrome of Rendu-Osler-Weber disease is characterized by multiple AVMs that may involve the skin, lips, gastrointestinal tract, urinary bladder, nose, central nervous system, and lungs. The most severe and life-threatening complication of pulmonary AVM is hemorrhage. In fact, hemoptysis is a common presentation. Associated gastrointestinal bleeding or signs of intracranial bleeding should suggest Rendu-Osler-Weber disease.

Absolute certainty in the clinical diagnosis of inflammatory nodules is rarely possible, but certain settings permit an accurate diagnosis. The common granulomatous infections, mainly tuberculosis, histoplasmosis, and coccidioidomycosis, are occasionally diagnosed as the cause of a nodule on the basis of clinical and laboratory data. When a patient is seen during the acute exudative phase of the disease, and serial roentgenograms reveal that the exudate has organized via the formation of a nodule, the etiology may be confirmed by growing the organism in culture from the acute exudate or by a definite rise in the patient's serologic titers. Cryptococcal infection is frequently an opportunistic infection that may require transbronchial, percutaneous, or open lung biopsy for diagnosis, but it may be associated with central nervous system symptoms, leading to a cerebrospinal fluid examination and identification of the infecting organism. *Nocardia* is another opportunistic organism that should be strongly considered when patients are known to be immunosuppressed, either for neoplastic disease or organ transplantation, and develop pulmonary nodules. The consideration of talc granuloma is largely reserved for drug abusers. In this clinical setting the development of either solitary or multiple pulmonary nodules is suggestive of septic emboli, which may frequently contain talc.

A pulmonary abscess is not clinically or radiologically suggested without evidence of a previous necrotizing pneumonia.

Age is a general clinical parameter that may be of considerable assistance in narrowing the differential diagnosis of a pulmonary nodule. Young et al.,[669] in their review of cases with atypical measles pneumonia, emphasized the more limited differential diagnosis of a solitary pulmonary nodule during childhood (Chart 20–3). They described a group of patients with an atypical form of measles characterized by a febrile illness with cough, headache, myalgias, abdominal pain, and a peripheral maculopapular rash. The rash was an inconsistent finding, making the diagnosis more difficult. A pneumonia developed in all of the patients, frequently associated with hilar adenopathy and pleural effusion. Resolution of the pneumonia was atypical in that a solitary pulmonary nodule was left as a residuum of the illness. The diagnosis of atypical measles was based on a rise in the hemagglutination inhibition and complement fixation titers of late convalescent sera. Young et al. emphasized that immunization for measles with inactivated virus vaccine preceded the atypical measles infection by a period of 3 to 4½ years.

Nodules that form as a result of an organizing infarct may be suspected in patients who have a preceding history of a pulmonary embolus weeks or months prior to the development of the nodule. This may be even more evident when the roentgenograms obtained during the period of the acute embolic episode show areas of increased radiologic opacity in the same area as the demonstrated pulmonary nodule. These nodules may safely be assumed to represent organized infarcts, and a more rigorous evaluation should not be necessary (see Fig 20–2).

Biopsy and Staging of Lung Cancer

After detection of a solitary pulmonary nodule and evaluation of all the discussed plain film features, comparison with prior film, and even HRCT, the etiology of a noncalcified solitary pulmonary nodule is often not confirmed. A biopsy procedure must be selected. Open lung biopsy should only be considered when there is a high probability of curative resection. Transbronchial biopsy is ideal for diagnosis of a central bronchial lesion, and image-guided percutaneous fine-needle aspiration biopsy is often the procedure of choice for peripheral nodules. The choice of fluoroscopic or CT guidance should be based on visibility and location of the nodule. Large peripheral nodules that are easily visualized may be more efficiently biopsied with fluoroscopic guidance, but precise localization of the needle is essential. CT provides the most accurate confirmation of needle position and is usually preferred for small nodules, especially when they are located near vascular structures. Cytologic evaluation should be done concurrently to ensure that the sample is diagnostic. The goal of the procedure is to provide the least-invasive technique for confirmation of suspected lung cancers and to provide an adequate specimen to permit the pathologist to distinguish small-cell carcinoma from non–small-cell carcinoma.

Prognosis and treatment of non–small-cell lung cancer is directly related to cell type (Chart 20–4) and stage at the time of diagnosis. The American Joint Committee on Cancer (AJCC) recommends staging of non–small-cell tumors according to the TNM system (Charts 20–5, 20–6, 20–7, and 20–8). Clinical staging is the best estimate of extent of tumor spread before any therapy and is often based on radiologic evaluations by plain film, CT, MRI, and radionuclide procedures including bone scans and positron emission tomography (PET) scans. The use of CT and MRI for lung cancer staging is controversial because neither modality provides tissue-specific information. Abnormalities are detected and evaluated primarily by size criteria. For example, hilar and mediastinal nodes may be measured in either short or long axis, but they are most often measured in their long axis. Nodes measuring more than 10 mm in long axis are usually defined as abnormal, but using this measurement has a sensitivity and specificity of only 65%. Recognizing this limitation, radiologists may find CT staging most useful for identifying those patients with very advanced disease and for determining the need for preoperative mediastinoscopy in patients who are candidates for surgical resection. Patients with negative CT for mediastinal adenopathy do not require mediastinoscopy, whereas patients with enlarged nodes should be preoperatively staged with biopsy confirmation.

Early studies evaluating PET suggest that it may be tissue specific for detection of regional and distant metastases. A solitary pulmonary nodule with no evidence of spread to regional nodes and no evidence of distant metastases is a Stage I tumor (TI, N0, M0).[453] Stage I tumors should be surgically resectable and have the best prognosis, with a 5-year survival of more than 50%. Patients with Stage IIIB tumors are rarely candidates for surgical resection, and patients with stage IV tumors present with distant metastases and should receive only palliative therapy, because their 12-month survival is less than 20%, and their 5-year survival approaches zero. Patients with Stage II and Stage IIIA tumors have evidence of local spread of tumor that may be extensive. These patients require careful staging to ensure an optimal treatment plan, which may include radical surgery, radiation therapy, and chemotherapy.

SUMMARY

1. Perception of the abnormality is the most important task of the radiologist in the management of the patient with a solitary nodule.

2. The optimal chest film is performed with high-kilovoltage techniques (120 kVp–150 kVp).

3. The only disadvantage of the high-kilovoltage technique is the decreased visualization of calcium. Calcium is best visualized at 68 kVp.

4. The differential diagnosis of a solitary nodule is lengthy, and the radiologist rarely makes a precise diagnosis.

5. Care must be taken to recognize artifacts, skin lesions (e.g., moles), rib lesions (e.g., fractures), calcified benign bone islands, and calcified granulomas.

6. Fluoroscopy is an expeditious way of localizing rib lesions and artifacts.

7. Examination of serial films is particularly useful for distinguishing pneumonias or infarcts from tumors. Infarcts regress in size; tumors grow.

8. Clinical correlation may confirm organizing infectious processes, infarcts, and metastases.

9. Pulmonary AVM and varix are suggested on the basis of shape and location. Confirmation may require pulmonary arteriography.

10. The ultimate diagnosis most commonly requires biopsy.

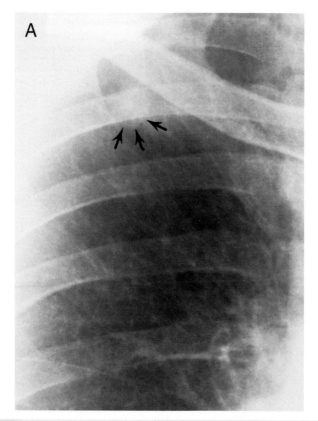

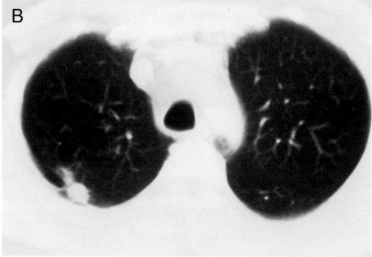

FIG 20–4
A, This peripheral lung cancer is minimally visible because of its size and position over a posterior rib. Note the rounded inferior border *(arrows).* **B,** CT confirms an irregular mass that extends to the pleura.

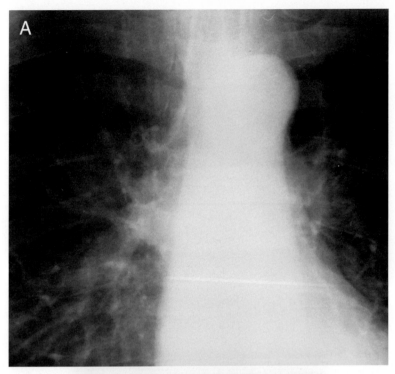

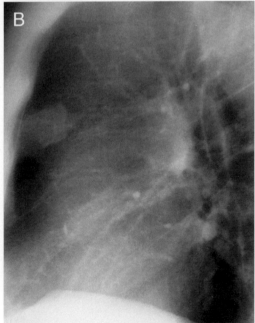

FIG 20–5
A, This central lung cancer projects over the right pulmonary artery and causes only a minimal change in opacity of the right hilum. This would have been missed if the exam had not included a lateral film. **B,** The corresponding lateral film shows an obvious mass in the retrosternal clear space. The lateral film is an essential part of the chest exam and often accounts for the detection of lung cancers that arise near the hilum or mediastinum.

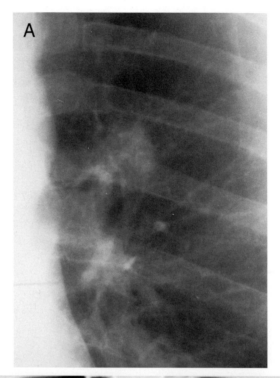

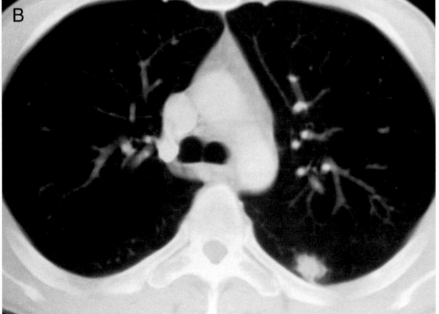

FIG 20–6
A, This poorly marginated opacity projects above the left hilum and is suggestive of a hilar mass. **B,** CT confirms the presence of a mass in the periphery of the superior segment of the left lower lobe, rather than the left hilum, as suggested by the plain film. CT is essential for confirmation and precise localization of suspected lung cancers.

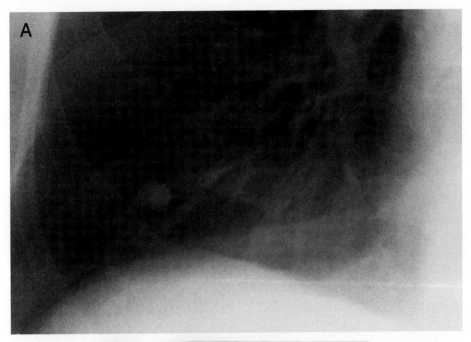

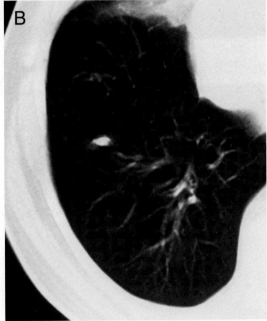

FIG 20–7
A, This right lower lobe nodule appears to be opaque, but the plain film is not adequate to confirm benign calcification. **B,** Thin-section CT is ideal for confirmation of central, laminated, or complete calcification of granulomas.

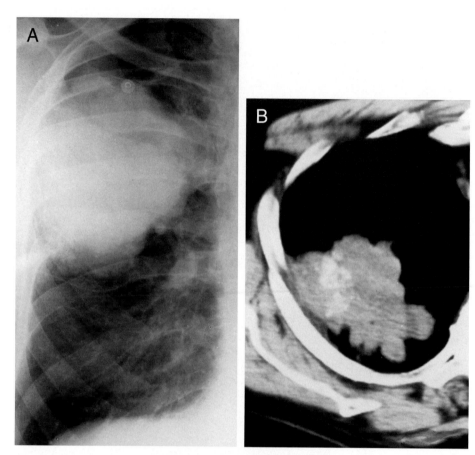

FIG 20–8
A, This large, lobulated adenocarcinoma appears to be homogenous on the plain film.
B, CT does show amorphous speckled areas of calcification in a large soft-tissue opacity mass. These calcifications should not be confused with the calcifications of a benign granuloma.

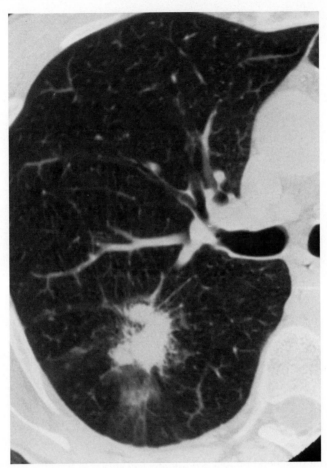

FIG 20–9
Spiculated masses have a high probability of malignancy. HRCT provides excellent characterization of the margins of this adenocarcinoma. The spiculations may represent either desmoplastic fibrosis or interstitial invasion by the tumor. Since inflammatory lesions and infarcts may cause spiculated masses, biopsy is required for diagnosis.

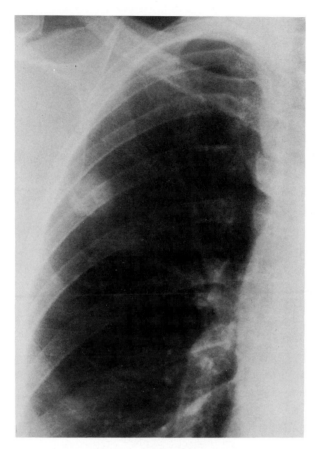

FIG 20–10
This very smooth peripheral nodule is a primary carcinoma of the lung. The smooth border raises the differential of primary vs. metastatic mass. Metastases are typically this smooth and would not be expected to produce the appearance seen in Figure 20–9.

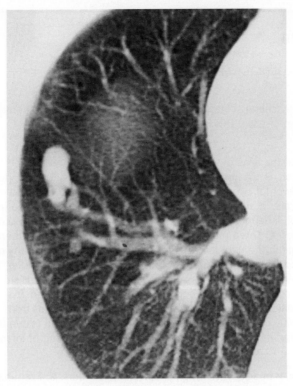

FIG 20–11
This arteriovenous malformation produced only a minimally visible nodular opacity on the plain film. Contrast-enhanced CT shows a contrasting nodule with direct connection with enhancing vessels and confirms the diagnosis.

ANSWER GUIDE

LEGENDS TO INTRODUCTORY FIGURES

FIG 20–1
This sharply circumscribed solitary pulmonary nodule requires consideration of both malignant and benign disease. This is a benign hamartoma.

FIG 20–2
A, PA film taken at the time of the patient's initial admission reveals left lower lobe air-space consolidation. **B,** PA film taken over 2 months after onset of the patient's illness reveals the left lower lobe air-space consolidation to have resolved, leaving linear opacities as residual scars. In addition, a new area of abnormality developed in the right lower lobe, consisting of ill-defined air-space consolidation and more-circumscribed opacities suggesting nodules. **C,** Three months after onset of the initial illness, there is a well-circumscribed nodule in the right lower lobe, which is consistent with any of the diagnostic possibilities considered in Chart 20–1. **D,** This is a coned view of the left lower lobe from the same film seen in **C.** The opacities in the left lower lobe are consistent with either linear scars or discoid atelectasis. When the sequence is considered, it should be obvious that the abnormalities considered in **C** and **D** are residual opacities from a process that has resolved, leaving linear scars and a solitary nodule. This is an example of pulmonary embolism. The residual nodule and linear opacities are the result of infarcts.

FIG 20–3
A, Note left perihilar opacity with irregular spiculated borders. **B,** Examination 5 months later revealed the opacity to be larger and more irregular. This is a classic growth pattern for primary carcinoma of the lung.

ANSWERS

   1, d; 2, c; 3, d; 4, c.

CHAPTER 21

Multiple Nodules and Masses

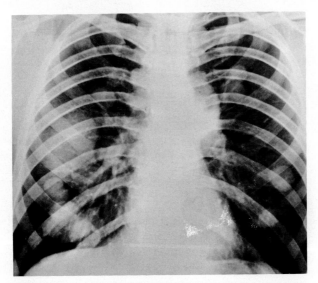

FIG 21–1

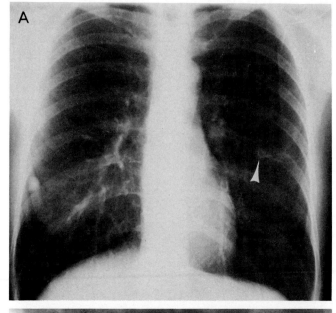

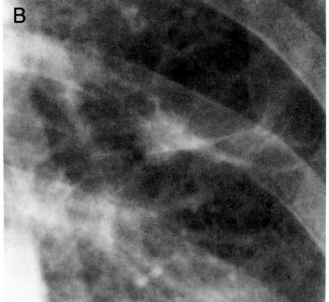

FIG 21–2

QUESTIONS

1. Figure 21–1 was the admission chest x-ray film of a 21-year-old man with a history of weight loss. Which of the following procedures would most likely determine the site of a primary tumor?
   a. Physical examination of the testis.
   b. CT scan of the pancreas.

c. Radionuclide bone scan.

d. CT scan of the brain.

e. CT scan of the chest.

2. Which of the following primary tumors is least likely to metastasize to the lung?

a. Melanoma.

b. Osteosarcoma.

c. Astrocytoma.

d. Adenocarcinoma of the colon.

e. Choriocarcinoma.

3. The patient with bilateral pulmonary nodules shown in Figure 21–2 most probably has:

a. Old calcified granuloma and carcinoma.

b. Metastatic osteosarcoma.

c. Histoplasmosis.

d. Metastatic melanoma.

e. Healed infarcts.

CHART 21–1.
Multiple Nodules and Masses With Sharp Borders

I. Neoplastic
    A. Malignant
        1. Metastases (kidney, gastrointestinal tract, uterus, ovary, testes; melanoma, sarcoma)
        2. Lymphoma[502]
        3. Post-transplant lymphoproliferative disorder[129,248]
    B. Benign
        1. Hamartoma[375,528]
        2. Arteriovenous malformation[277] or hemangioma[375]
        3. Amyloidosis[271,618]
        4. Pseudolymphoma[263]
II. Inflammatory
    A. Fungal[390]
        1. Histoplasmosis[306]
        2. Coccidioidomycosis[306]
        3. Cryptococcosis[217]
        4. Invasive aspergillosis[248]
    B. Nocardiosis[26,232]
    C. Tuberculosis[412] (typical and atypical)
    D. Parasites[370]
        1. Hydatid cysts[27]
        2. Paragonimiasis[289,291]
    E. Septic emboli
    F. Atypical measles[93]
    G. Inflammatory pseudotumors[375] (fibrous histiocytoma, plasma cell granuloma,[306] hyalinizing pulmonary nodules)
    H. Q fever[407]
III. Vascular
    A. Rheumatoid nodules and Caplan's syndrome[306]
    B. Wegener's granulomatosis and Wegener's variants[2,342,377]
    C. Organizing infarcts[21,244]
IV. Post-traumatic (organizing hematoma)[519]
V. Chronic renal failure (calcified nodules)[89]

DISCUSSION

One of the first decisions in the evaluation of the film showing multiple pulmonary opacities is to distinguish multiple areas of pulmonary infiltration from multiple nodules. The problems with identifying multiple areas of infiltration were considered in Chapter 16. A major criterion for distinguishing infiltrative lesions from nodules and masses is the border characteristic of the opacity. As a general rule, nodules or masses should be sharply defined from the surrounding lung parenchyma. Loss of definition of the border implies that the process is spreading into the lung parenchyma, either following interstitial planes or actually spilling into the alveolar spaces. Loss of definition is therefore more consistent with the concept of an infiltrative process. HRCT has been used to better characterize the borders of a variety of metastatic nodules and has shown that metastases may be locally invasive.[272] This would account for the phenomenon of nodules growing and becoming less circumscribed. Another radiologic characteristic that helps in the identification of nodules is homogeneity; that is, the opacity has neither aerated alveoli nor air-containing bronchi and therefore appears to be solid.

A second major problem confronting the radiologist in the evaluation of the patient with multiple pulmonary nodules is the perception of the nodules. Small peripheral pulmonary nodules are often not detectable on the plain film. These nodules are obscured by surrounding vascular opacities or may be incompletely surrounded by aerated lung. They are also obscured by overlying ribs. CT detects peripheral subpleural nodules and nodules obscured by the heart, mediastinum, and vessels. Spiral CT with a single-breath-hold technique reduces artifacts and has reduced the risk of missing small nodules that change position with respiratory motion. CT is currently the most-sensitive procedure available for detecting pulmonary nodules. By increasing the sensivity of the procedure, it has become the optimal technique for staging a variety of cancers, but as the sensitivity increases, the specificity decreases. While CT detects more metastatic nodules than the plain film, it also detects more benign nodules caused by granulomas and unrelated scars. The decision to perform a CT scan should be based on the primary diagnosis and the plan of therapy. When the plain films show multiple bilateral pulmonary nodules, the value of detecting an additional number of nodules depends on the mode of therapy planned for the patient. If the therapy will not be influenced by the detection of additional nodules, it is doubtful whether the more expensive and complicated procedure is justified. If resection of multiple nodules is contemplated, the value of detecting the additional nodules is obvious.

Neoplasms

From the preceding discussion, it should be apparent that metastatic disease is the most common cause of multiple pulmonary nodules in today's practice. The list of primary tumors that metastasize to the lung is long.[214,381] In most cases, multiple pulmonary metastases are detected after the primary lesion, thus making the presumptive diagnosis of metastases from the known primary lesion a very secure diagnosis (Fig 21–3). Although this is a reliable assumption for larger masses that are detected by plain film, very small occult opacities detected by CT may often represent benign nodules. These very small opacities must be cautiously evaluated when their detection may influence choices of therapy, sometimes even justifying biopsy. Multiple pulmonary metastases constitute a relatively unusual presenting complaint that is sometimes followed by an extensive search for an occult primary tumor. One primary tumor that is well known for this presentation is testicular carcinoma. When a young male patient's chest film shows multiple pulmonary nodules and masses of varying size, testicular carcinoma should be one of the first considerations. Physical exam may confirm the diagnosis, but detection of very small occult tumors often requires testicular ultrasound. Other primary tumors that may be occult but which metastasize to the lungs include melanoma, ovarian carcinoma, breast cancer, renal cell carcinoma, colon cancer, and other gastrointestinal tumors. Most other tumors that have a high rate of pulmonary metastases have local findings and are less likely to present as an occult primary. Spontaneous pneumothorax and multiple pulmonary nodules[111] together are an unusual combination that is nearly diagnostic of osteosarcoma (Fig 21–4), although it has been encountered with other tumors (e.g., Wilm's tumor).[309] This combination should suggest the diagnosis of osteosarcoma, but primary bone tumors are rarely occult. They usually cause pain and are diagnosed with plain films and combinations of CT, MRI, and radionuclide bone scans. Patients with primary bone tumors are more likely to have occult pulmonary metastases at the time of diagnosis. The unsuspected metastases may be diagnosed by plain film or may require CT. Some tumors that frequently metastasize to the chest often produce patterns other than nodules. Patients with late stages of pancreatic carcinoma frequently have malignant pleural effusions and pulmonary interstitial spread with either a reticular or fine nodular pattern, but they infrequently have multiple larger nodules and masses. Central nervous system tumors are distinctive for their rarity as a cause of metastases to the lung. Furthermore, the rare pulmonary metastases from these tumors apparently occur only after the blood-brain barrier has been violated. Of all the malignant conditions considered in Chart 21–1, lymphoma may be the least likely to present with multiple well-circumscribed masses. This is because lymphoma tends to be infiltrative and spreads along the alveolar walls and interlobular septae. Lymphoma, therefore, usually has a more ill-defined appearance. (Answer to question 1 is *a*, and question 2 is *c*.)

Benign neoplasms presenting as multiple masses are rare. The two such neoplasms best known for this presentation are multiple pulmonary hamartomas and multiple AVMs.[375] As mentioned in the discussion of solitary nodules, hamartomas occasionally have a characteristic cartilage calcification, but they more commonly appear as a homogeneous nodule, requiring biopsy confirmation for a specific diagnosis. Multiple AVMs may be even more characteristic than the solitary AVM, since there are more opportunities for the radiologist to identify the feeding and draining vessels. As with solitary lesions, the diagnosis may be strongly suggested by CT with identification of the vessels. The diagnosis of multiple AVMs may be further suggested by the family history. Hereditary telangiectasia (Rendu-Osler-Weber syndrome) is a rare autosomal dominant condition. Patients with this condition may have cyanosis, hemoptysis, and cerebrovascular accidents.[338]

Inflammatory Diseases

Histoplasmosis may be one of the most easily confirmed causes of multiple inflammatory nodules. A case of the epidemic form of histoplasmosis, with a chest film showing multiple ill-defined opacities during the acute stage of the disease, followed by healing of the nodules to well-circumscribed nodules, is the model for studying the evolution of multiple inflammatory nodules. This appearance may be even more specific when the nodules are subsequently noted to calcify. The diagnosis of histoplasmosis may be confirmed by the conversion of skin tests and by positive serologic studies for histoplasmosis. Coccidioidomycosis is another fungal disease that can occasionally be diagnosed during its acute phase, at which time the patient has a febrile illness associated with a flulike syndrome and chest roentgenography demonstrates multiple patchy opacities similar to those of bronchopneumonia. These opacities may resolve over a period of weeks or may undergo organization, leading to the pattern of multiple nodules. Some of the nodules may undergo central necrosis and subsequent cavitation. If the patient is in an endemic area and serologic tests demonstrate rising titers, the diagnosis is easily documented.

Cryptococcus is another fungal agent that may cause the formation of multiple pulmonary nodules. However, neither the clinical course nor serial x-ray films are adequate for confirming the diagnosis of pulmonary cryptococcosis. As in histoplasmosis and coccidioidomycosis, serial x-ray films may show patchy areas of ill-defined opacity similar to those in bronchopneumonia. This pattern may be followed by the development of nodules, but the clinical setting is rarely so characteristic as that seen in histoplasmosis and coccidioidomycosis. Short of lung biopsy, one associated finding that makes the diagnosis possible is the association of cryptococcal meningitis. Cryptococcosis should therefore be strongly considered in patients who are seen with multiple pulmonary opacities and central nervous system disturbances. This is best documented by demonstration of the fungus in cerebrospinal fluid. In contrast to histoplasmosis and coccidioidomycosis, cryptococcosis is most commonly encountered as an opportunistic infection in patients who are immunosuppressed.

Pulmonary nocardiosis is another infectious cause of pulmonary nodules that is rarely seen in the general population but is not rare in the immunologically compromised patient. The agent *Nocardia asteroides* is a soil contaminant that was once classified as a fungus but is currently classified as a gram-positive bacterium. The radiologic manifestations of pulmonary nocardiosis are, as in the other granulomatous diseases, predictably variable. Balikian et al.[26] described six cases with the following presentations: (1) a tiny solitary nodule, (2) multiple nodules, (3) cavitary pneumonias, (4) bilateral, patchy bronchopneumonias, (5) a subpleural plaquelike infiltrate, and (6) empyema. One of these patients even had a bronchopleural fistula. Therefore, multiple pulmonary nodules constitute only one of the manifestations of nocardiosis. The diagnosis is most appropriately suggested in the immunosuppressed patient and confirmed either by identification of the organism from sputum or fluid samples or by biopsy. The use of percutaneous needle biopsy and transbronchial biopsy has greatly increased the confirmation of this diagnosis. Since specific antibiotic therapy is essential for cure, an aggressive approach and early diagnosis are essential.

Tuberculosis is an uncommon cause of multiple pulmonary nodules. As in histoplasmosis, central calcification is one of the most diagnostic features of an old, healed tuberculous nodule. Calcification does not indicate a precise bacteriologic diagnosis, but it does indicate that the histology is one of a granuloma that has undergone central necrosis and calcification, thus limiting the differential to histoplasmoma vs. tuberculoma. A major problem in evaluating patients with known previous tuberculosis and multiple pulmonary nodules is identifying coexistent tumors. Since tuberculomas may vary in size and shape, and calcium may not be detectable in all of the nodules, the evaluation of old films is essential. A change in one of the nodules or the development of a new nodule indicates either reactivation of the tuberculosis or a new process, such as carcinoma. Because of the frequency of carcinoma arising around old tuberculous scars, even calcified nodules must be carefully evaluated. Eccentric calcification in a nodule is not adequate for confirming that the nodule is a completely benign process; neither can the coexistence of calcified and noncalcified nodules be accepted as evidence that all of the nodules are benign. The cases in Figures 21–2 and 21–5 illustrate this problem. In Figure 21–2, note that the right lower lobe nodule is densely calcified, while the nodule on the left lung is homogeneous and has irregular, spiculated borders suggestive of a primary carcinoma of the lung. (Answer to question 3 is *a*.)

Sarcoidosis is frequently described as having a nodular presentation, but the descriptive terminology must be carefully chosen. The fine miliary nodules (see Chapter 17) are not generally considered to represent the nodular form of sarcoidosis, and the larger opacities seen in sarcoidosis commonly have ill-defined borders that make them rather distinct from the pattern seen in patients with multiple metastases. This pattern is more like that discussed in Chapter 16. Occasional patients do have moderately discrete opacities that are the result of sarcoidosis (Fig 21–6, *A* and *B*). The histologic character of these nodules is somewhat variable. Heitzman[260] has shown that patients with sarcoidosis may have massive accumulations of interstitial granulomas that may account for the large opacities. These large accumulations of granulomas may understandably present in a more circumscribed manner than the obstructive pneumonia that was described in Chapter 16 as a cause of the ill-defined opacities more typical of sarcoidosis. The most diagnostic radiologic information is obtained by comparison with old films, which may reconstruct the course of a process that initially entailed bilateral and symmetric hilar adenopathy followed by the development of multiple pulmonary nodules. Again, there may be a marked disparity between the radiologic severity and the clinical severity of the disease, with the patient appearing to be relatively asymptomatic at a time when there may be many large opacities in the lung. This is very helpful in excluding metastatic and lymphomatous processes.

Parasites[370] as a cause of multiple pulmonary opacities are relatively uncommon in the United States but are of great importance in the worldwide population. The classic parasite to produce either single or multiple well-circumscribed pulmonary opacities is *Echinococcus granulosus* (dog tapeworm), which causes hydatid disease. Since hydatid disease results in the formation of fluid-filled cysts, the presentation may be that of multiple opacities; more commonly, some of the cysts will have drained their watery fluid, leading to the radiologic appearance of thin-walled circumscribed lucencies (see Chapter 24). On histologic examination, the wall of a hydatid cyst has three layers. The inner layer is a very thin unicellular layer from which arise the scolices; the middle layer is a laminated chitinous layer, which is the parasite (endocyst); while the third layer is a fibrous reaction of the host to the parasite. When a cyst develops a communication with a bronchus, the radiologic appearance will change. Introduction of air into the cyst causes separation of the fibrous and laminated layers of the cyst. A small amount of air between the two layers leads to a lucent crescent, or the air meniscus sign. This appearance might be mimicked by the development of a fungus ball in a pre-existing cavity, but examination of previous films should resolve this differential, because the previous existence of a homogeneous circumscribed opacity would be evidence against the diagnosis of a fungus ball. When the endocyst ruptures, the fluid drains into the tracheobronchial tree, leading to the radiologic appearance of an air-fluid level in a sharply defined lucency. After the fluid has partially drained, the laminated chitinous middle layer of the cyst separates from the fibrous layer and may appear to float in the remaining fluid. This radiologic presentation has been described as the "water lily" sign and is distinctive for hydatid disease. A history of having lived in an area of the world where hydatid disease is endemic is essential if the diagnosis is to be suspected. The incidence of the disease is particularly high in Russia, Eastern Europe, Italy, Greece, Iran, the Middle East, Spain, North Africa, Argentina, Uruguay, Australia, New Zealand, and Ireland. In North America the disease is seen mainly in Canada, Alaska, and the southwestern United States, particularly New Mexico, Arizona, and Nevada.

Paragonimiasis[289,291,445] is another parasitic disease that is reported to be the cause of multiple pulmonary opacities. Paragonimiasis is rare in the Western world but is encountered in patients who have traveled extensively. Elsewhere it is a widespread, endemic disease with a low mortality, occurring in Korea, Japan, China, the Philippine Islands, Indonesia, New Guinea, and Thailand. An African variety of paragonimiasis is found in eastern Nigeria and Zaire. Paragonimiasis is also encountered in Peru, Ecuador, Brazil, and Venezuela. The most likely patient population in the United States to contract paragonimiasis is the military population, in particular those who have been in Southeast Asia. The life cycle of the adult fluke includes humans, snails, and certain crayfish and crabs. Crabs are the usual source of human infection. The fluke normally burrows into the lungs of humans and animals to form small granulomatous cysts. Eggs are shed from the cysts into the air passages upon coughing or swallowing and are excreted in the feces. When these eggs contaminate fresh water, snails become infected, developing a sporocyst and radial stage, followed by the liberation of cercariae. The latter are actively motile parasites that penetrate the soft periarticular tissues of crayfish and crabs. These parasites are consumed by humans when the crabs are eaten. An adult cercaria is liberated in the bowel and penetrates the wall of the jejunum, crossing the peritoneal cavity to the tendinous portion of the diaphragm, which it burrows through into the pleural space. It crosses the pleural space, penetrates the visceral pleura, and burrows into the lung. It then reaches maturity and begins to produce eggs, thus beginning the life cycle of the parasite once again. Patients with paragonimiasis clinically have chronic hemoptysis, slight dyspnea, mild fever, severe anorexia, and weight loss. They gradually become accustomed to their symptoms and may have hemoptysis for years. The radiologic consequence of the disease is the emergence of multiple pulmonary opacities which, as in hydatid disease, may appear as masses or as cystic or cavitary lesions.

Septic emboli are another important cause of inflammatory nodules. Like many of the inflammatory conditions described herein, septic emboli frequently present with multiple ill-defined opacities that gradually become more circumscribed as the process heals. The nodular phase should be regarded as a later phase of the process. The nodules actually represent organized infarcts. Clinical correlation is essential in suggesting and confirming this diagnosis. Most patients have an identifiable source of infection, such as osteomyelitis, cellulitis, or extrapulmonary abscess. Another source of septic emboli is bacterial endocarditis involving the right side of the heart. This is particularly common in intravenous drug abusers.

Vascular and Collagen Vascular Diseases

The vascular diseases that result in multiple pulmonary opacities include venous thromboembolism and the collagen vascular diseases. As just indicated, the nodules that appear following thromboembolism are organizing infarcts. This diagnosis is usually verified by a history of documented emboli weeks to months prior to the development of the nodules. Roentgenograms obtained at the time of the acute embolic event reveal areas of ill-defined opacity. Since the infarcts heal by organization of the nodules, the nodules should be smaller than the preceding ill-defined opacities, which were caused primarily by hemorrhagic edema.

Wegener's granulomatosis and the Wegener's variants (limited Wegener's and lymphomatoid granulomatosis)[156,363] result in a diffuse vasculitis involving most of the vessels of the lung. As these vessels become occluded, infarcts develop in the areas of vascular occlusion, with the radiologic result of multiple areas of increased opacity. These opacities are ill-defined in the early phases of the process and become circumscribed as the infarcts organize. Clinical correlation is extremely helpful when a history of coexistent renal or sinus disease is uncovered. The classic triad of Wegener's granulomatosis consists of lung, kidney, and sinus disease. The limited form of Wegener's granulomatosis is usually confined to the lung and requires biopsy for confirmation.

Rheumatoid nodules[156,186] are the least common of the various thoracic manifestations of rheumatoid disease, but they do constitute a significant cause of multiple pulmonary nodules. These nodules tend to occur in the periphery of the lung, are frequently pleural-based, and occasionally cavitate. Histologically, they are necrobiotic nodules, similar to the subcutaneous nodules of rheumatoid arthritis.

SUMMARY

1. Multiple pulmonary nodules are distinguished from multifocal infiltrative diseases by their homogeneous appearance and sharply defined borders.

2. Multiple pulmonary nodules are most frequently the result of metastatic disease.

3. The list of primary tumors that metastasize to the lung is long. Central nervous system tumors least commonly lead to pulmonary metastases.

4. The presence of calcification may be virtually diagnostic of a benign granuloma, but this must be carefully considered. The presence of one calcified granuloma does not prove that other nodules are benign granulomas.

5. Evaluation of old films is imperative. The pattern of large, multifocal ill-defined opacities evolving to smaller, sharply defined nodules over a period of weeks to months indicates either healing granulomas or organizing infarcts to be the cause of the nodules. The evolution excludes the diagnosis of metastases.

6. Clinical correlation is essential in suggesting parasitic diseases as a cause of pulmonary nodules.

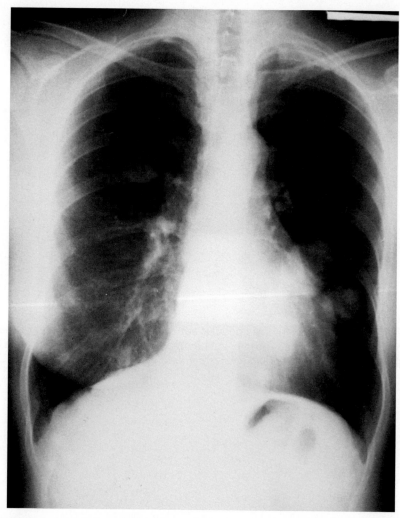

FIG 21–3
The combination of multiple well-circumscribed pulmonary masses in a patient who has had a left mastectomy virtually ensures the diagnosis of metastatic breast cancer.

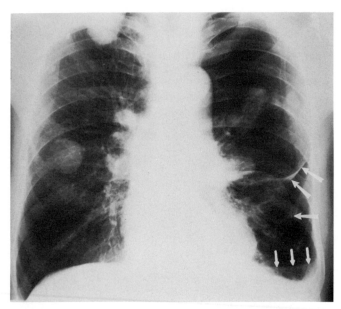

FIG 21–4
Combination of multiple pulmonary nodules and spontaneous pneumothorax is nearly diagnostic of metastatic osteosarcoma. Pneumothorax is detected by identification of pleural line *(large arrows)*. Air-fluid level *(small arrows)* indicates hydropneumothorax.

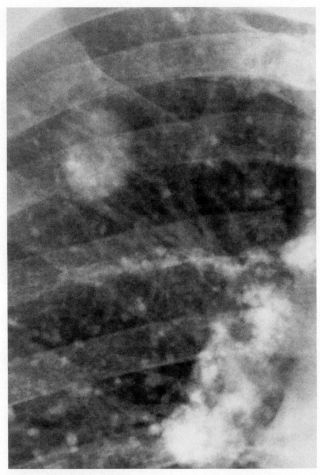

FIG 21–5
Multiple small, scattered nodules with calcified hilar nodes are consistent with prior granulomatous infection. As in the case shown in Figure 21–2, the presence of granulomas does not ensure that the larger soft-tissue mass in the right upper lobe is benign. This patient has multiple granulomas and a primary carcinoma of the lung.

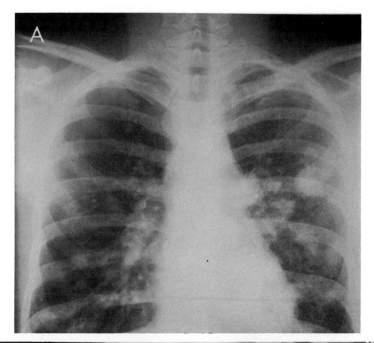

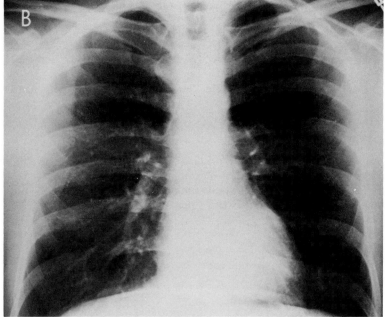

FIG 21–6
A, Combination of multiple nodules and bilateral hilar and mediastinal adenopathy could suggest metastases, but ill-defined borders are not typical of metastases. Lymphoma would not be easily excluded by the radiologic presentation. Clinical correlation revealing an asymptomatic patient would strongly support the diagnosis of sarcoidosis. **B,** Follow-up examination 18 months later, revealing complete spontaneous resolution of the nodules, essentially confirms the diagnosis of sarcoidosis.

ANSWER GUIDE

LEGENDS FOR INTRODUCTORY FIGURES

FIG 21–1

These nodules are distinguished from the multifocal opacities seen in Chapter 16 by their sharp borders. Metastatic disease is the most common cause of this pattern. The primary tumor in the case of this young man is testicular carcinoma.

FIG 21–2

A, Note the difference in these two nodules. The nodule on the right is more opaque than the ribs and is sharply defined. The patient has calcified granuloma on the right. **B,** Left lower lobe nodule is less opaque and has irregular, spiculated borders. This is a primary carcinoma of the lung.

ANSWERS

1, a; 2, c; 3, a.

PART III

HYPERLUCENT ABNORMALITIES

CHAPTER 22

Hyperlucent Thorax

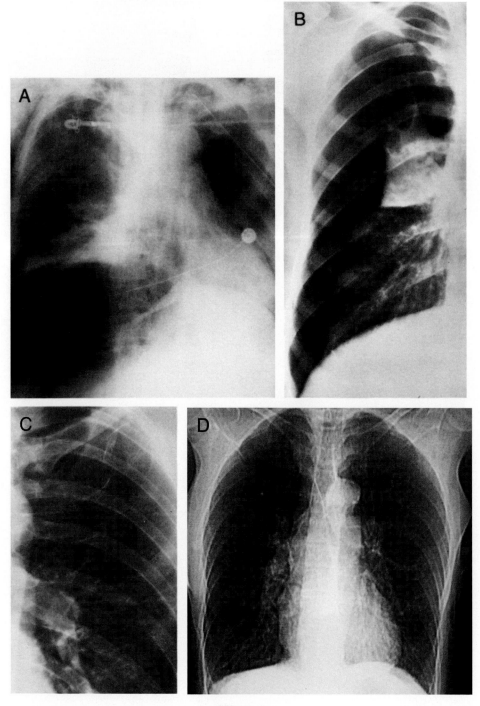

FIG 22–1

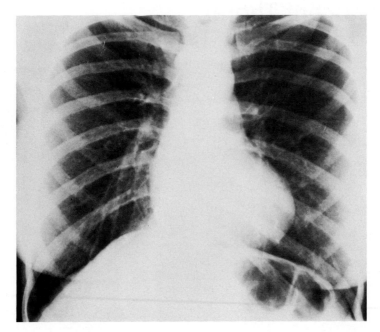

FIG 22–2

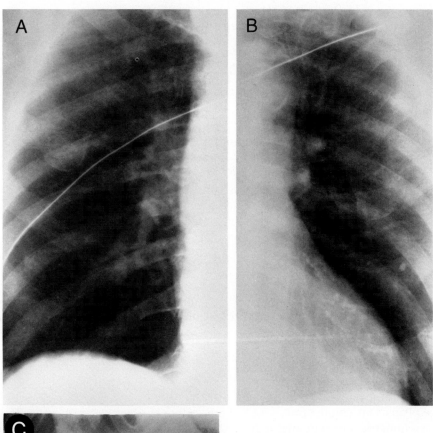

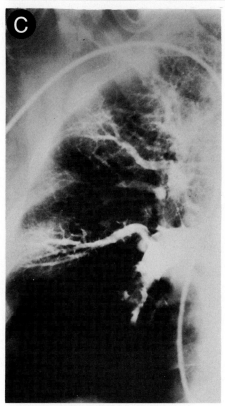

FIG 22–3

QUESTIONS

1. Match the abnormal thoracic lucencies seen in Figures 22–1, *A–D*, with the following diagnoses.
   ____ Centrilobular emphysema.
   ____ Subpulmonic tension pneumothorax.
   ____ Bullous emphysema.
   ____ Ruptured subpleural bulla.
2. Decreased peripheral vascularity is consistent with all of the following diagnoses, but the small proximal vessels are suggestive of only one. Which is the most likely diagnosis in the case illustrated in Figure 22–2?
   a. Tetralogy of Fallot.
   b. Pulmonary embolism.
   c. Eisenmenger's complex.
   d. Panacinar emphysema.
   e. Acute asthma.
3. Which is the most likely cause for loss of lower lobe vasculature in the case illustrated in Figure 22–3?
   a. Tetralogy of Fallot.
   b. Pulmonary embolism.
   c. Bronchiolitis obliterans.
   d. Chronic obstructive pulmonary disease.
   e. Panacinar emphysema.
4. Asymmetric air trapping may be confirmed by which of the following techniques?
   a. Lateral decubitus film.
   b. Forced inspiratory film.
   c. Forced expiratory film.
   d. Overpenetrated Bucky film.
   e. Oblique film.

CHART 22–1.
Hyperlucent Lungs
_____

   I. Bilateral
      A. Faulty radiologic technique (overpenetrated film)
      B. Thin body habitus
      C. Bilateral mastectomy
      D. Right-to-left cardiac shunts (e.g., tetralogy of Fallot, pseudotruncus, truncus type IV)
      E. Pulmonary embolism[423]
      F. Emphysema[182,185,225,260,612]
      G. Acute asthmatic attack[186]
      H. Acute bronchiolitis (usually in pediatric patients)[229,476]
      I. Interstitial emphysema[504,660]
  II. Unilateral
      A. Mastectomy
      B. Absent pectoralis muscles
      C. Faulty radiologic technique including rotation of patient
      D. Extrapulmonary air collections (e.g., pneumothorax, mediastinal emphysema, subcutaneous emphysema)
      E. Pulmonary embolism (acute or chronic)[668]
      F. Emphysema (particularly bullous emphysema)[260]

(Continued.)

CHART 22–1.   (cont.).

   G. Atrophy of trapezius muscle (after radical neck dissection)[591]
   H. Bronchial obstruction
      1. Neoplastic
         a. Bronchogenic carcinoma
         b. Metastatic (rare, but most common primary sites are breast, thyroid, pancreas, colon,
           melanoma)[36]
      2. Granulomatous masses including broncholith
      3. Bronchial mucocele[597]
      4. Foreign body (common in children)
   I. Hilar mass (e.g., adenopathy, bronchogenic cyst)
   J. Bronchiolitis obliterans (Swyer-James, or Macleod, syndrome)[556]
   K. Compensatory overaeration
   L. Congenital lobar emphysema
   M. Cardiomegaly (left lower lobe)

DISCUSSION

The first step in the evaluation of the apparently hyperlucent lung is to check on radiologic technique. A high-contrast, low-kilovoltage technique may result in a high-contrast chest film and thus obscure the normal vascular markings of the lung, leading to the false impression of hyperlucent lungs. Such highly contrasted films are readily identified by the marked contrast between the soft-tissue opacities and the lucency of the lung. This is a particularly common problem with the portable film, for which high-kilovoltage techniques are more difficult to obtain. Radiologic technique may also result in a unilateral hyperlucent lung when the patient is rotated. Rotation produces the unilateral hyperlucent appearance by projecting soft tissues over one side of the chest while rotating the soft tissues off the opposite side of the chest. This latter problem is particularly noticeable in female patients with large, pendulous breasts, which add considerably to the opacity over the lower lung fields. Improper centering of the x-ray beam may also cause asymmetric exposure.

Anatomic variations also result in the appearance of hyperlucent lungs. The best-known example is the patient with a very thin body habitus, which results in an overpenetrated chest film. As in the evaluation of other overpenetrated films, the hot light should reveal normal branching pulmonary vascularity and thus confirm lack of soft tissues rather than a true hyperlucent lung. Asymmetric absence of soft tissues can likewise result in unilateral hyperlucent lungs. Radical mastectomy is the most common source of this problem. Rarely, congenital asymmetry of the chest wall results in a similar appearance. This is noted in patients who have either hypoplastic or absent pectoralis muscles.

Extrapulmonary air collections, including subcutaneous emphysema, mediastinal emphysema, and pneumothoraces (Fig 22–1, *A* and *B*) all produce lucent abnormalities that are usually recognized on the basis of their location and are not usually confused with hyperlucent lungs.

Most of the above conditions result in differences in the opacity of the lung because of overlying soft tissues or their absence. It is important to remember that the radiologic opacity of the normal lung is produced by the pulmonary vascularity. The pulmonary vessels are radiologically identifiable because they contain blood, which is of soft tissue opacity, and are surrounded by air. Therefore, any loss of opacity of the lung reflects a change in the pulmonary vascularity. This should be detected by noting diminution in the size and number of radiologically identifiable vessels (Fig 22–4). The size and number of radiologically visible vessels are directly related to pulmonary blood flow, supporting the observation that a truly hyperlucent lung is a reflection of decreased blood flow through the lung. This may be the result of either cardiac or primary pulmonary disease.

Emphysema

Emphysema is a very important cause of loss of pulmonary vascularity (see Fig 22–1, *C* and *D*).[182,185] Severe cases of emphysema will produce marked attenuation and stretching of pulmonary vessels. This process may be diffuse to such an extent that there may even be nearly complete absence of vessels. The diagnosis of emphysema by evaluation of the pulmonary vascularity requires a subjective evaluation of the vascular patterns. Thurlbeck and Simon[612] divided vascular patterns into three main categories of abnormality: (1) the vessels are present but narrowed in most of the lung, (2) there is a normal axial pathway but fewer side branches, and (3) there may be complete absence of vessels. Simon also introduced the concept of marker vessels, which he described as normal or enlarged vessels in areas of less-extensive involvement. Although these vascular alterations may be subtle on plain film, HRCT is very sensitive for detection of variations in regional perfusion (Fig 22–5).

There is hardly any aspect of chest disease that generates more controversy than the role of the radiologist in the diagnosis of emphysema, but most agree that the alterations in pulmonary vascularity are the most reliable radiologic criteria for this diagnosis. Thurlbeck and Simon[612] evaluated 700 patients in an effort to correlate paper-mounted whole-lung sections with PA and lateral view roentgenograms to determine the accuracy of radiologic diagnosis of emphysema. They measured lung length and width, the size of the retrosternal clear space, heart size, and position of the diaphragm. They observed that lung length and the size of the retrosternal clear space increased, the level of the diaphragm was lowered, the heart size decreased, and the lung width was unchanged as emphysema became more severe. They believed that lung length and diaphragm level were the most discriminating measurements for diagnostic accuracy, followed by size of the retrosternal clear space. However, they identified no combination of these radiologic variables that identified emphysema better than the subjective diagnosis of the disease based on arterial deficiency. They also emphasized that radiologic lung dimensions are related to stature and must therefore be cautiously interpreted. For example, kyphosis of the thoracic spine will cause an increase in the AP diameter of the chest.

When the foregoing criteria are applied, the plain chest film (Fig 22–6) is highly specific for the diagnosis of emphysema in patients with advanced disease, but it is not sensitive. HRCT has been shown to be much more sensitive for the diagnosis of early emphysema in demonstrating vascular attenuation, areas of hyperlucency, and small bullae that are not detectable by plain film radiography[204,336,611] (Figs 22–5 and 22–7).

It is important to emphasize that emphysema is an anatomic diagnosis. The morphologic definition of emphysema requires the presence of destruction of alveolar walls and obstruction of small airways. This destruction results in increased size of the distal air spaces. Emphysema is further subdivided into two types: panlobular (panacinar) and centrilobular (centriacinar). An emphysematous process that destroys all of the lung distal to the terminal bronchiole is termed panlobular, while incomplete destruction of lung distal to the terminal bronchiole is termed centrilobular emphysema. The destruction in centrilobular emphysema may occur in the center of the lobule, but may also be eccentrically located. Of the two types, centrilobular is the more common. Other terms frequently confused in the discussion of emphysema are *bulla* and *bleb.* A bleb is a collection of air within the layers of visceral pleura, and a bulla is an emphysematous space in the lung parenchyma with a diameter of more than 1 cm; however, these terms are frequently used interchangeably. Heitzman[260] states that a bulla represents a distended secondary pulmonary lobule or group of lobules involved by panacinar emphysema. Bullous lesions have a rounded or oval configuration indicating that there is a significant element of air trapping in the bulla (see Fig 22–8, *A* and *B*). Bullae may rupture, causing pneumothorax and a bronchopleural communication, which may be difficult to manage without a thoracotomy (see Fig 22–1, *B*).

Radiologic distinction of the types of emphysema is frequently impossible, but there are differences in the distribution. Centriacinar emphysema (Fig 22–1, *D*) tends to involve the upper lobes, while panacinar emphysema tends to be more severe in the bases (see Fig 22–9, *A* and *B*). Bullous emphysema may accompany panacinar emphysema, but it also occurs in a localized form (Fig 22–1, *B*).

The term *chronic obstructive pulmonary disease* (COPD) should not be used interchangeably with *emphysema.*[182,185,260] The diagnosis of COPD is a clinical diagnosis encompassing the entire group of obstructive pulmonary diseases, including chronic bronchitis, asthma, bronchiolitis obliterans, bronchiectasis, and emphysema.[260] Of these entities, only emphysema results in chronic bilateral loss of pulmonary vascularity and thus in hyperlucent lungs.

In contrast to the foregoing situation, a severe acute asthmatic attack may cause bilateral air trapping with depression of the diaphragm and hyperlucent lungs, but these changes are reversible.

Air Trapping

Air trapping is an important cause of hyperlucent lung. Air trapping has the effect of stretching the alveoli, compressing the capillaries and arterioles, and thus decreasing the pulmonary blood flow. However, this is undoubtedly an oversimplification of the pathologic mechanisms by which air trapping leads to a decrease in the size of pulmonary vessels.

The acute asthmatic attack is one of the most striking examples of transient air trapping. It is well known that bronchial asthma usually produces little radiologic abnormality except during acute attacks, at which time there may be significant air trapping with hyperlucency, attenuation of the vascular markings, and depression of the diaphragm. Acute bronchiolitis is another important cause of diffuse air trapping, but it is primarily a disease of the pediatric age group. In both of these situations, the air trapping is transient. Confirmation of air trapping is established with films taken during the expiratory phase of respiration.

Pulmonary Embolism

Massive pulmonary emboli may obstruct blood flow through the main pulmonary artery, producing bilaterally hyperlucent lungs, but fortunately this is a rare occurrence. More localized areas of hyperlucency (Westermark's sign)[668] may result from smaller pulmonary emboli (see Fig 22–3, *A–C*). These areas of hyperlucency may be segmental, lobar, or involve an entire lung. The diagnosis is usually suggested by the clinical setting. These patients frequently present with acute pleuritic chest pain, dyspnea, and extreme apprehension. A ventilation and perfusion scan may confirm the diagnosis by demonstrating that the hyperlucent areas on the chest x-ray film are poorly perfused but normally ventilated. The combination of perfusion and ventilation scanning is extremely important in distinguishing pulmonary emboli from emphysema, another important cause of hyperlucent lung and poor pulmonary vascular perfusion. In the case of emphysema, the ventilation scan will demonstrate significant trapping of the radionuclide imaging agent, with delayed activity. Pulmonary arteriography is currently the most definitive procedure for the diagnosis of pulmonary embolism.[574] There is often good correlation of the hyperlucent areas on the chest roentgenogram, with the larger arterial obstructions demonstrated by arteriography. (Answer to question 3 is *b*.)

Cardiac Disease

The cardiac diseases that result in decreased pulmonary blood flow are the right-to-left cardiac shunts. These shunts usually occur in combination with obstruction of pulmonary blood flow from the right side of the heart at the pulmonary valve, right ventricle, or tricuspid valve. The most common of these conditions is the tetralogy of Fallot. The combination of infundibular pulmonary stenosis with a ventricular septal defect forms a bypass for the blood to enter directly into the high-pressure left ventricular system, thereby bypassing the pulmonary circulation. With this arrangement, both the peripheral and proximal pulmonary vessels will be abnormally small (see Fig 22–2). Although the vascularity is decreased, this appearance is not often perceived as hyperlucent lungs. (Answer to question 2 is *a*.) None of the other considerations should cause the proximal pulmonary arteries to be abnormally small. Tetralogy of Fallot is a congenital heart disease that results clinically in cyanosis and is usually identified in early childhood. Other right-to-left shunts, such as pseudotruncus arteriosus, type 4 truncus arteriosus, Ebstein's malformation of the tricuspid valve, and tricuspid atresia, may produce decreased pulmonary vasculature by a similar mechanism. Cardiac catheterization is essential for accurate diagnosis of these congenital heart lesions.

In addition to the right-to-left shunts, long-standing left-to-right shunts may result in the Eisenmenger's complex, an endarteritis obliterans of the small pulmonary arteries that decreases peripheral vasculature and thus may cause hyperlucent lungs. Eisenmenger's complex can be radiologically distinguished from right-to-left shunts by observing progressive enlargement of the proximal pulmonary arteries. Frequently, the Eisenmenger response to a left-to-right shunt results in pulmonary arteries that are massively dilated proximally and may even suggest bilateral hilar masses. The dilated proximal vessels are caused by increased resistance in the peripheral pulmonary vascular bed. Serial roentgenograms should therefore reveal a striking contrast between the primary right-to-left shunts (tetralogy) and the left-to-right shunts (atrial septal defect, ventricular septal defect, patent ductus arteriosus) that precipitate the Eisenmenger response. For example, a roentgenogram obtained early in the course of ventricular septal defect demonstrates large peripheral and proximal pulmonary vessels. As the obliterative arteritis develops, the peripheral vessels gradually diminish in size, while the proximal vessels enlarge. In this late stage the shunt may reverse. The latter complication is recognized by the clinical observation of cyanosis.

Unilateral Hyperlucent Lung

The preceding discussion of hyperlucent lung focused primarily on diseases that result in bilaterally hyperlucent lungs, comprising cardiac shunts with decreased vascularity, acute asthmatic attacks, acute bronchiolitis, emphysema, and pulmonary embolism. It must be emphasized, however, that pulmonary embolism and emphysema may be bilateral diseases but frequently lead to the radiologic appearance of unilaterally hyperlucent lungs (see Figs 22–3 and 22–8). In such cases roentgenography is unfortunately not sensitive enough to detect all areas of involvement, but it can be assumed that areas of hyperlucency reflect areas of severe involvement.

The nonpulmonary causes of hyperlucent lung, including faulty radiologic technique, mastectomy, absent pectoralis muscles, and extrapulmonary air collections, are more likely to be unilateral than bilateral. Besides excluding the nonpulmonary causes of hyperlucent lung, the radiologic evaluation of a unilateral hyperlucent lung requires the additional determination of whether the lucent lung or the opaque lung is abnormal. This is particularly true in the case of large airway obstruction, which may result in air trapping. Since the overdistention of the lung in these cases results in decreased perfusion of the vascular bed, the additional flow is directed to the normal lung, with the result of a truly increased opacity of the normal lung. In addition, the bronchial obstruction results in overinflation of the lung with a shift of the mediastinum toward the normal side in a manner resembling compensatory overaeration, as is seen in cases of atelectasis. Flattening of the diaphragm on the side of the hyperlucency should be a clue that the bronchial obstruction is producing air trapping rather than atelectasis with compensatory overaeration of the opposite side. The presence of air trapping can be readily confirmed by a number of procedures, including (1) an expiratory film that reveals the volume of the hyperlucent lung to be unchanged, (2) fluoroscopy, which likewise reveals the volume of the hyperinflated lung to be unchanged, and (3) a lateral decubitus film with the hyperinflated side down. The lateral decubitus film is particularly helpful in infants, small children, and uncooperative patients, since it has the effect of splinting the side that is down and is therefore the equivalent of an expiratory film for that side. A suspected endobronchial mass may result in either bronchial obstruction with atelectasis or bronchial obstruction with air trapping. It is generally agreed that collateral air drift contributes to air trapping beyond bronchial obstructions. This collateral air drift is irreversible and therefore permits air to enter the area of lung distal to the obstruction, where the air is then trapped, resulting in hyperexpansion. Atelectasis probably occurs distally to bronchial obstructions in those patients who have underlying diseases that prevent normal collateral air drift. Felson and others have emphasized that bronchial obstruction in an adult is more likely to result in atelectasis, while bronchial obstruction in a child most frequently leads to air trapping. The primary diagnostic considerations are quite different in these two cases. An endobronchial mass is the most frequent tumor in an adult, while a foreign body is the most common endobronchial mass in a child. (Answers to question 4 are *a* and *c*.)

Swyer-James syndrome, or Macleod syndrome,[219,587] deserves special mention because it was originally described as a radiologic syndrome consisting of a unilaterally hyperlucent lung (Fig 22–10, *A*). There is considerable evidence that cases of the syndrome are the late sequelae of a viral pneumonia, particularly an adenoviral bronchiolitis. Histologic examinations of patients with this diagnosis have demonstrated a bronchiolitis obliterans (Fig 22–10, *B*). To date there has been no satisfactory explanation for the predominantly unilateral involvement. The radiologic appearance may be quite striking. The unilateral hyperlucent lung may be associated with varying signs of air trapping. The most exaggerated cases of air trapping may demonstrate flattening of the diaphragm and herniation of lung through the mediastinum, and even compression of the normal lung. This degree of air trapping is in fact uncommon. Early case reports suggested that air trapping was not a feature of the syndrome.

The observation of a hilar mass with associated air trapping is rare. Because of the frequency of bronchial obstruction by carcinoma of the lung, hyperlucent lung might be an anticipated abnormality, but, as stated previously, atelectasis is much more commonly observed. Because of the possibility of detecting air trapping from an early bronchogenic carcinoma, studies using inspiratory and expiratory films have been performed as a possible means for the early detection of bronchogenic tumor, but this approach has not been of particular value.

Other hilar and mediastinal lesions, including adenopathy, fibrosing mediastinitis, and, very rarely, benign masses such as this bronchogenic cyst, may result in a unilateral hyperlucent lung (Fig 22–11, *A* and *B*).

SUMMARY

1. Hyperlucency of the lung may be a bilateral or unilateral process. If unilateral, it may involve an entire lung, a lobe, a segment, or even a lobule.

2. Artifactual causes of unilateral hyperlucent lung, including faulty radiologic technique, must always be excluded.

3. Mastectomy is probably the most common cause of unilateral hyperlucency of the chest.

4. The true pulmonary diseases that result in hyperlucent lung are a reflection of decreased pulmonary blood flow. The causes for decreased pulmonary blood flow are diverse and include cardiac shunts, pulmonary emboli, emphysema, endobronchial masses, and bronchiolitis obliterans.

5. The radiologic diagnosis of emphysema is controversial but most agree that the vascular changes correlate well with the pathologic diagnosis of emphysema. Most of the controversies concern the sensitivity of chest roentgenography for detecting early emphysema. HRCT is very specific and very sensitive for the diagnosis of early emphysema.

6. The term *chronic obstructive pulmonary disease* should be used as a clinical term, since it includes emphysema, chronic bronchitis, bronchial asthma, bronchiolitis obliterans, and bronchiectasis. The radiologic features of these diseases are diverse. The areas of hyperlucency are the result of destruction of lung parenchyma. The radiologic result is the appearance of decreased pulmonary vasculature. Loss of pulmonary vascularity is a reliable radiologic sign of emphysema.

7. Although pulmonary emboli are frequently multiple and bilateral, they may result in localized areas of hyperlucency (Westermark's sign).

8. In the case of large airway obstruction, the first decision is to determine whether the hyperlucent or the opaque side is abnormal. This is easily accomplished by confirming air trapping with expiratory films, fluoroscopy, or lateral decubitus films.

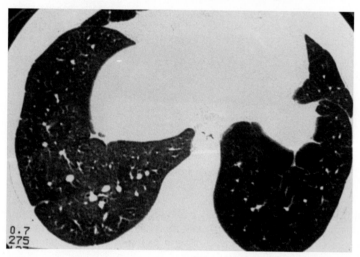

FIG 22–4
HRCT of a patient with a unilateral hyperlucent left lower lobe. Note the asymmetry of the pulmonary vessels, with decreased size and number of vessels in the hyperlucent area.

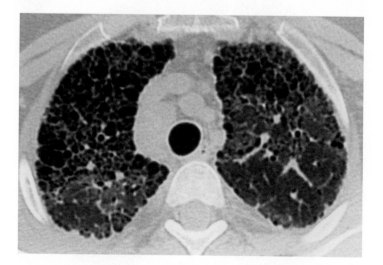

FIG 22–5
HRCT of a patient with centrilobular emphysema shows multiple lucent spaces and minimal vascularity in the anterior lungs, although there are moderately large vessels in the posterior lungs. Also compare the hyperlucent areas with the opacity of the more normally perfused areas.

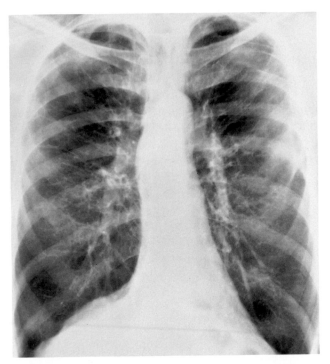

FIG 22–6
Depression of the diaphragm, a vertically positioned small heart, and hyperlucent lungs caused by loss of normal vasculature constitute a highly specific appearance for emphysema. These findings indicate advanced disease and are not sensitive for the diagnosis of early emphysema by plain film radiography.

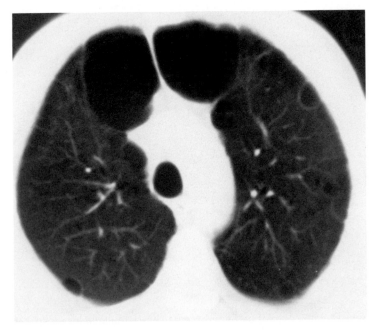

FIG 22–7
CT scan shows multiple avascular areas of emphysema and is more sensitive than plain film radiography for the early diagnosis of emphysema.

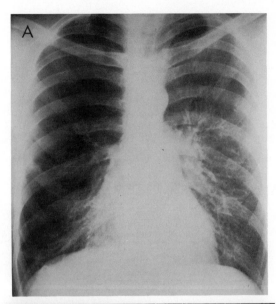

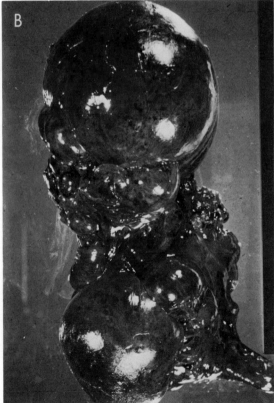

FIG 22–8
A, Bullous emphysema is a common cause of unilateral or localized hyperlucency. Note attenuation of right upper vasculature and compression of right lower lobe. **B,** Gross specimen from another case illustrates large, balloon-like structures that may fill an entire hemithorax.

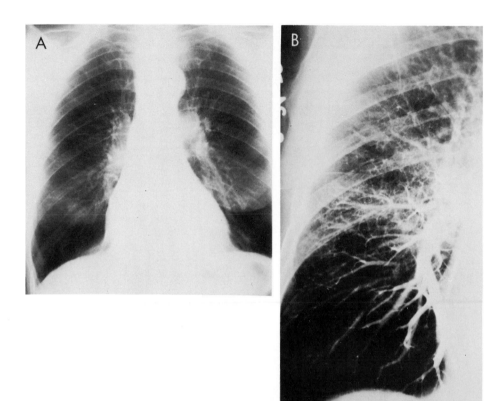

FIG 22–9
A, Hyperlucency of lung bases is suggestive of decreased vascularity. **B,** Pulmonary arteri-ogram from case seen in **A** confirms impression of decreased vascularity to the bases. Note stretching of vessels. This is an example of panacinar emphysema. Basilar distribu-tion is typical.

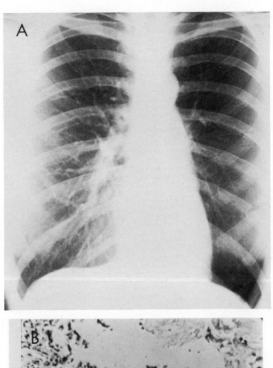

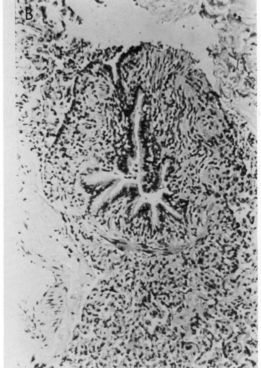

FIG 22–10
A, Swyer-James syndrome was originally described as unilateral hyperlucent lung. This condition appears to be a late complication of viral infection of the bronchi and bronchioles. **B,** Histologic section from another case of Swyer-James syndrome reveals narrowing of a bronchiole by chronic inflammatory cellular reaction. This is bronchiolitis obliterans.

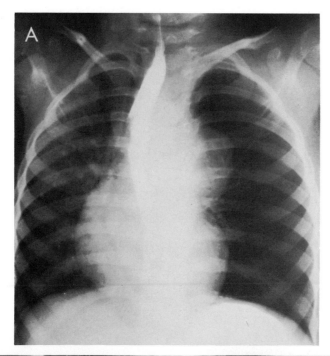

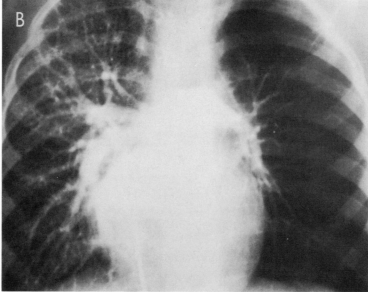

FIG 22–11
A, Combination of mediastinal mass and hyperlucent lung might suggest a malignant mass with invasion of the pulmonary artery, but this was a young asymptomatic patient. (Case courtesy of H. D. Rosenbaum, M.D., University of Kentucky.) **B,** Pulmonary arteriogram documents that hyperlucent lung is the result of decreased vascularity. This is a bronchogenic cyst, which appears to compress the pulmonary artery.

ANSWER GUIDE

LEGENDS FOR INTRODUCTORY FIGURES

FIG 22–1

A, Subpulmonic tension pneumothorax has produced a large lucent area in the lower right thorax. The heart is shifted to the left and the diaphragm is depressed. This patient had staphylococcal pneumonia and developed a bronchopleural fistula that led to the fatal pneumothorax. **B,** Subpleural bullae are a frequent cause of spontaneous pneumothorax. This patient has cystic fibrosis with early development of apical bullae. **C,** Bullous emphysema causes loss of pulmonary vasculature and hyperlucent lungs. The bullae have very thin walls that appear as linear opacities. Very large bullae may sometimes be difficult to distinguish from a loculated pneumothorax. **D,** Centrilobular emphysema is the most common type of emphysema. It is usually diffuse but may be most severe in the upper lobes. This is an advanced case with enlargement of both lungs, flattening of the diaphragm, and loss of vascularity, causing bilateral hyperlucent lungs.

FIG 22–2

The combination of small peripheral vessels and small proximal pulmonary arteries indicates decreased flow through the pulmonary circulation. Entities that cause pulmonary arterial hypertension would result in an increase in size of proximal pulmonary arteries. Note the elevated apex of the heart. This is the "boot-shaped" heart that indicates right ventricular enlargement, the classic appearance for tetralogy of Fallot.

FIG 22–3

A, Development of hyperlucent right lower lobe with any of the clinical signs of pulmonary embolic disease should strongly suggest the correct diagnosis. This is the classic Westermark's sign of pulmonary embolism. **B,** Compare the vascular markings of the normal left lung with the hypovascular right lower lobe. **C,** Pulmonary arteriogram from same case documents a large right lower lobe embolus.

ANSWERS

1, d, a, c, b; 2, a; 3, b; 4, a, c.

CHAPTER 23

Solitary Lucent Defect

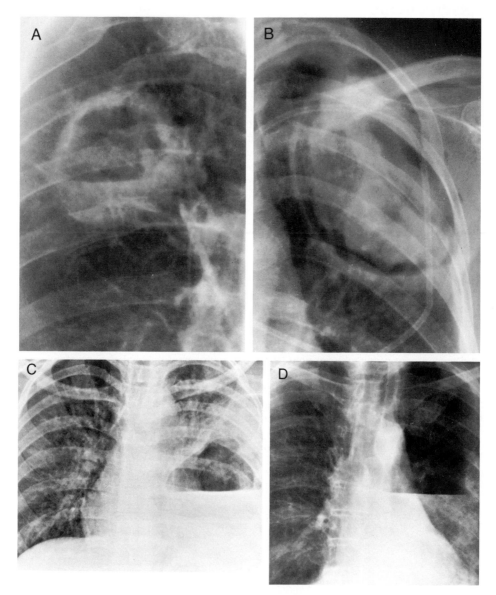

FIG 23–1

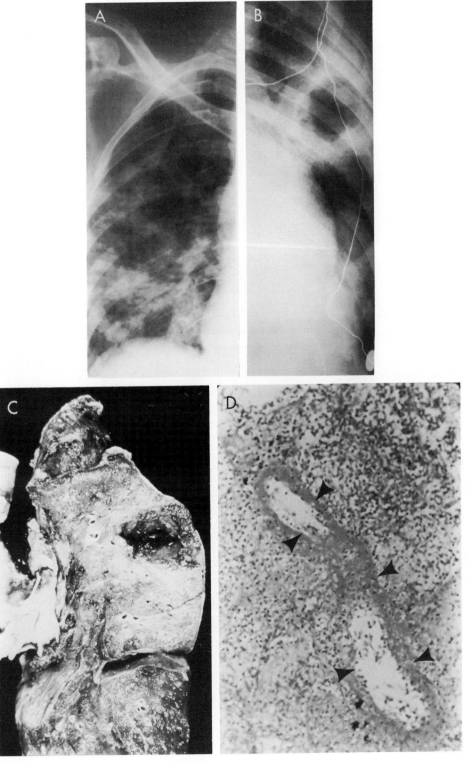

FIG 23–2

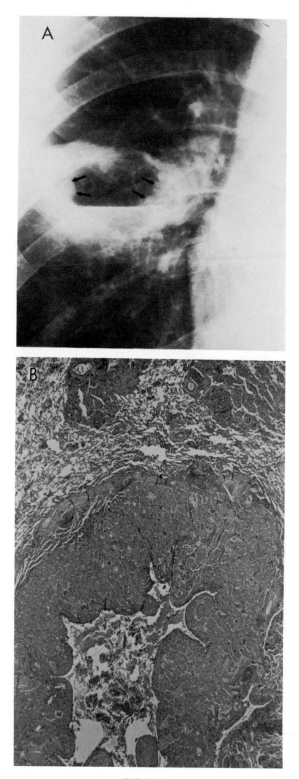

FIG 23–3

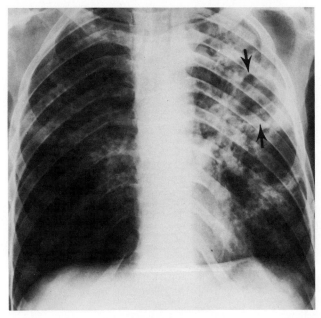

FIG 23–4

QUESTIONS

1. Match the cases shown in Figure 23–1, *A–D,* with the following diagnoses.
   ____ Bronchogenic carcinoma.
   ____ Pneumonia with abscess.
   ____ Bronchopleural fistula with hydropneumothorax.
   ____ Pulmonary gangrene.
2. Which of the following pulmonary infections is least likely in the case illustrated in Figure 23–2?
   a. *Streptococcus pneumoniae.*
   b. *Pseudomonas.*
   c. *Klebsiella.*
   d. *Staphylococcus aureus.*
   e. Mixed gram-negative.
3. Refer to Figure 23–3. Which one of the following diagnoses is least likely?
   a. Bronchogenic carcinoma.
   b. Metastatic nasopharyngeal carcinoma.
   c. Chronic anaerobic abscess.
   d. Bronchogenic cyst.
   e. Tuberculous cavity.
4. Which of the following best explains the radiologic presentation in Figure 23–4?
   a. Metastatic melanoma.
   b. Tuberculosis with bronchogenic spread.
   c. Bronchogenic carcinoma.
   d. Coccidioidomycosis.
   e. Metastatic nasopharyngeal carcinoma.

CHART 23–1.
Solitary Lucent Defect

I. Cavity
   A. Inflammation
      1. Abscess, acute or chronic
         a. Pyogenic infection[31,231,260] (staphylococcal and gram-negative pneumonia)
         b. Aspiration pneumonia[31] (common source of anaerobes)
      2. Fungal infection[390,478]
         a. Histoplasmosis[104,117]
         b. Coccidioidomycosis[392]
         c. Blastomycosis[242,474]
         d. Cryptococcosis[217,252]
         e. Mucormycosis[32,671]
      3. Mycobacterial infection
         a. Tuberculosis (typical and atypical)[64,91,412]
         b. Nocardiosis[26,232]
   B. Neoplasms
      1. Primary lung tumor[605]
      2. Metastases (usually multiple)[128]
         a. Squamous cell (nasopharynx, esophagus, cervix)
         b. Adenocarcinoma (lung, breast, gastrointestinal tract)
         c. Osteosarcoma (rare)
         d. Melanoma
   C. Vascular (commonly multiple)
      1. Rheumatoid[156,492]
      2. Wegener's granulomatosis[342,377]
      3. Infarct (thromboemboli or septic emboli)[121]
   D. Inhalation
      1. Silicosis and coal-worker's pneumoconiosis (most commonly owing to complicating tuberculosis)
II. Pneumatocele (infectious and traumatic)[16,127,139,250]
III. Congenital cyst[487,488] (bronchogenic cyst[13] and intrapulmonary sequestration[160,162,256])
IV. Bronchiectatic cyst[488]
V. Bullous emphysema[182]

DISCUSSION

The radiologic presentation of a localized, avascular, lucent lung defect surrounded by a band of opacity might best be described as a hole in the lung, although this is a nonmedical term. Chart 23–1 lists a number of causes for a solitary hole in the lung that differ considerably in their pathogenesis. For this reason, such terms as cavity, cyst, and pneumatocele in fact constitute the differential diagnosis for a hole in the lung.[331] This chapter examines differences in the pathogenesis of these lesions as a basis for understanding the similarities and differences in their radiologic presentations.

Cavity

The radiologic appearance of a pulmonary cavity is the result of necrosis of lung parenchyma with evacuation of the necrotic tissue via the tracheobronchial tree. A communication with the tracheobronchial tree permits air to enter the area of necrosis, with the radiologic result of a lucent defect. The necrosis results in near-complete destruction of the alveolar walls, interlobular septa, and bronchovascular bundles in the area of the cavity, resulting in loss of normal vascular markings throughout the area of lucency. The surrounding normal lung parenchyma reacts to the necrosis by forming a band of inflammation around the necrotic material, with local edema and hemorrhage. When the cavity expands under tension, as frequently happens in patients who are on positive-pressure ventilator therapy, there may even be compression of normal surrounding lung. The surrounding inflammatory cellular infiltrate, edema, hemorrhage, and compressed normal lung all contribute to the cavity wall. Central necrosis of a preexisting nodule with drainage of its liquefied contents is a second mechanism for the development of a cavity. Central necrosis with liquefaction of a pulmonary lesion cannot be detected by either plain films or conventional tomograms prior to drainage of a portion of the liquid. However, CT is sensitive to the difference in opacity caused by liquefaction and may be useful for detecting early necrosis of either a pulmonary infection or neoplasm (Fig 23–5, *A* and *B*).

The radiologic characteristics of the wall of a cavity are determined by the reaction of the lung parenchyma to the pathologic process. A surrounding air-space consolidation indicates acute edema, hemorrhage, or exudate, while irregular reticular strands are suggestive of chronic fibrotic scars. Therefore, wall characteristics may be helpful in establishing the age of the cavity. In addition, necrosis of either an inflammatory or neoplastic mass may leave thick nodular walls (see Figs 23–1, *A* and 23–6, *A–C*).

PYOGENIC INFECTION

The term *abscess* is usually reserved for cavities that are the result of pyogenic infections. This complication indicates a virulent process that results in vasculitis with thrombosis of small vessels, which leads to necrosis of lung tissue. The abscess, which is made up of necrotic material, will appear to be of tissue opacity until communications with airways are established. These communications permit drainage of the necrotic debris. This liquefied necrotic material is coughed up, with the radiologic result of a lucent defect or cavity. The presence of cavitation in the acute phase of a pulmonary infection is a significant radiologic finding that narrows the differential considerations; viral and mycoplasma pneumonia are virtually eliminated, and pneumococcal pneumonia (infection with *Streptococcus pneumoniae*) would be a rarity. The organisms most likely to lead to cavitation are *Staphylococcus*, β-hemolytic *Streptococcus*, *Klebsiella*, *Pseudomonas*, *Escherichia coli*, the mixed gram-negative organisms, and anaerobes. (Answer to question 2 is *a*.)

Aspiration is frequently the source of the mixed gram-negative and anaerobic infections.[31] This may be the result of subclinical aspiration and has been described as gravitational pneumonia. Aspiration pneumonia should be particularly suspected when the cavity occurs in a dependent portion of the lung. The clinical setting of a condition such as poor oral hygiene, alcoholism, or a tumor in the nasopharynx, larynx, or mouth would support the diagnosis. The patient typically experiences a febrile response with productive cough, like that of other patients with necrotizing pneumonia.

On occasion the cavities resulting from a necrotizing pneumonia will rupture, forming a bronchopleural fistula. This leads to the radiologic appearance of a hydropneumothorax, which is usually recognized by an air-fluid level in the pleural space. Pleural air-fluid collections are elliptical, lack an identifiable wall, and have air-fluid levels that differ in length depending on the radiographic projection. Abscesses tend to have spherical thick walls and air-fluid levels that are equal in length regardless of the radiographic projection[482,537,578] (see Figs 23–1, C and D, and 23–7, A and B). The clinical correlations of pyogenic pneumonia are usually dramatic, with the patient being profoundly ill, running a toxic febrile course, and having an elevated white blood cell count. Because of the necrosis of lung tissue, hemoptysis is not a rare complication of these more virulent infections. Culture of the organism is required for definitive diagnosis.

Pulmonary gangrene[443,671] results from very acute ischemic necrosis of lung tissue. It differs from lung abscess in that a region of lung undergoes necrosis, detaches from viable lung, and forms a mass of devitalized tissue lying within a cavity. Organisms to be considered when gangrene is identified include *Staphylococcus aureus, Streptococcus* species, *Klebsiella pneumoniae, Haemophilus influenzae, Mucor* fungi, and *Aspergillus*. The characteristic radiographic appearance is that of a mass surrounded by eccentric lucency (see Fig 23–1, B). Radiographically, pulmonary gangrene may resemble a fungus ball in a cavity, but the latter is due to a solid mass of fungus that has colonized a preexisting cavity or cystic space. CT may be helpful in demonstrating that the intracavitary mass consists of lung. Early diagnosis of gangrene is important because it often requires surgical resection.

GRANULOMATOUS DISEASE

Tuberculosis is the prototypical cause of an infectious pulmonary cavity. The cavitary phase of tuberculosis rarely occurs at the time of the initial infection but is a secondary phenomenon resulting from a hyperimmune response.[91,654] The necrosis of lung tissue liberates organisms previously isolated by a surrounding fibrotic reaction. The cavities of tuberculosis are usually quite distinctive because of their proclivity to either the apical or the posterior segments of the upper lobes. About 10% of tuberculous cavities are found in atypical locations. A cavity in an anterior segment of an upper lobe as the sole manifestation of pulmonary tuberculosis is very rare. Isolated lower lobe cavities are rarely caused by tuberculosis, but lower lobe tuberculosis in association with upper lobe disease is not rare. While these latter locations should be considered more suggestive of some of the other causes of cavitary disease, such as acute necrotizing pneumonias or fungal infections, an unusual location should not be cause for rejecting the diagnosis of tuberculosis (Fig 23–6).[64,91,240,412]

Other radiologic features that aid in the identification of a tuberculous cavity include (1) associated reticular pulmonary scars, (2) volume loss in the involved lobe, (3) pleural thickening, (4) pleural calcification, and (5) calcified hilar or mediastinal lymph nodes. These are all the result of a long-standing inflammatory response. The reticular or linear scars cause a very irregular margin of the outer wall of the cavity. These linear opacities are the result of both granulomas and fibrotic scarring. The fibrotic scars are also the cause of the volume loss, which is radiologically detected by noting elevation of the hilum and shift of the mediastinum (see discussion of cicatrizing atelectasis, in Chapter 13). Calcified nodular opacities in the area of the cavity indicate previous granulomatous infection; however, homogeneous nodules are of less diagnostic value.

As suggested previously, the presence of a tuberculous cavity indicates a failure in host defenses. This results in liberation of organisms that may have been isolated for years. Therefore, the presence of cavitation indicates active infectious disease. Exposure during this stage of the disease accounts for the majority of new cases of tuberculosis. In addition to the possibility of spreading the infection to others, patients in this phase of tuberculosis are at considerable risk of developing disseminated infection, which may be bronchogenic or hematogenous.

The distinction of hematogenous and bronchogenic spread is greatly assisted by assessment of the clinical course. Involvement of multiple organs indicates hematogenous or miliary infection. As described in Chapter 17, the radiologic presentation of miliary tuberculosis is that of a diffuse fine nodular pattern, with the nodules sharply defined. The association of cavitary tuberculosis with disseminated larger opacities in the range of 2 mm to 5 mm and which have ill-defined borders is more suggestive of bronchogenic spread, with the opacities representing peribronchial inflammatory infiltrates and exudation into the terminal air-spaces. The latter has been termed "acinar" tuberculosis.[186] Figure 23–4 illustrates a case of bronchogenic, disseminated tuberculosis. The combination of a large, irregular upper-lobe cavity and multiple ill-defined opacities in the lower lobe strongly suggests the diagnosis. Primary or secondary tumor would be unlikely to produce such a pattern; the irregular nodules with ill-defined borders are certainly not typical metastatic nodules. Bronchogenic carcinoma might produce a similar cavity but would be an unlikely cause for the disseminated opacities. Coccidioidomycosis is a granulomatous infection that can mimic tuberculosis and cannot be entirely eliminated in this case by radiologic criteria alone, but the case shown in Figure 23–4 certainly does not represent a classic appearance for cavitary coccidioidomycosis. (Answer to question 4 is *b*.)

When conventional laboratory examinations fail to isolate the cause of an apical cavity, atypical mycobacteria must be considered. There are cases of atypical mycobacterial infection suggesting that the radiologic features of the cavity may be identical to those in typical tuberculosis, but some differences in the radiologic presentation of the two infections have been described. The atypical organisms are more likely to produce multiple thin-walled apical cavities with only minimal surrounding parenchymal disease and with minimal or no pleural reaction. Surrounding nodules are likewise uncommon. An apical cavity in a patient who fails to respond to a purified protein derivative (PPD) skin test requires consideration of the atypical mycobacteria and the fungi, such as *Histoplasma*.

Histoplasmosis[104,117,390] is another consideration in the differential diagnosis of an apical cavity that may completely mimic the appearance of tuberculosis. There may even be extensive associated parenchymal scarring, volume loss, and calcifications involving both the lung parenchyma and hilar lymph nodes. This diagnosis should be considered most likely in patients who have negative reactions to skin or serologic tests for tuberculosis and positive reactions to skin or serologic tests for histoplasmosis.

Cavitary coccidioidomycosis[392] is much more variable in terms of location of the cavities than is either tuberculosis or histoplasmosis. In contrast to tuberculosis, coccidioidomycotic cavities may occur in the anterior segment of the upper lobes as well as in the lower lobes, but these cavities, like those of tuberculosis, are more common in the upper lobes. The cavities of coccidioidomycosis frequently form in areas of a preexisting nodule. The classic evolution of a coccidioidomycotic cavity begins with a parenchymal infiltrate that organizes into a nodule. The nodule undergoes necrosis, leading to the formation of a cavity when communications with small airways are established to permit drainage of the necrotic material. It has been stated that the very thin-walled cavity is classic of coccidioidomycosis, but this is a relatively late stage of cavitary coccidioidomycosis. In fact, the thick-walled cavity is at least as common as the classic "grape skin," or thin-walled, cavity (Fig 23–8, *A* and *B*).

Clinical correlation is helpful in evaluating patients with cavities. As expected, hemoptysis is a nonspecific finding and is consistent with any cavitary process. A history of having been in an area where coccidioidomycosis is endemic supports the diagnosis. In fact, patients who have not been in an endemic area are usually not suspected of having this infection, but on occasion the organism can be transported to the patient. This has been documented in patients working with cotton, wool, and other farm products from the desert Southwest. The results of skin and serologic tests add valuable data to the diagnosis of coccidioidomycosis.

Other fungal[478] agents, including *Blastomyces dermatitidis* (North American blastomycosis), *Cryptococcus neoformans* (cryptococcosis), and actinomycosis are less common causes of pulmonary cavities that produce patterns similar to those of tuberculosis and histoplasmosis. These diagnoses require laboratory confirmation. *Nocardia* species are gram-positive organisms that were previously classified as fungi. Nocardiosis frequently results either in consolidation or in pulmonary nodules, which may cavitate. It is rarely encountered in normal patients but is not rare in patients who are immunologically suppressed. Nocardiosis is a well-known cause of pulmonary infection in renal transplant patients and in patients with alveolar proteinosis. It should not lead to chronic cavities, with the surrounding scars typical of both tuberculosis and histoplasmosis.

Neoplasm

Cavitation of pulmonary neoplasms[605] is not rare. About 16%[605] of all peripheral primary carcinomas show radiologic evidence of cavitation. This is most frequent in epidermoid carcinomas, with approximately 30% of the peripheral epidermoid carcinomas showing cavitation. The second most common cell type of tumor to undergo cavitation is bronchioloalveolar cell carcinoma, which is a very well-differentiated adenocarcinoma.[636,638]

The radiologist's first responsibility in the assessment of a possible cavitating neoplasm is to verify the presence of cavitation. This is frequently accomplished by simple identification of a large hole in a mass. When there is doubt about cavitation, the presence of an air-fluid level on a film taken with the patient upright should be confirmatory. When such views cannot be obtained, the lateral decubitus film is an adequate substitute. CT is very sensitive for the detection of cavitation and often reveals liquefaction of a mass before the lesion appears cavitary on the plain film.

It has been suggested that the presence and size of fluid levels may be helpful in distinguishing carcinomas from abscesses. While it is true that many cavitating carcinomas do not contain a significant amount of fluid and thus have either no air-fluid level or only modest fluid levels, fluid levels do occur in carcinomas and are not a trustworthy sign for distinguishing between a cavitating neoplasm and an abscess. Theros[605] emphasized that bleeding into a neoplasm may result in a high air-fluid level, thus mimicking the appearance of an abscess. Cavitating carcinomas may become secondarily infected, leading to the development of air-fluid levels. The location of the cavity within the mass has been cited as another feature for distinguishing carcinomas from abscesses. The presence of eccentric cavitation might indicate malignancy, but an Armed Forces Institute of Pathology study identified an equal number of eccentric and central cavities in more than 1,200 patients with carcinoma.[605] A lobulated or nodular wall is another radiologic feature of cavities that has been evaluated in an effort to distinguish neoplasms from abscesses. This nodularity may be observed at the interface of the cavity with either the lung or with the inner cavity wall. The walls of abscesses tend to be smoother,[578] but it must be emphasized that both tuberculous cavities and abscesses may produce a nodular margin. In fact, nodular walls may be seen in any cavity that has resulted from a necrotic process. The radiologic features of the wall of a cavity cannot be used to reliably distinguish a neoplasm from an abscess.[663] The cases shown in Figures 23–1, *A,* and 23–3, *A* and *B,* are squamous cell carcinomas of the lung. Compare their borders with the tuberculosis case shown in Figure 23–6, *A–C.* All of the possibilities offered in question 3 are plausible except bronchogenic cyst, which should have smooth, thin walls. (Answer to question 3 is *d.*) Additionally, it must be emphasized that a smooth, thin wall does not exclude the presence of tumor. Dodd and Boyle[128] emphasized that cavitating neoplasms may have thin walls. By now it should be obvious that the radiologic features of a cavity are infrequently diagnostic of tumor. The identification of a cavity therefore requires complete bacteriologic and cytologic evaluation. If a positive diagnosis cannot be established by either technique, biopsy is frequently mandatory to exclude tumor.

The distinction of primary lung tumor from metastasis as the cause of a solitary cavity is also not easily accomplished.[128] It should be emphasized that metastatic cavities are more commonly multiple or at least associated with multiple pulmonary nodules. A solitary metastasis may present a particularly difficult diagnostic problem, since metastases that cavitate are frequently of squamous cell origin and may therefore mimic the histologic features of a primary lung tumor. Cavitary lung metastases are most likely to be from the head and neck in men and the gynecologic tract in women.

Vascular Lesions

Wegener's granulomatosis[342,377] and rheumatoid arthritis[492] are the two most likely collagen vascular diseases to result in a perivascular inflammatory reaction[364] and to thus cause necrosis of lung tissue with subsequent cavitation. Both of these entities are likely to result in either multiple pulmonary opacities or multiple cavities. These lesions are considered in greater detail in the chapters on multiple opacities and multiple cavities (Chapters 16 and 24).

Thromboemboli[121] and septic emboli[674] also produce vascular occlusion that may lead to ischemic necrosis with cavitation. They are also more likely to produce multiple areas of opacity with multiple cavities.

Inhalational Diseases

Both silicosis and coal-worker's pneumoconiosis have been reported to result in cavitation, most often in one of the conglomerate masses seen in these diseases. These cavities have been postulated to result from ischemic necrosis of the center of the mass. This is a rare complication of silicosis. The most likely cause of a cavity occurring in a patient with silicosis is complicating tuberculosis. In fact, tuberculosis must be ruled out in all patients with silicosis who develop subsequent cavitation. The associated reticular changes in these patients may also result from the primary disease or the associated tuberculosis. Serial films documenting a change require complete clinical evaluation to exclude active tuberculosis.

Pneumatoceles

Pneumatoceles could appropriately have been discussed with the pyogenic infections that result in holes in the lung, but it is important to distinguish pneumatoceles from true cavities.[12,127,150,250] The appearance of a lucency in the midst of extensive air space consolidation does not always indicate a necrotic cavity. The development of pneumatoceles, particularly in staphylococcal and hydrocarbon aspiration pneumonias, represents a well-known example of a lucency that mimics the radiologic appearance of cavitation. In the early stages of infection, these cystic spaces are virtually indistinguishable from cavities. Clinical and laboratory correlation are frequently the only way to establish the correct cause of the holes. The pneumatoceles characteristically occur in the healing phase of the disease, and they radiologically appear to enlarge and increase in number while the patient appears to be clinically improving. They are more frequently multiple than solitary. The pathologic mechanism for the development of pneumatoceles has not been clearly defined. One postulate is that they are secondary to small airway obstructive disease with a sleeve valve mechanism that results in localized air trapping. Other researchers believe that pneumatoceles result from an alteration of the normal pulmonary elasticity. Their importance is that they do not indicate destruction of lung parenchyma and are usually transient, although their resolution may take weeks to months.

The term *traumatic pneumatocele*[150] is applied to those lesions that follow blunt injury to the chest (Fig 23–9). These injuries initially result in an area of pulmonary contusion. The development of a cystic structure following resolution of the pulmonary contusion is generally believed to result from laceration of the lung. The situation is therefore somewhat different from the pneumatocele that results from an infectious process and is clearly different from a true cavity in its pathogenesis. A history of trauma and serial x-ray films usually confirm the origin of the cyst. Computed tomography has been useful in the diagnosis of post-traumatic pneumatoceles.[211,224,624]

Congenital Cyst

The congenital lesions that may result in the radiologic appearance of a solitary hole in the lung include the bronchogenic[488] cyst and bronchopulmonary sequestration. Although these structures are considered to be congenital or developmental, they are frequently seen in young adults.

The bronchopulmonary sequestration may assume a very characteristic radio-logic appearance[162] (see Fig 23–10, A). It is a complex foregut anomaly found me-dially in either lower lobe, almost always in the posterior basal segment.[256,533] It is somewhat more frequent on the left and may present as a cavity posterior to the heart.[186] This appearance may casually resemble that of a hiatal hernia except that a hiatal hernia is usually more of a midline structure. The distinction is eas-ily made after a barium swallow. There are two types of bronchopulmonary se-questration: intralobar and extralobar. The extralobar variety is totally isolated from the lung by its own pleura and is therefore unlikely to present as a cavitary or cystic lesion. The development of a lucent defect requires the development of a communication with airways that will permit the drainage of fluid from the cys-tic structure. This is a common presentation for the intralobar sequestration that may occur spontaneously or as a result of superimposed infection. Prior to devel-opment of the communication, the sequestration is more likely to have the radi-ologic appearance of a mass or ill-defined opacity. The clinical presentation is of-ten that of recurrent infection in the area of sequestration. This may suggest the differential diagnosis of chronic recurrent lower lobe infection, including cystic bronchiectasis, chronic abscess, and intrapulmonary sequestration. Radiologic ev-idence of the diagnosis requires aortography for demonstration of the anomalous artery from the aorta to the sequestered lung (see Fig 23–10, B). Histologically, the sequestration consists of a multicystic structure. The linings of the cysts fre-quently contain multiple elements that resemble alveolar walls, bronchioles, and even bronchi. The bronchuslike structures do not have normal communications with the tracheobronchial tree. Occasionally some of the cyst may continue to be fluid filled and may even give rise to the appearance of a mass within a cystic structure. Because of the multicystic nature of the lesion, the radiologic appear-ance of the hole in the lung may be that of a large cystic structure with multiple loculations and even multiple air-fluid levels.

The bronchogenic cyst,[488] in contrast to the pulmonary sequestration, is a simple cyst (Fig 23–11). The majority of bronchogenic cysts occur as mediastinal opacities. Of the small number that occur in the lung (approximately 14%), the radiologic presentation is usually that of a well-circumscribed, homogeneous soft tissue opac-ity. Approximately 36% of bronchogenic cysts occurring in the lung will be air-con-taining and therefore present a lucent defect. The differentiation of these cysts from acquired inflammatory cysts usually presents a diagnostic dilemma, with the latter being either chronic lung abscesses or a dominant cyst of cystic bronchiectasis. Bronchogenic cysts are not expected in the apices and are therefore unlikely to be confused with a tuberculous cavity. Since the inflammatory causes of a hole in the lung are much more common, bronchogenic cyst frequently becomes a diagnosis of exclusion. It is often easier for the radiologist to reject the diagnosis of a bron-chogenic cyst than to actually make the diagnosis. Ill-defined borders with surrounding irregular infiltrate, reticular strands radiating away from the hole, loculations (coarse bands of opacity) within the hole, and associated pleural reac-tions all strongly suggest an infectious etiology rather than a congenital cyst. Only those cases with very thin, sharply defined walls should be considered as possible bronchogenic cysts. This appearance might be mimicked by coccidioidomycosis and may also be confused with a pneumatocele or bullous lesion. It must be empha-sized that bullous lesions are frequently multiple and associated with stretching and attenuation of the pulmonary vasculature. Pneumatocele is best excluded on the basis of history, since it typically follows staphylococcal pneumonia, hydrocarbon pneumonia, or trauma. Bronchogenic cyst is therefore suggested by exclusion of the more likely causes of a localized lucency.

Bronchiectatic Cysts

Cystic bronchiectasis is not a rare cause of multiple holes in the lung and is considered in detail in Chapter 24. Occasionally a very large dominant cyst may result from cystic bronchiectasis and mimic an abscess or a congenital cyst.[488]

Bullous Emphysema

Bullous emphysema[260] is another process that rarely presents with a solitary cystic structure or hole in the lung, but these defects may vary considerably in size and result in the appearance of a large hole in the lung. Other associated bullae may produce only minimal changes on the roentgenogram. These holes tend to have very thin walls and are frequently surrounded by attenuated, elongated pulmonary vessels. The cyst itself should appear to be avascular. Cysts of bullous emphysema may be distinguished from thin-walled bronchogenic cysts by their peripheral location, as opposed to a more central location for the bronchogenic cyst. They are commonly encountered in either the apices or the bases of the lungs and are often the cause of recurrent pneumothoraces.

SUMMARY

1. Holes in the lung may be caused by cavities, pneumatoceles, bronchiectatic cysts, bullous emphysema, and even congenital cysts, including bronchogenic cysts and intrapulmonary sequestration.

2. True cavities are the result of infection, tumor, or vascular insufficiency with ischemic necrosis.

3. The processes that lead to infectious cavities may be divided into two categories: (1) pyogenic infection and (2) granulomatous inflammation. The clinical course is usually quite distinct for each category. Pyogenic infections produce an acute febrile illness with elevation and a shift to the left of the white blood cell count and the radiologic appearance of extensive air-space consolidation followed by cavitation. In contrast, cavitary diseases resulting from granulomatous infection follow a more indolent course, with low-grade temperatures, less sputum production, and mildly elevated white blood cell counts.

4. The granulomatous infections produce associated radiologic findings of chronic disease, including pleural thickening, reticular opacities in the lung, cicatrizing atelectasis, and pulmonary nodules. Careful clinical correlation and laboratory diagnosis usually confirm the suspicion of a granulomatous process.

5. Both primary and secondary neoplasms may cavitate. Multiple pulmonary nodules with cavitation strongly suggest metastatic disease. A solitary cavity with thick nodular walls must be considered tumorous until proved otherwise. Approximately two-thirds of cavitating tumors will be of squamous cell origin and either primary in the lung or secondary.

6. Of the vascular diseases that result in ischemic necrosis and thus a solitary cavity, thromboembolism is the most common. These diseases frequently produce multiple radiologic opacities, although they may occasionally produce only one cavity. Clinical correlation is particularly important. For example, Wegener's granulomatosis may be associated with renal disease or sinus disease that virtually confirms the diagnosis. Although the clinical setting of thromboemboli can be nonspecific, an association of thrombophlebitis, pleuritic chest pain, and pleural effusion followed by the development of a cavity is virtually diagnostic.

7. Cavitation of a conglomerate mass of silicosis may result from ischemic necrosis, but this complication must be considered to be superimposed tuberculosis until proved otherwise.

8. Infectious pneumatoceles must be distinguished from abscesses. Both result from a necrotizing pneumonia. Clinical correlation is essential, since pneumatoceles tend to occur in the healing phases of pneumonia, when the patient appears to have passed the crisis. Differentiating between an abscess and a pneumatocele is definitely important, since pneumatoceles resolve spontaneously after a period of weeks to months without any notable residual effect. Abscesses may persist as a source of recurrent infection or leave parenchymal scars.

9. Traumatic pneumatocele is the result of pulmonary laceration with the development of a cystic space.

10. Intrapulmonary sequestration is a complex foregut anomaly that may result in a cystic lesion in the base of the lung. It frequently appears as a localized multilocular cyst and may be associated with recurrent basilar pulmonary infections. It may therefore be confused with cystic bronchiectasis. Aortography is the confirmatory diagnostic procedure. Bilateral pulmonary sequestrations are very rare.[652]

11. Cystic bronchiectasis is more commonly the cause of multiple holes in the lung; however, one cystic structure may be dominant and therefore mimic the appearance of a solitary cyst. Of the entities considered in this differential diagnosis, sequestration most closely mimics cystic bronchiectasis, since both occur in the bases of the lung.

12. Bullous emphysema may also result in a dominant cyst with very thin walls. There is usually an associated attenuation of pulmonary vasculature. The cysts tend to be in the periphery of the lung and are frequently pleural-based. Because of their characteristic location and associated findings, they should not be easily confused with the other entities considered in this chapter.

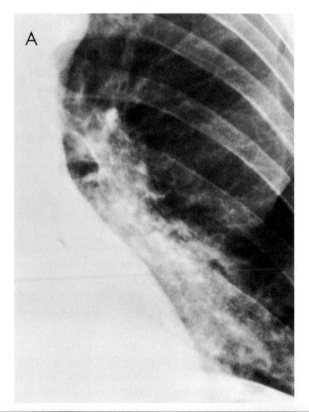

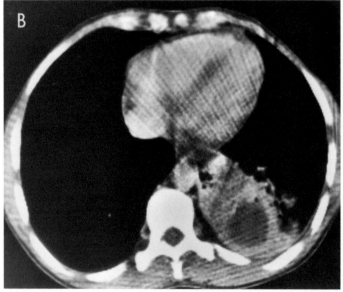

FIG 23–5
A, PA film demonstrates consolidation of the left lower lobe in an early phase of a necrotizing pneumonia. **B,** CT scan reveals a well-localized area of liquefaction of tissue, which is consistent with an early stage of a developing pulmonary abscess. Note the low-attenuation necrotic material surrounded by the more-opaque consolidated lung.

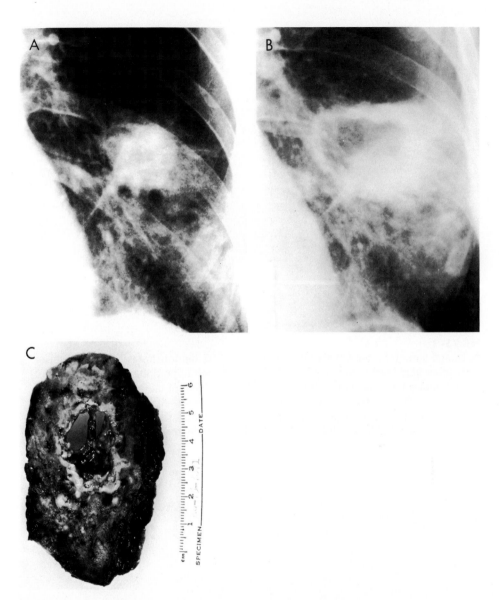

FIG 23–6
A, Irregular spiculated mass is suggestive of a primary lung tumor. **B,** Follow-up examination 6 weeks later, however, reveals the mass to have rapidly enlarged and cavitated. Cavitation of an apparent mass would appear to support the diagnosis of tumor, but such a rapid increase in size opposes this diagnosis. This is a tuberculous abscess that has drained its liquefied center, with the radiologic result of a cavity. **C,** Gross specimen from another case reveals how tuberculosis occasionally results in cavities with nodular walls, thus resembling a tumor.

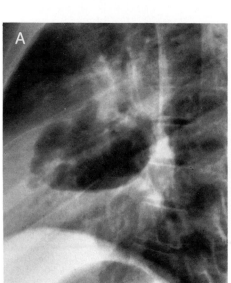

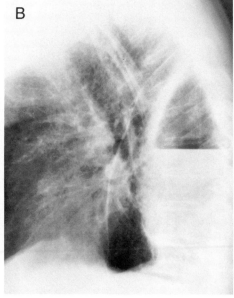

FIG 23–7
A, Lateral film of the patient shown in Figure 23–1, C, demonstrates a spherical cavity with an air-fluid level in the lingular segment of the left upper lobe. This confirms the diagnosis of pneumonia with lung abscess. **B,** Lateral film of the patient seen in Figure 23–1, D, demonstrates a posterior vertically oriented elliptical structure with an air-fluid level. This confirms a pleural air-fluid collection consistent with hydropneumothorax. This resulted from pneumonia with a bronchopleural fistula.

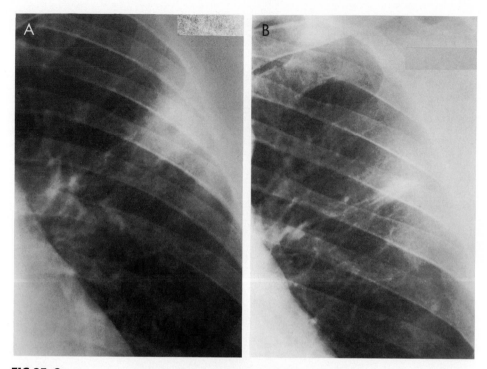

FIG 23–8

A, Atypical case of coccidioidomycosis: (1) Cavity occurred in a large focal opacity with ill-defined borders. It is not a thin-walled cavity, but this is probably more common than sometimes suggested. (2) The patient had never been in the southwestern United States. The organism was brought to the patient, who worked with cotton and wool from the Southwest. **B,** Cavity did not completely resolve but left a nodular residual, a well-known result of any granulomatous infection.

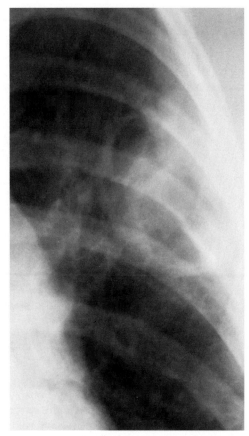

FIG 23–9
This lucency developed in an area of consolidation that resulted from pulmonary contusion following a crush injury to the left chest. This is a so-called traumatic lung cyst or pneumatocele.

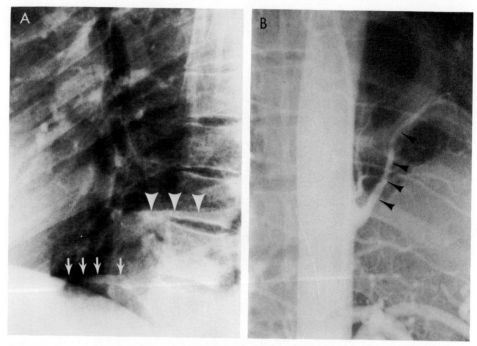

FIG 23–10
A, Lateral chest film reveals air-fluid level in left lower lobe *(large arrowheads).* Note that posterior portion of left hemidiaphragm is obscured, confirming the location. Anterior left hemidiaphragm is outlined by *small white arrows.* This raises the differential diagnosis of a hiatal hernia, abscess, cystic bronchiectasis, or intralobar sequestration.
B, Aortogram from same case reveals large artery arising from abdominal aorta and feeding to left lower lobe cyst. This confirms the diagnosis of pulmonary sequestration.

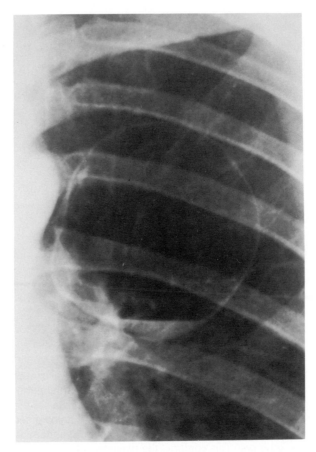

FIG 23–11
Very thin-walled, circumscribed lucent lesion is typical appearance for a congenital bronchogenic cyst that has drained its fluid content. (From Reed JC, Sobonya RE: RPC from the AFIP. *Radiology* 1975; 117:315–319. Used by permission.)

ANSWER GUIDE

LEGENDS FOR INTRODUCTORY FIGURES

FIG 23–1

A, Squamous cell carcinoma of the lung caused this cavity with thick nodular walls and a low air-fluid level. Compare its appearance with the tuberculosis case seen in Figure 23–6, *A–C.* **B,** Another cavity with thick irregular walls contains a large soft-tissue mass. This is the expected appearance for pulmonary gangrene. It results from a virulent infection that has invaded the pulmonary vessels. This is a case of mucormycosis. (From Zagoria RJ, Choplin RH, Karstaedt N: Pulmonary gangrene as a complication of mucormycosis. *AJR* 1985; 114:1195–1196. Used by permission.) **C,** A large, lucent lesion with a long air-fluid level is surrounded by a large area of air-space consolidation. An earlier lateral film (Fig 23–7, *A*) confirmed the location of the lesion to be in the lingula. This is a necrotizing pneumonia with pulmonary abscess. **D,** Compare this lucent lesion with the one shown in Figure 23–1, *C.* It also contains a high fluid level but lacks either a well-defined wall or surrounding pulmonary consolidation. These are clues to a loculated hydropneumothorax. The lateral view (Fig 23–7, *B*) confirmed the extrapulmonary location of the lesion. This is an empyema with a bronchopleural fistula.

FIG 23–2

A, Note multifocal, ill-defined opacities in right lung. **B,** Left lung has sharply defined cavity. This case is radiologically similar to that illustrated in Figure 23–4, but patient had a high temperature, elevated blood count, and short course of illness. This is also an example of bronchogenic spread of pulmonary infection. The inner wall of the cavity was smooth because it was under tension produced by the respirator. This is staphylococcal pneumonia. **C,** Gross specimen from same case as **B** reveals large cavity surrounded by consolidation. **D,** Histologic examination of lung around the periphery of the cavity reveals narrowing of small arterioles *(arrowheads)* by inflammatory reaction. Ischemia secondary to vasculitis and thrombosis is the cause of the necrosis and thus of the cavity.

FIG 23–3

A, Nodularity of inner wall *(arrows)* of cavity should suggest a necrotic tumor. This is a primary carcinoma of the lung. **B,** Histologic section from this primary carcinoma of the lung reveals central necrosis and nodular inner walls of the mass. (From Theros EG: Varying manifestations of peripheral pulmonary neoplasms: A radiologic-pathologic correlative study. *AJR* 1977; 128:893–914. Used by permission.)

FIG 23–4

Combination of left upper lobe cavity *(arrows)* and multifocal, ill-defined opacities in both lungs is very suggestive of an infectious process with bronchogenic spread. It is helpful to know whether this is an acute or chronic process. The patient had tuberculosis with bronchogenic dissemination.

ANSWERS

1, a, c, d, b; 2, a; 3, d; 4, b.

C H A P T E R   2 4

Multiple Lucent Lesions

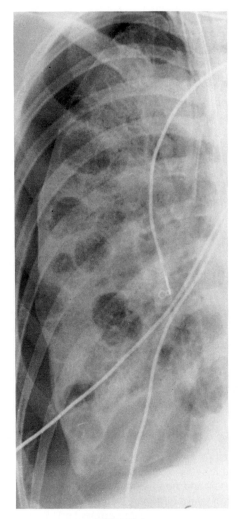

FIG 24–1

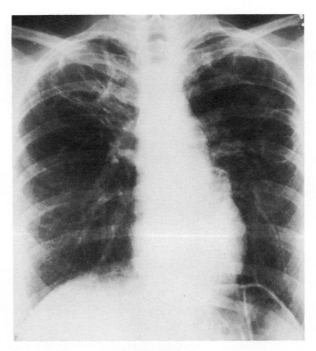

FIG 24–2

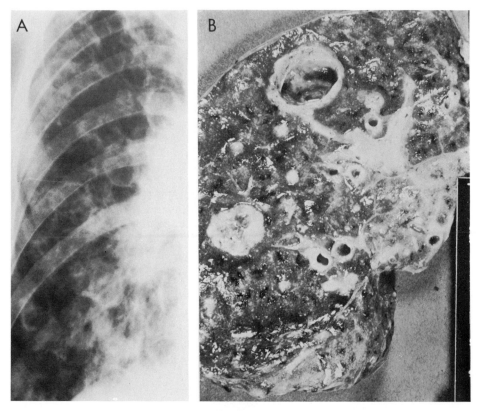

FIG 24–3

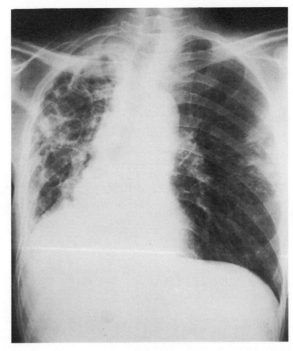

FIG 24–4

QUESTIONS

1. Refer to Figure 24–1. Which of the following is the best diagnosis?
   a. Adult respiratory distress syndrome.
   b. Pneumatoceles.
   c. Multiple abscesses.
   d. Bronchopleural fistula.
   e. Necrotizing pneumonia, abscesses, and bronchopleural fistula.
2. The multiple cavities with surrounding reticular opacities shown in Figure 24–2 are consistent with which of the following diagnoses?
   a. *Klebsiella* pneumonia.
   b. Tuberculosis.
   c. *Mycoplasma* pneumonia.
   d. Coccidioidomycosis.
   e. *Pseudomonas* pneumonia.
3. Which of the following is *least* likely to cause the multiple cavities shown in Figures 24–3, *A* and *B*?
   a. Carcinoma of the esophagus.
   b. Bronchogenic carcinoma.
   c. Nasopharyngeal carcinoma.
   d. Carcinoma of the uterine cervix.
   e. Carcinoma of the tongue.

4. Which is the most likely diagnosis in the case illustrated in Figure 24–4?
   a. Metastatic squamous cell carcinoma.
   b. *Klebsiella* pneumonia.
   c. Tuberculosis.
   d. Staphylococcal pneumonia.
   e. *Mycoplasma* pneumonia.

CHART 24–1.
Multiple Lucent Lesions

I. Cavities
  A. Infection
    1. Bacterial pneumonias[231] (*Staphyloccus, Klebsiella,* other gram-negative organisms, anaerobes, and *Nocardia*)
    2. Fungal
      a. Histoplasmosis[104,117]
      b. Blastomycosis[474]
      c. Coccidioidomycosis[392]
      d. Cryptococcosis[217,252,315]
      e. Mucormycosis[32]
      f. Sporotrichosis[100]
      g. Aspergillosis[478]
    3. Tuberculosis[64]
    4. Parasites (echinococcal disease)[370]
  B. Neoplasms
    1. Metastases[22,107,113,128,309]
    2. Lymphoma (rare)[374]
    3. Bronchioloalveolar cell carcinoma[636,638]
  C. Vascular
    1. Rheumatoid disease[492]
    2. Wegener's granulomatosis[377]
    3. Infarcts[121]
    4. Septic emboli[241,674]
II. Cystic bronchiectasis (recurrent pneumonias, tuberculosis, cystic fibrosis, agammaglobulinemia, allergic aspergillosis)
III. Pneumatoceles[16,127,150,250]
IV. Bullous emphysema (see Chapter 22)
V. Honeycomb lung (see Chapter 19)
VI. Cystic adenomatoid malformation (newborn)[376,641]
VII. Herniation of small bowel (congenital or traumatic)

CHART 24–2.
Cavitating Nodules

I. Neoplasms
   A. Primary lung
      1. Squamous cell carcinoma
      2. Adenocarcinoma
      3. Bronchioloalveolar cell carcinoma[636,638]
   B. Metastasis
      1. Squamous cell (e.g., head and neck, cervix, esophagus)
      2. Adenocarcinoma
      3. Melanoma
      4. Sarcoma (e.g., osteosarcoma)
   C. Lymphoma[374]
II. Infections
   A. Septic emboli[241,674] *(Staphylococcus aureus)*
   B. Nocardiosis
   C. Cryptococcosis[286,315]
   D. Coccidioidomycosis
   E. Aspergillosis
III. Vascular and collagen vascular diseases
   A. Pulmonary embolism with infarction[121]
   B. Vasculitis (e.g., Wegener's granulomatosis,[377] Wegener's variants)
   C. Rheumatoid nodules and Caplan's syndrome[156,492]

CHART 24–3.
Ill-defined Opacities With Holes

I. Infections
   A. Necrotizing pneumonias[31,231]
      1. *Staphylococcus aureus*
      2. β-Hemolytic streptococcus
      3. *Klebsiella pneumoniae*
      4. *Escherichia coli*
      5. *Proteus, Aerobacter*
      6. *Pseudomonas*
      7. Anaerobes
   B. Aspiration pneumonia (usually mixed gram-negative organisms)
   C. Septic emboli
   D. Fungus
      1. Histoplasmosis
      2. Blastomycosis
      3. Coccidioidomycosis
      4. Cryptococcosis[281,315]
   E. Tuberculosis
II. Neoplasms
   A. Primary carcinomas
   B. Bronchioloalveolar cell carcinoma[638]
   C. Lymphoma
III. Vascular and collagen vascular diseases
   A. Emboli with infarction
   B. Wegener's granulomatosis
IV. Trauma
   A. Contusion with pneumatoceles[150,418]

CHART 24–4.
Pulmonary Lucent Lesions Related to AIDS

1. PCP-related lung cysts[90]
2. Premature bullous emphysema[237,330] (periphery of upper lobe)
3. Pneumatoceles[237]
4. Necrotizing pneumonias (pyogenic bacteria and *Pneumocystis*[167,320,368])
5. Tuberculosis[215]
6. Atypical mycobacterial infection
7. Fungal infections (fewer than 5% of AIDS patients[434])
   a. Cryptococcosis
   b. Coccidioidomycosis
   c. Nocardiosis (not a true fungus)
   d. Histoplasmosis
8. Mixed infections (common)

DISCUSSION

Many of the entities considered in Chapters 19, 22, and 23 also result in multiple lucent lesions. In fact, some entities more typically produce multiple lesions. The latter include cystic bronchiectasis, pneumatoceles, bullous emphysema, honeycomb lung, and metastatic tumor. Although the precise location of the solitary lucent defect is important, the distribution of multiple lucencies assumes an even greater importance in their radiologic analysis.

Cavities

INFECTION

As in solitary cavities, infection is the most common cause of multiple cavities in the lung. The acute pyogenic infections are radiologically characterized by extensive areas of air-space consolidation, a clinical course of elevated temperature, and often diagnostic laboratory findings, including elevation of the white blood cell count with an associated shift to the left and positive sputum cultures. The development of multiple lucencies in the midst of an acute pneumonia raises the differential of (1) resolution of the process with intervening normal lung, (2) necrosis of tissue with multiple cavities, and (3) pneumatoceles (see Figs 24–1 and 24–5). The pathogenesis of these processes was considered in Chapter 23. Clinical correlation is extremely valuable in making this distinction. When the patient appears to be recovering from illness, the holes most certainly represent either normal aerated lung or pneumatoceles. The radiologic observation of a round, sharply defined lucency with a discrete, smooth wall suggests that the lucencies represent pneumatoceles. Ill-defined lucencies without a distinct margin are more typical of reaerated lung. The development of air-fluid levels in the midst of an area of consolidation indicates the development of spaces in the lung parenchyma that are most probably the result of tissue necrosis and abscess formation. Air-fluid levels are not encountered in either normally aerated lung or pneumatoceles; they are likely to appear when the patient is profoundly ill. In such cases, they are diagnostic of a virulent necrotizing pneumonia. The most common organisms to result in such a process include *Staphylococcus, Klebsiella, Pseudomonas,* anerobes,[31] and other gram-negative organisms. As emphasized earlier, it is exceptional for pneumococcal pneumonia, *Mycoplasma* pneumonia, or viral pneumonias to cavitate.[358,561]

The chronic granulomatous infections, including tuberculosis, histoplasmosis, blastomycosis, and coccidioidomycosis, may all result in multiple cavities. The course of these infections is substantially different from that of the acute necrotizing pneumonias, making both the clinical presentation and the radiologic progression distinctively different. The radiologic appearance of these four entities may be identical; in particular, histoplasmosis, blastomycosis, and tuberculosis are frequently indistinguishable radiologically. Although the cavities from these three infectious processes may be associated with considerable parenchymal reaction, the parenchymal reaction is often a reticular or reticulonodular reaction that is usually distinctive when compared with the consolidations of acute necrotizing pneumonias (see Fig 24–2). (Answers to question 2 are *b* and *d*.) The marked tendency to apical distribution is likewise characteristic but not absolutely diagnostic of these infections. In tuberculosis and histoplasmosis, cavities may develop months to years after the primary infection. There is, however, a rare form of tuberculosis (primary progressive tuberculosis) in which there is progression from primary air-space consolidation to cavitary tuberculosis over a short period without an asymptomatic interval between the two phases of the disease.

Blastomycosis and coccidioidomycosis, in contrast to histoplasmosis and tuberculosis, are more difficult to define in terms of primary and secondary disease. Rabinowitz[474] has emphasized that the cavities of blastomycosis may be apical and mimic the appearance of tuberculosis, but he has also described cases in which cavitation occurred during the acute alveolar exudative phase of the disease and thus might have mimicked the appearance of a necrotizing pneumonia. Rabinowitz emphasized that the radiologic course of such cases of blastomycosis is more protracted than that of necrotizing pneumonia and that clearing of the exudate sometimes requires 2 to 3 months. The clinical course is also more indolent than that of the necrotizing pneumonias, with characteristic low-grade temperatures.

Coccidioidomycosis is known for producing very thin-walled cavities that may lack the surrounding parenchymal reaction that is expected in the other granulomatous infections. The radiologic presentation of thin-walled cavities occurs as a late sequela of the infection. In the early stages of the process, cavities may occur in areas of air-space consolidation. This early acute cavitation results from central necrosis and liquefaction of parenchyma. As the infection is contained, there is organization with circumscription of the opacity. The radiologic sequence may thus be that of a process that begins with an air-space consolidation followed by cavitation leading to the appearance of a thick-walled cavity. When air is trapped in the cavity, it will expand under tension. As the surrounding inflammatory response resolves, the characteristic thin-walled cavity appears. The cavities of coccidioidomycosis are also much less likely to follow the characteristic apical distribution of tuberculosis or histoplasmosis.

The combination of a typical radiologic presentation of multiple thin-walled cavities and a definite history of exposure to *Coccidioides*, with positive serologic studies, frequently makes possible a precise diagnosis.

NEOPLASMS

The pattern of multiple cavities is not rare in patients with pulmonary metastases (see Figs 24–3, *A* and *B*). This radiologic pattern virtually eliminates the diagnosis of primary bronchogenic carcinoma but has been reported as a rare presentation of bronchioloalveolar cell carcinoma.[636,638] The diagnosis of metastasis is frequently aided by knowledge of a distant primary tumor. The typical radiologic appearance is that of sharply circumscribed multiple opacities, with some having central lucencies. These cavities frequently have thick nodular walls, although occasionally the wall may be very thin and smooth. Wall characteristics are not reliable for distinguishing metastases from other causes of multiple cavities. Approximately two-thirds of cavitating metastases are of the epidermoid variety. Tumors of the head and neck,[113] esophagus, and uterine cervix are best known for producing cavitary metastases, but as many as one-third of cavitary metastases may be from adenocarcinoma. Primary carcinoma of the lung is well known as a cause of cavitation but does not often cause multiple cavities. (Answer to question 3 is *b*.) Even malignant melanoma and osteosarcoma have been reported to cavitate. Lymphoma is an infrequent cause of cavitary pulmonary nodules. The exact pathologic mechanism for cavitation of metastases is not always easily determined, but most cavitating metastases seem to represent tumors that have undergone central necrosis.

VASCULAR DISEASES

We have already suggested that true cavities represent ischemic necrosis of lung tissue; however, cavitation is generally considered to be a secondary result of the infectious and neoplastic diseases. Primary diseases of the pulmonary blood vessels also result in cavitation. These include thromboembolism, from venous thrombosis and septic sources, and the collagen vascular diseases, which cause vasculitis and thus result in small vessel occlusions.

The radiologic diagnosis of thromboembolism with infarction is not easily achieved. The majority of patients with venous thromboemboli may in fact have normal chest x-ray films. Those patients who do exhibit radiologic abnormalities have extremely variable patterns that include (1) localized areas of hyperlucency that result from decreased perfusion of an area of lung (Westermark's sign), (2) nonspecific areas of atelectasis, (3) air-space consolidation by hemorrhage and edema, (4) pleural effusion, and (5) cavitation. Of these radiologic presentations, only cavitation can be considered diagnostic of true infarction of lung tissue. Patients with significant amounts of hemorrhage and edema may have had infarction of lung tissue. Infarction cannot be detected during the acute phase of the illness, but the development of cavitation indicates necrosis of lung tissue. It has been stated that cavitating infarcts are usually secondarily infected, but sterile infarcts have been observed to cavitate. It is true that septic emboli from other sources of infection, such as intravenous drug abuse, osteomyelitis, or cellulitis more frequently undergo cavitation than do venous thromboemboli. The diagnosis of septic embolism is most commonly made by combining the radiologic presentation of multiple cavitating lesions with one of the clinical histories described above.

The two collagen-vascular diseases most likely to result in multiple cavitary lesions are Wegener's granulomatosis (Fig 24–6, *A* and *B*) and rheumatoid arthritis (Fig 24–7, *A* and *B*). The pulmonary radiologic patterns of classic Wegener's granulomatosis and the Wegener's variants (limited Wegener's and lymphomatoid granulomatosis) are identical. These entities were all mentioned as causes of solitary cavities, but they are more likely to result in multiple parenchymal opacities with one or more of the opacities progressing to cavitation. In Wegener's granulomatosis, the process frequently results in pulmonary hemorrhage with multifocal areas of ill-defined consolidation that may undergo cavitation. However, in other cases the cavitating lesions may be observed as discrete, well-defined cavities, some of which have thick walls and resemble cavitating nodules. These cavities all result from the diffuse vasculitis and localized areas of ischemic necrosis in these diseases.

Cysts

CYSTIC BRONCHIECTASIS

Cystic bronchiectasis is a complication of either recurrent or chronic infection that may completely mimic the appearance of multiple cavities. This is not true cavitation, but rather dilation of multiple bronchi with the appearance of cystic spaces. One of the most common underlying causes for severe cystic bronchiectasis is cystic fibrosis. Patients with cystic fibrosis have a defect in mucus production, with an unusually thick mucus that predisposes to recurrent pulmonary infections. The recurrent pulmonary infections lead to extensive inflammatory reaction in the bronchial walls (chronic bronchitis), which is followed by cystic bronchiectasis. Ring shadows around the hila are an important radiologic clue to a bronchial origin for the cystic spaces. These rings represent abnormally dilated and thickened bronchi rather than true cavitation. They are frequently more obvious in the upper lobes and may be associated with signs of air trapping in the lower lobes, including loss of peripheral vascularity and flattening of the diaphragm. Another process that may produce a similar effect is agammaglobulinemia. Patients with agammaglobulinemia are also predisposed to recurrent bacterial infections and may have secondary obstructive airway disease and bronchiectasis.

Other patients who have recurrent bacterial pneumonias even with no apparent underlying predisposing condition are prone to the development of bronchiectasis. In the early phases this bronchiectasis may be cylindric and even reversible, but after many episodes of pneumonia, the bronchial damage may progress to the form of bronchiectasis described as varicose or cystic bronchiectasis. This is most characteristically encountered in the lower lobes. During the early phases of this process, roentgenograms obtained during the intervals between infection may be normal. This is followed by the gradual accumulation of linear opacities in the bases. At this stage, HRCT may reveal cylindric bronchiectasis. As the bronchiectasis progresses, there may be saccular dilation of the bronchi, with lucent areas appearing in the bases as ring shadows, again representing abnormally dilated and thickened bronchi. Multiple thin-walled lucencies with low air-fluid levels are very suggestive of cystic bronchiectasis. In essence, HRCT has replaced bronchography and is a useful method for confirming the etiology of these lucent areas. HRCT has the added advantage of showing the extent of the disease.

Tuberculosis is another cause of cystic bronchiectasis. When multiple cavities are encountered in either the apices or throughout a lung after long-standing infection with tuberculosis, the possibility that these lucencies represent bronchiectasis in addition to necrotic cavities must be considered. This distinction can occasionally be made by plain films demonstrating tubular lucencies that appear to connect with the hila. Such an appearance may be verified by HRCT. When the cystic spaces are very large, the distinction of true cavities from dilated bronchi may be virtually impossible radiologically and even confusing for the histologist. In the case presented in Figure 24–4, there is severe destruction of the right lung, with both necrotic cavities and tuberculous cystic bronchiectasis. The associated loss of volume and apical pleural reaction should help make the diagnosis of tuberculosis. (Answer to question 4 is *c*.)

Allergic bronchopulmonary aspergillosis occurs primarily in asthmatic patients and is often associated with bronchiectasis. The perihilar cystic spaces that may develop in these patients are often the result of a unique form of cystic bronchiectasis that involves the proximal bronchi but appears to spare the smaller distal bronchi. Mucus plugs in these dilated bronchi will produce areas of increased density that often have a typical branching pattern. If the plugs are coughed up, cystic spaces are often seen. A history of chronic asthma and laboratory identification of elevated precipitin levels to *Aspergillus fumigatus* should confirm the diagnosis.

PNEUMATOCELES

Pneumatoceles are an unusual cause of a solitary lucency in the lung. Pneumatoceles are usually multiple and most commonly result in multiple lucent defects (Fig 24–8). The most typical radiologic appearance for pneumatoceles is therefore that of multiple thin-walled cystic structures occurring in an area of previous air-space pneumonia. These spaces may persist for weeks or even months, but they do not represent necrosis of lung tissue. Paramediastinal pneumatoceles that follow mechanical ventilation differ from other pneumatoceles in location and etiology. They have previously been assumed to be air collections in the inferior pulmonary ligament.[625] Godwin has reported evidence, based on CT examinations of these patients, that these medial air collections are in either the medial pleural space or the posterior mediastinum.[211] Traumatic pneumatoceles result from pulmonary lacerations that may involve the pleura. The spaces initially fill with blood or hematoma, with the lucent lesions appearing as the blood is replaced with air.[224,624]

CONGENITAL LESIONS

Congenital causes of circumscribed lucencies in the lung are relatively rare; reports of multiple bronchogenic cysts are exceedingly rare. Intralobar pulmonary sequestrations are frequently seen as multicystic structures in one area, particularly in the lower lobe, but, like bronchogenic cysts, they rarely entail multiple areas of involvement. Congenital cystic adenomatoid malformation (CCAM) is possibly the only true multicystic congenital disease of the lung. The most typical radiologic presentation of CCAM is that of multiple large lucencies that have walls of varying thickness and that commonly fill one hemithorax. These cystic structures may have air-fluid levels. This entity is seen in the newborn and is infrequently encountered after early childhood. It is rare for the cysts to be completely filled with fluid and appear as solid lesions, but such cases have been reported. The radiologic appearance of these lesions is quite distinctive and should not be confused with lobar emphysema, which may produce a unilateral hyperlucent lung during the newborn period but which lacks the thick reticular bands separating the multicystic spaces of cystic adenomatoid malformation. Radiologically, CCAM is most likely to be confused with herniation of the small bowel through a congenital hernia of the diaphragm, but the abdominal findings in herniation of the small bowel are usually distinctive because of the absence of gas-containing bowel loops in the abdomen. Staphylococcal pneumonia with multiple cystic spaces might also mimic the appearance of CCAM (see Fig 24–5), but pleural effusion, which commonly accompanies staphylococcal pneumonia, has not been reported with CCAM. The clinical history of high fever and sepsis in staphylococcal pneumonia makes distinction of these entities relatively simple.

AIDS-Related Lucent Lesions

A variety of lucent lesions have been observed in patients with AIDS and have been described as bullae, pneumatoceles, cysts, and cavities.[90,167,237,320,330,368,434,527] Pyogenic pneumonias are most common in the early stages of HIV infection. The patterns of pyogenic pneumonia in patients with HIV are essentially the same as those seen in patients with normal immunity. Virulent organisms such as staphylococcus are not frequent but are likely to cause necrosis. Lung abscesses (Fig 24–9) occur in the acute stages of necrotizing pneumonias, whereas pneumatoceles occur during the healing phase. Postprimary tuberculosis is another cause of necrotic cavities. This manifestation of tuberculosis is identical to postprimary tuberculosis in patients with normal immunity and, like the pyogenic pneumonias, occurs during the early stages of HIV infection. This is most often before the onset of AIDS. Other granulomatous infections, including nocardiosis, coccidioidomycosis, cryptococcosis, and *Mycobacterium avium-intracellulare,* are less frequent causes of cavities. *Pneumocystis carinii* pneumonia is a reported cause of localized opacities that may undergo necrosis and cavitate, but this is uncommon. *Pneumocystis* more typically causes diffuse interstitial or air-space opacities that may develop cystic-appearing lucent spaces. Like necrotizing cavities, these spaces are often randomly scattered throughout the lungs. They rarely contain fluid and in many cases probably represent pneumatoceles. These lucent spaces may be obscured by the diffuse opacities and are therefore not well visualized on plain film, but they are often confirmed with CT (Fig 24–10). When PCP fails to clear, it may leave a coarse reticular pattern with intervening cystic spaces and a radiologic appearance resembling the pattern of honeycombing fibrosis (Fig 24–11). Bullous lesions have also been reported as a late complication of PCP. These lesions are usually distinguished from postinflammatory cysts and pneumatoceles by their locations. Cysts and pneumatoceles are randomly scattered throughout the lungs, whereas bullae are subpleural and most frequently found in the apices (Fig 24–12). This complication appears to be particularly common in patients with recurrent *Pneumocystis* infections. The pathologic mechanism for this so-called premature bullous emphysema has not been well defined, but the complication has also been observed in intravenous drug abusers. There is a high incidence of pneumothorax, which is often complicated by a persistent air-leak caused by rupture of bullae into the pleural space.

SUMMARY

1. Multiple cavities most commonly result from pulmonary infections that lead to necrosis of lung tissue. Acute necrotizing pneumonias usually result in multiple cavities in one area of the lung, with associated air-space consolidation and an acute toxic febrile course.

2. The granulomatous infections, including tuberculosis, histoplasmosis, blastomycosis, and coccidioidomycosis, follow a more indolent course with low-grade temperatures. Cavities in these diseases are usually seen in the secondary hyperimmune phases of the disease and may develop from months to years after the primary infection.

3. Metastases are the most common neoplasms to result in multiple cavities. These cavities may vary in size and shape. Wall thickness is not a good criterion for distinguishing benign from malignant cavitary lesions, although it is true that thick nodular walls favor a neoplastic process rather than an inflammatory reaction.

4. True cavities also result from vascular occlusions. This differential diagnosis includes thromboembolism with infarction, septic embolism with infarction, and vasculitis with infarction. The most common cause of vasculitis that may lead to necrotic cavities is Wegener's granulomatosis. This is less frequently encountered in rheumatoid arthritis.

5. Cystic bronchiectasis is a severe form of end-stage bronchiectasis that may result in multiple holes in the lung. It is frequently associated with a history of recurrent infection. Predisposing factors may include agammaglobulinemia and cystic fibrosis.

6. Tuberculosis and histoplasmosis may also result in cystic bronchiectasis. These diagnoses should be particularly considered when the lucencies are primarily in the upper lobes and when there are other radiologic findings of previous granulomatous infection.

7. Pneumatoceles typically present with multiple thin-walled cystic spaces in the lung. They occur during the healing phases of acute necrotizing pneumonias, particularly staphylococcal pneumonia.

8. AIDS-related lucent lesions include abscesses, pneumatoceles, and bullae. Pneumothorax is a frequent complication.

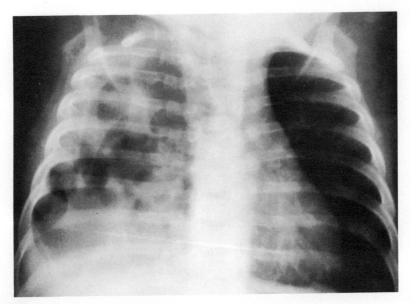

FIG 24–5
Multiple thin-walled lucent lesions in an infant suggest the differential diagnosis of cystic adenomatoid malformation, diaphragmatic hernia, and staphylococcal pneumonia. Associated pleural reaction is strong evidence in favor of staphylococcal pneumonia. Clinical presentation of a toxic febrile reaction should confirm the diagnosis. During the acute phase of the disease, lucencies may represent both cavities and pneumatoceles.

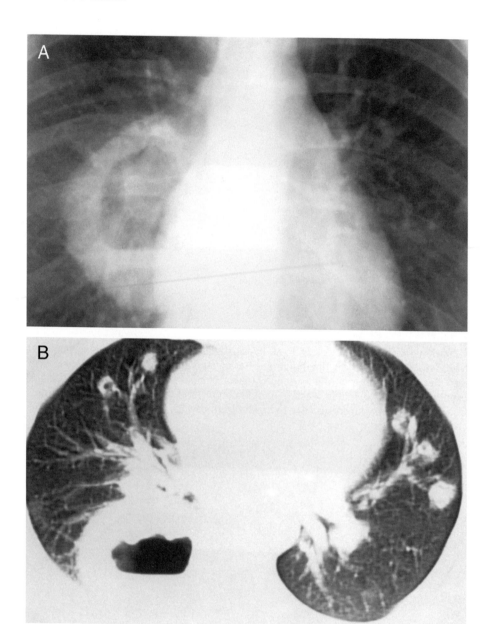

FIG 24–6
A, Wegener's granulomatosis is the cause of this large, thick-walled cavity with an air-fluid level. Additional nodules are minimally visible on the plain film. **B,** CT of the same patient shows additional nodules, some of which are cavitary. This appearance of multiple cavitary nodules with a large dominant cavity is more typical of Wegener's than a solitary cavity would be.

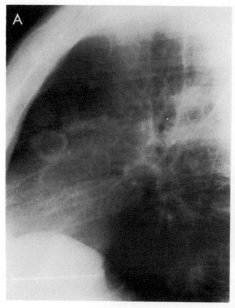
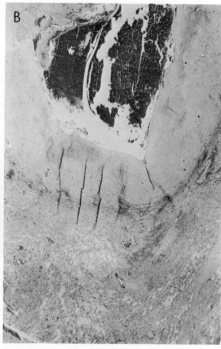

FIG 24–7
A, Rheumatoid arthritis is a well-recognized cause of pulmonary nodules, particularly cavity nodules. **B,** Histologic section from rheumatoid nodule reveals central necrosis, which accounts for tendency toward cavitation. (From Reeder MM, Hochholzer L: RPC of the month from the AFIP. *Radiology* 1969; 92:1106–1111. Used by permission.)

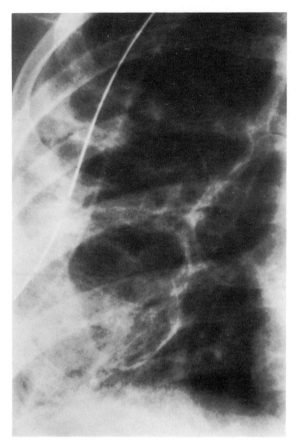

FIG 24–8
Large lucencies developed during the recovery phase of adult respiratory distress syndrome. They are not true cavities. They were transient and might therefore be considered to represent pneumatoceles, but more probably they are localized areas of interstitial emphysema.

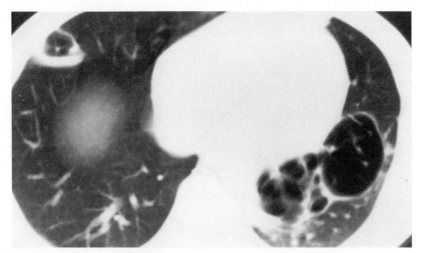

FIG 24–9
AIDS-related lucent lesions include abscesses, pneumatoceles, and premature bullous emphysema. CT shows a peripheral lucent lesion in the right lung, with an air-fluid level and multiple thin-walled lucent lesions in the left lower lobe. This patient had a necrotizing pneumonia with abscesses and pneumatoceles.

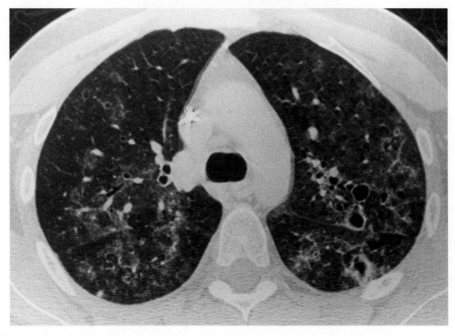

FIG 24–10
CT of a patient with AIDS and PCP shows scattered areas of ground-glass and reticular opacities. There are also multiple lucent cystic spaces, with some variation in wall thickness.

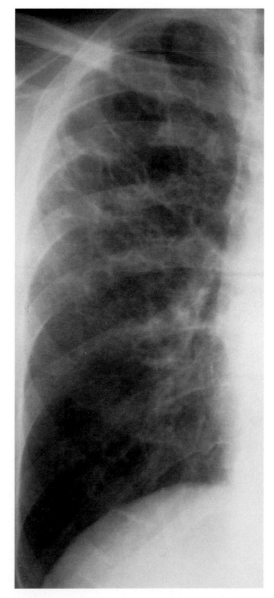

FIG 24–11
Coned view of a film taken 1 month after the acute onset of PCP shows coarse reticular opacities with intervening lucent spaces. This appearance resembles the pattern of honeycombing fibrosis but probably represents a combination of inflammatory infiltrate and cystic spaces or pneumatoceles. The patient was treated with pentamidine, accounting for the upper lobe predominance.

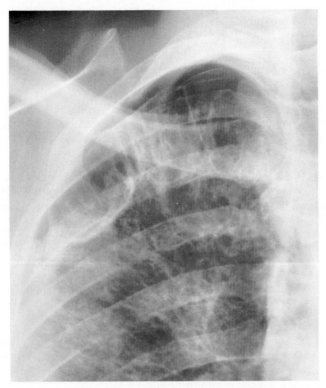

FIG 24–12
Premature bullous emphysema in AIDS patients causes subpleural, apical lucent lesions and is often complicated by recurrent pneumothoraces.

ANSWER GUIDE

LEGENDS FOR INTRODUCTORY FIGURES

FIG 24–1
Diffuse coalescent opacities with multiple interspersed circumscribed lucent lesions and a spontaneous pneumothorax are the result of necrotizing staphylococcal pneumonia with abscesses and bronchopleural fistula.

FIG 24–2
Multiple bilateral upper lobe cavities with surrounding reticular opacities are nearly diagnostic of a granulomatous process. Infections that lead to this response include tuberculosis, histoplasmosis, and coccidioidomycosis. This patient had coccidioidomycosis.

FIG 24–3
A, Squamous cell carcinomas are well-known causes of cavitary lung tumors. Multiple cavitary tumors could result from primary tumors of the esophagus, nasopharynx, tongue, and uterine cervix. This patient had carcinoma of the esophagus. **B,** Gross specimen from case illustrated in **A** emphasizes that cavities are the result of central necrosis of multiple masses. Note multiple small solid nodules.

FIG 24–4
Combination of multiple cavities, pleural thickening, and loss of volume (note shift of mediastinum to right) is most consistent with chronic granulomatous infection. The patient had both cavities and cystic bronchiectasis as the result of long-standing tuberculosis. Volume loss was the result of cicatrizing atelectasis.

ANSWERS

1, e; 2, b, d; 3, b; 4, c.

Bibliography

1. Abdallah PS, Mark JBD, Merigan TC: Diagnosis of cytomegalovirus pneumonia in compromised hosts. *Am J Med* 1976; 61:326–332.
2. Aberle DR, Gamsu G, Lynch D: Thoracic manifestations of Wegener granulomatosis: diagnosis and course. *Radiology* 1990; 174:703–709.
3. Aberle DR, Gamsu G, Ray CS, et al: Asbestos-related pleural and parenchymal fibrosis: detection with high-resolution CT. *Radiology* 1988; 166:729–734.
4. Aberle DR, Wiener-Kronish JP, Webb WR, et al: Hydrostatic versus increased permeability pulmonary edema: diagnosis based on radiographic criteria in critically ill patients. *Radiology* 1988; 168:73–79.
5. Ackerman LV, Taylor FH: Neurogenous tumors within the thorax. *Cancer* 1951; 4:669–691.
6. Adler B, Padley S, Miller RR, et al: High-resolution CT of bronchioloalveolar carcinoma. *Am J Roentgenol* 1992; 159:275–277.
7. Ahn JM, Im J-G, Ryoo JW, et al: Thoracic manifestations of Behçet syndrome: radiographic and CT findings in nine patients. *Radiology* 1995; 194:199–203.
8. Alazraki NP, Friedman PJ: Posterior mediastinal "pseudo-mass," of the newborn. *Am J Roentgenol* 1972; 116:571–574.
9. Alexander E, Clark RA, Colley DP, et al: CT of malignant pleural mesothelioma. *Am J Roentgenol* 1981; 137:287–291.
10. Altman AR: Thoracic wall invasion secondary to pulmonary aspergillosis: a complication of chronic granulomatous disease of childhood. *Am J Roentgenol* 1977; 129:140–142.
11. Amendola MA, Shirazi KK, Brooks J, et al: Transdiaphragmatic bronchopulmonary foregut anomaly: "dumbbell" bronchogenic cyst. *Am J Roentgenol* 1982; 138:1165–1167.
12. Anderson LS, Forrest JV: Tumors of the diaphragm. *Am J Roentgenol* 1973; 119:259–265.
13. Andrews NC, Pratt PC, Christoforidis AJ: Bronchogenic cysts in patients presumed to have pulmonary tuberculosis. *Dis Chest* 1959; 36:353–360.
14. Aronchick JM, Gefter WB: Drug-induced pulmonary disease: an update. *J Thorac Imaging* 1991; 6(1):19–29.
15. Arroliga AC, Podell DN, Matthay RA: Pulmonary manifestations of scleroderma. *J Thorac Imaging* 1992; 7(2):30–45.
16. Asmar BI, Thirumoorthi MC, Dajani AS: Pneumococcal pneumonia with pneumatocele formation. *Am J Dis Child* 1978; 132:1091–1093.
17. Austin JHM, Romney BM, Goldsmith LS: Missed bronchogenic carcinoma: radiographic findings in 27 patients with a potentially resectable lesion evident in retrospect. *Radiology* 1992; 182:115–122.
18. Austin JHM, Yount BG Jr, Thomas HM III, et al: Radiologic assessment of pulmonary arterial pressure and blood volume in chronic diffuse, interstitial pulmonary disease. *Invest Radiol* 1979; 14:9–17.
19. Bachman AL, Macken K: Pleural effusions following supervoltage radiation for breast carcinoma. *Radiology* 1959; 72:699–709.
20. Baker RG: The primary pulmonary lymph node complex of cryptococcosis. *Am J Clin Pathol* 1976; 65:83–92.
21. Balakrishnan J, Meziane MA, Siegelman SS, et al: Pulmonary infarction: CT appearance with pathologic correlation. *J Comput Assist Tomogr* 1989; 13:941–945.
22. Baldry PE: Cavitation in pulmonary sarcomatous metastases with hypertrophic osteoarthropathy. *Br J Dis Chest* 1959; 53:173–176.
23. Balikian JP, Cheng TH, Costello P, et al: Pulmonary actinomycosis. *Radiology* 1978; 128:613–616.
24. Balikian JP, Herman PG: Non-Hodgkin lymphoma of the lungs. *Radiology* 1979; 132:569–572.
25. Balikian JP, Herman PG, Godleski JJ: Serratia pneumonia. *Radiology* 1980; 137:309–311.
26. Balikian JP, Herman PG, Kopit S: Pulmonary nocardiosis. *Radiology* 1978; 126:569–573.

27. Balikian JP, Mudarris FF: Hydatid disease of the lungs. *Am J Roentgenol* 1974; 122: 692–707.
28. Balthazar EJ, Naidich DP, Megibow AJ, et al: CT evaluation of esophageal varices. *Am J Roentgenol* 1987; 148:131–135.
29. Baron RL, Stark DD, McClennan BL, et al: Intrathoracic extension of retroperitoneal urine collections. *Am J Roentgenol* 1981; 137:37–41.
30. Barry WF Jr: Infrapulmonary pleural effusion. *Radiology* 1956; 66:740–743.
31. Bartlett JG: Anaerobic bacterial pneumonitis. *Am Rev Respir Dis* 1979; 119:19–23.
32. Bartrum RJ Jr, Watnick M, Herman PG: Roentgenographic findings in pulmonary mucormycosis. *Am J Roentgenol* 1973; 117:810–815.
33. Bar-Ziv J, Nogrady MB: Mediastinal neuroblastoma and ganglioneuroma. *Am J Roentgenol* 1975; 125:380–390.
34. Bashist B, Ellis K, Gold RP: Computed tomography of intrathoracic goiters. *Am J Roentgenol* 1983; 140:455–460.
35. Basset F, Corrin B, Spencer H, et al: Pulmonary histiocytosis X. *Am Rev Respir Dis* 1978; 118:811–820.
36. Baumgartner WA, Mark JBD: Metastatic malignancies from distant sites to the tracheobronchial tree. *J Thorac Cardiovas Surg* 1980; 79:499–503.
37. Becklake MR: Asbestos-related diseases of the lung and other organs: their epidemiology and implications for clinical practice. *Am Rev Respir Dis* 1976; 114:187–227.
38. Bein ME: Plain film diaphragm view as adjunct to full lung tomography. *Am J Roentgenol* 1979; 133:217–220.
39. Bein ME, Putman CE, McLoud TC, et al: A reevaluation of intrathoracic lymphadenopathy in sarcoidosis. *Am J Roentgenol* 1978; 131:409–415.
40. Ben-Menachem Y, Kuroda K, Kyger ER III, et al: The various forms of pulmonary varices. *Am J Roentgenol* 1975; 125:881–889.
41. Benton C, Silverman FN: Some mediastinal lesions in children. *Semin Roentgenol* 1969; 4:91–101.
42. Berg HK, Petrelli NJ, Herrera L, et al: Endobronchial metastasis from colorectal carcinoma. *Dis Colon Rectum* 1984; 27:745–748.
43. Berger HW, Samortin TG: Miliary tuberculosis: diagnostic methods with emphasis on the chest roentgenogram. *Chest* 1970; 58:586–589.
44. Bergin CJ, Castellino RA: Mediastinal lymph node enlargement on CT scans in patients with usual interstitial pneumonitis. *Am J Roentgenol* 1990; 154:251–254.
45. Bergin CJ, Coblentz CL, Chiles C, et al: Chronic lung diseases: specific diagnosis by using CT. *Am J Roentgenol* 1989; 152:1183–1188.
46. Bergin CJ, Müller NL: CT in the diagnosis of interstitial lung disease. *Am J Roentgenol* 1985; 145:505–510.
47. Berkmen YM: The many faces of bronchiolo-alveolar carcinoma. *Semin Roentgenol* 1977; 12:207–214.
48. Berne AS, Heitzman ER: The roentgenologic signs of pedunculated pleural tumors. *Am J Roentgenol* 1962; 87:892–895.
49. Birnberg FA, Webb WR, Selch MT, et al: Thymic carcinoid tumors with hyperparathyroidism. *Am J Roentgenol* 1982; 139:1001–1004.
50. Black LF: The pleural space and pleural fluid. *Mayo Clin Proc* 1972; 47:493–506.
51. Blum J, Reed JC, Pizzo SV, et al: Miliary aspergillosis associated with alcoholism. *Am J Roentgenol* 1978; 131:707–709.
52. Bor DH, Rose RM, Modlin JF, et al: Mediastinitis after cardiovascular surgery. *Rev Infect Dis* 1983; 5:885–897.
53. Borow M, Conston A, Livornese L, et al: Mesothelioma following exposure to asbestos: a review of 72 cases. *Chest* 1973; 64:641–646.
54. Boushea DK, Sundstrom WR: The pleuropulmonary manifestations of ankylosing spondylitis. *Semin Arthritis Rheum* 1989; 18:277–281.
55. Bradsher RW Jr: Overwhelming pneumonia. *Med Clin North Am* 1983; 67:1233–1250.
56. Bragg DG, Chor PJ, Murray KA, et al: Lymphoproliferative disorders of the lung: histopathology, clinical manifestations and imaging features. *Am J Roentgenol* 1994; 163:273–281.

57. Bragg DG, Janis B: The radiographic presentation of pulmonary opportunistic inflammatory disease. *Radiol Clin North Am* 1973; 11:357–369.
58. Bragg DG, Janis B: The roentgenographic manifestations of pulmonary opportunistic infections. *Am J Roentgenol* 1973; 117:798–809.
59. Bramson RT, Mikhael MA, Sagel SS, et al: Recurrent Hodgkin's disease manifesting roentgenographically as a pleural mass. *Chest* 1974; 66:89–91.
60. Brereton HD, Johnson RE: Calcification in mediastinal lymph nodes after radiation therapy of Hodgkin's disease. *Radiology* 1974; 112:705–707.
61. Brettner A, Heitzman R, Woodin WG: Pulmonary complications of drug therapy. *Radiology* 1970; 96:31–38.
62. Brogdon BG, Kelsey CA, Moseley RD Jr: Factors affecting perception of pulmonary lesions. *Radiol Clin North Am* 1983; 21:633–654.
63. Bryk D: Infrapulmonary effusion. Effect of expiration on the pseudodiaphragmatic contour. *Radiology* 1976; 120:30–36.
64. Buckner CB, Walker CW: Radiologic manifestations of adult tuberculosis. *J Thorac Imag* 1990; 5:28–37.
65. Buckner CB, Walker CW, Purnell GL: Pulmonary embolism: chest radiographic abnormalities. *J Thorac Imag* 1989; 4:23–27.
66. Buff SJ, McLelland R, Gallis HA, et al: *Candida albicans* pneumonia: radiographic appearance. *Am J Roentgenol* 1982; 138:645–648.
67. Burdon JGW, Sinclair RA, Henderson MM: Small cell carcinoma of the lung. *Chest* 1979; 76:302–304.
68. Burgener FA, Hamlin DJ: Intrathoracic histiocytic lymphoma. *Am J Roentgenol* 1981; 136:499–504.
69. Buschman DL, Gamsu G, Waldron JA Jr, et al: Chronic hypersensitivity pneumonitis: use of CT in diagnosis. *Am J Roentgenol* 1992; 159:957–960.
70. Bynum LJ, Wilson JE III: Radiographic features of pleural effusions in pulmonary embolism. *Am Rev Respir Dis* 1978; 117:829–833.
71. Caceres J, Mata JM, Alegret X, et al: Increased density of the azygos lobe on frontal chest radiographs simulating disease: CT findings in seven patients. *Am J Roentgenol* 1993; 160:245–248.
72. Capitanio MA, Kirkpatrick JA Jr: *Pneumocystis carinii* pneumonia. *Am J Roentgenol* 1966; 97:174–180.
73. Cardenose G, Deluca SA: Rounded atelectasis. *Am Fam Physician* 1989; 39:135–136.
74. Carey LS, Ellis FH Jr, Good CA, et al: Neurogenic tumors of the mediastinum: a clinicopathologic study. *Am J Roentgenol* 1960; 84:189–205.
75. Carilli AD, Ramanamurty MV, Chang Y, et al: Noncardiogenic pulmonary edema following blood transfusion. *Chest* 1978; 74:310–312.
76. Carmody TJ, Wergowske GL, Joffe CD: Unusual nodular pulmonary lesions associated with thrombolytic therapy. *Cathet Cardiovasc Diagn* 1984; 10:485–488.
77. Carr DT, Mayne JG: Pleurisy with effusion in rheumatoid arthritis, with reference to the low concentration of glucose in pleural fluid. *Am Rev Respir Dis* 1962; 85:345–350.
78. Carrington CB, Gaensler EA, Contu RE, et al: Natural history and treated course of usual and desquamative interstitial pneumonia. *N Engl J Med* 1978; 298:801–809.
79. Carvalho PM, Carr DH: Computed tomography of folded lung. *Clin Radiol* 1990; 41:86–91.
80. Castellino RA, Blank N: Adenopathy of the cardiophrenic angle (diaphragmatic) lymph nodes. *Am J Roentgenol* 1972; 114:509–515.
81. Cayea PD, Rubin E, Teixidor HS: Atypical pulmonary malaria. *Am J Roentgenol* 1981; 137:51–55.
82. Chaffey MH, Klein JS, Gamsu G, et al: Radiographic distribution of *Pneumocystis carinii* pneumonia in patients with AIDS treated with prophylactic inhaled pentamidine. *Radiology* 1990; 175:715–719.
83. Chan T, Palevsky HI, Miller WT: Pulmonary hypertension complicating portal hypertension: findings on chest radiographs. *Am J Roentgenol* 1988; 151:909–914.
84. Chang CH(J): The normal roentgenographic measurement of the right descending pulmonary artery in 1,085 cases. *Am J Roentgenol* 1962; 87:929–935.

85. Chang CH(J), Zinn TW: Roentgen recognition of enlarged hilar lymph nodes: an anatomical review. *Radiology* 1976; 120:291–296.
86. Charan NB, Myers CG, Lakshminarayan S, et al: Pulmonary injuries associated with acute sulfur dioxide inhalation. *Am Rev Respir Dis* 1979; 119:555–560.
87. Chen JTT: *Essentials of cardiac roentgenology.* Boston, Little, Brown and Company, 1987.
88. Chen JTT, Dahmash NS, Ravin CE, et al: Metastatic melanoma to the thorax: report of 130 patients. *Am J Roentgenol* 1981; 137:293–298.
89. Chinn DH, Gamsu G, Webb WR, et al: Calcified pulmonary nodules in chronic renal failure. *Am J Roentgenol* 1981; 137:402–405.
90. Chow C, Templeton PA, White CS: Lung cysts associated with *Pneumocystis carinii* pneumonia: radiographic characteristics, natural history, and complications. *Am J Roentgenol* 1993; 161:527–531.
91. Choyke PL, Sostman HD, Curtis AM, et al: Adult-onset pulmonary tuberculosis. *Radiology* 1983; 148:357–362.
92. Christensen EE, Dietz GW, Murry RC, et al: Effect of kilovoltage on detectability of pulmonary nodules in a chest phantom. *Am J Roentgenol* 1977; 128:789–793.
93. Chun PKC: Multiple pulmonary nodules in a young man. *Chest* 1978; 73:527–528.
94. Cimmino CV: Contacts of the left lung with the mediastinum. *Am J Roentgenol* 1975; 124:412–416.
95. Citro LA, Gordon ME, Miller WT: Eosinophilic lung disease (or how to slice P.I.E.). *Am J Roentgenol* 1973; 117:787–797.
96. Cohen M, Grosfeld J, Baehner R, et al: Lung CT for detection of metastases: solid tissue neoplasms in children. *Am J Roentgenol* 1982; 138:895–898.
97. Collins JD, Pagani JJ: Extrathoracic musculature mimicking pleural lesions. *Radiology* 1978; 129:21–22.
98. Collins VP, Loeffler RK, Tivey H: Observations on growth rates of human tumors. *Am J Roentgenol* 1956; 76:988–1000.
99. Communications to the editor. *Chest* 1978; 74:319–321.
100. Comstock C, Wolson AH: Roentgenology of sporotrichosis. *Am J Roentgenol* 1975; 125:651–655.
101. Conant EF, Fox KR, Miller WT: Pulmonary edema as a complication of interleukin-2 therapy. *Am J Roentgenol* 1989; 152:749–752.
102. Conant EF, Wechsler RJ: Actinomycosis and nocardiosis of the lung. *J Thorac Imaging* 1992; 7(4):75–84.
103. Conces DJ, Kraft JL, Vix VA, et al: Apical *Pneumocystis carinii* pneumonia after inhaled pentamidine prophylaxis. *Am J Roentgenol* 1989; 152:1192–1194.
104. Connell JV Jr, Muhm JR: Radiographic manifestations of pulmonary histoplasmosis: a 10-year review. *Radiology* 1976; 121:281–285.
105. Coppage L, Shaw C, Curtis AMcB: Metastatic disease to the chest in patients with extrathoracic malignancy. *J Thorac Imaging* 1987; 2:24–37.
106. Cordier J-F, Loire R, Brune J: Idiopathic bronchiolitis obliterans organizing pneumonia. Definition of characteristic clinical profiles in a series of 16 patients. *Chest* 1989; 96:999–1004.
107. Coussement AM, Gooding CA: Cavitating pulmonary metastatic disease in children. *Am J Roentgenol* 1973:117:833–839.
108. Crowe JK, Brown LR, Muhm JR: Computed tomography of the mediastinum. *Radiology* 1978; 128:75–87.
109. Crystal RG, Fulmer JD, Roberts WC, et al: Idiopathic pulmonary fibrosis. *Ann Intern Med* 1976; 85:769–788.
110. Cushing H, Wolbach SB: The transformation of a malignant paravertebral sympathicoblastoma into a benign ganglioneuroma. *Am J Pathol* 1927; 3:203–216.
111. D'Angio GJ, Iannaccone G: Spontaneous pneumothorax as a complication of pulmonary metastases in malignant tumors of childhood. *Am J Roentgenol* 1961; 86:1092–1102.
112. Daley CL: Pyogenic bacterial pneumonia in the acquired immunodeficiency syndrome. *J Thorac Imaging* 1991; 6(4):36–42.

113. Daly BD, Leung SF, Cheung H, et al: Thoracic metastases from carcinoma of the na-sopharynx: high frequency of hilar and mediastinal lymphadenopathy. *Am J Roentgenol* 1993; 160:241–244.

114. Dandy WE Jr: Incomplete pulmonary interlobar fissure sign. *Radiology* 1978; 128:21–25.

115. Darling ST: A protozoan general infection producing pseudotubercles in the lungs and focal necroses in the liver, spleen and lymph nodes. *JAMA* 1906; 46:1283–1285.

116. Dashiell TG, Payne WS, Hepper NGG, et al: Desmoid tumors of the chest wall. *Chest* 1978; 74:157–162.

117. Davies SF, Sarosi GA: Acute cavitary histoplasmosis. *Chest* 1978; 73:103–105.

118. Davis JM, Mark GJ, Greene R: Benign blood vascular tumors of the mediastinum. *Radiology* 1978; 126:581–587.

119. Davis SD, Henschke CI, Chamides BK, et al: Intrathoracic Kaposi sarcoma in AIDS patients: radiographic-pathologic correlation. *Radiology* 1987; 163:495–500.

120. Davis SD, Yankelevitz MD, Wand A, et al: Juxtaphrenic peak in upper and middle lobe volume loss: assessment with CT. *Radiology* 1996, 198(1) 143–149.

121. Davison K: Lung abscess following aseptic pulmonary embolism. *Br J Tuberc Dis Chest* 1958; 52:149–153.

122. DeBeer RA, Garcia RL, Alexander SC: Endobronchial metastasis from cancer of the breast. *Chest* 1978; 73:94–96.

123. DeJournette RL: Rocket propellant inhalation in the Apollo-Soyez astronauts. *Radiology* 1977; 125:21–24.

124. DeLorenzo LJ, Huang CT, Maguire GP, et al: Roentgenographic patterns of *Pneumocystis carinii* pneumonia in 104 patients with AIDS. *Chest* 1987; 91:323–327.

125. Dennis LN, Rogers LF: Superior mediastinal widening from spine fractures mimicking aortic rupture on chest radiographs. *Am J Roentgenol* 1989; 152:27–30.

126. Dietrich PA, Johnson RD, Fairbank JT, et al: The chest radiograph in Legionnaires' disease. *Radiology* 1978; 127:577–582.

127. Dines DE: Diagnostic significance of pneumatocele of the lung. *JAMA* 1968; 204:79–82.

128. Dodd GD, Boyle JJ: Excavating pulmonary metastases. *Am J Roentgenol* 1961; 85:277–293.

129. Dodd GD III, Ledesma-Medina JL, Baron RL, et al: Posttransplant lymphoproliferative disorder: intrathoracic manifestations. *Radiology* 1992:184:65–69.

130. Donlan CJ Jr, Reid JW: Endobronchial Hodgkin's disease. *JAMA* 1978; 239:1061–1062.

131. Dorff GJ, Rytel MW, Farmer SG, et al: Etiologies and characteristic features of pneumonias in a municipal hospital. *Am J Med Sci* 1973; 266:349–358.

132. Dyke PC, Mulkey DA: Maturation of ganglioneuroblastoma to ganglioneuroma. *Cancer* 1967; 20:1343–1349.

133. Dynes MC, White EM, Fry WA, et al: Imaging manifestations of pleural tumors. *Radiographics* 1992; 12:1191–1201.

134. Ecker MD, Jay B, Koehane MF: Procarbazine lung. *Am J Roentgenol* 1978; 131:527–528.

135. Effman EL, Merten DF, Kirks DR, et al: Adult respiratory distress syndrome in children. *Radiology* 1985; 157:69–74.

136. Eklof O, Gooding CA: Intrathoracic neuroblastoma. *Am J Roentgenol* 1967; 100:202–207.

137. Ekstrom D, Weiner M, Baier B: Pulmonary arteriovenous fistula as a complication of trauma. *Am J Roentgenol* 1978; 130:1178–1180.

138. Ellis AR, Mayers DL, Martone WJ, et al: Rapidly expanding pulmonary nodule caused by Pittsburgh pneumonia agent. *JAMA* 1981; 245:1558–1559.

139. Ellis K: The adult respiratory distress syndrome (ARDS). *Comtemp Diagn Radiol* 1978; 1:1–6.

140. Ellis K, Wolff M: Mesotheliomas and secondary tumors of the pleura. *Semin Roentgenol* 1977; 12:303–311.

141. Ellis R: Incomplete border sign of extrapleural masses. *JAMA* 1977; 237:2748.
142. Engeler CE, Tashjian JH, Trenkner SW, et al: Ground-glass opacity of the lung paenchyma: a guide to analysis with high-resolution CT. *Am J Roentgenol* 1993; 160:249–251.
143. England DM, Hochholzer L, McCarthy MJ: Localized benign and malignant fibrous tumors of the pleura. A clinicopathologic review of 223 cases. *Am J Surg Pathol* 1989; 13:640–658.
144. Epler GR, McLoud TC, Gaensler EA, et al: Normal chest roentgenograms in chronic diffuse infiltrative lung disease. *N Engl J Med* 1978; 298:934–939.
145. Epstein BS, Epstein JA: Extrapleural intrathoracic apical traumatic pseudomeningocele. *Am J Roentgenol* 1974; 120:887–892.
146. Epstein DM, Gefter WB, Miller WT: Lobar bronchioloalveolar cell carcinoma. *Am J Roentgenol* 1982; 139:463–468.
147. Faer MJ, Burnan RE, Beck CL: Transmural thoracic lipoma: demonstration by computed tomography. *Am J Roentgenol* 1978; 130:161–163.
148. Fagan CJ, Swischuk LE: Dumbbell neuroblastoma or ganglioneuroma of the spinal canal. *Am J Roentgenol* 1974; 120:453–460.
149. Fagan CJ, Swischuk LE: The opaque lung in lobar emphysema. *Am J Roentgenol* 1972; 114:300–304.
150. Fagan CJ, Swischuk LE: Traumatic lung and paramediastinal pneumatoceles. *Radiology* 1976; 120:11–18.
151. Fairbank JT, Mamourian AC, Dietrich PA, et al: The chest radiograph in Legionnaires' disease. *Radiology* 1983; 147:33–34.
152. Fairbank JT, Tampas JP, Longstreth G: Superior vena cava obstruction in histoplasmosis. *Am J Roentgenol* 1972; 115:488–494.
153. Fawcitt J, Parry HE: Lung changes in pertussis and measles in childhood. *Br J Radiol* 1957; 30:76–82.
154. Feigin DS: Misconceptions regarding the pathogenicity of silicas and silicates. *J Thorac Imaging* 1989; 4:68–80.
155. Feigin DS: Nocardiosis of the lung: chest radiographic findings in 21 cases. *Radiology* 1986; 159:9–14.
156. Feigin DS: Vasculitis in the lung. *J Thorac Imaging* 1988; 3:33–48.
157. Feigin DS, Eggleston JC, Siegelman SS: The multiple roentgen manifestations of sclerosing mediastinitis. *Johns Hopkins Med J* 1979; 144:1–8.
158. Feigin DS, Fenoglio JJ, McAllister HA, et al: Pericardial cysts: a radiologic-pathologic correlation and review. *Radiology* 1977; 125:15–20.
159. Feigin DS, Seigelman SS, Theros EG, et al: Nonmalignant lymphoid disorders of the chest. *Am J Roentgenol* 1977; 129:221–228.
160. Felker RE, Tonkin ILD: Imaging of pulmonary sequestration. *Am J Roentgenol* 1990; 154:241–249.
161. Felman AH, Rhatigan RM, Pierson KK: Pulmonary lymphangiectasis. *Am J Roentgenol* 1972; 116:548–558.
162. Felson B: *Chest roentgenology.* Philadelphia, WB Saunders, 1973.
163. Felson B: Lung torsion: radiographic findings in nine cases. *Radiology* 1987; 162:631–638.
164. Felson B: The extrapleural space. *Semin Roentgenol* 1977; 12:327–333.
165. Felson B, Jacobson HG: Chest wall lesions mimicking intrapulmonary pathological conditions. *JAMA* 1978; 239:535–536.
166. Ferguson DD, Westcott JL: Lipoma of the diaphragm. *Radiology* 1976; 118:527–528.
167. Feuerstein IM, Archer A, Pluda JM, et al: Thin-walled cavities, cysts, and pneumothorax in *Pneumocystis carinii* pneumonia: further observations with histopathologic correlation. *Radiology* 1990; 174:697–702.
168. Fink IJ, Kurtz DW, Cazenave L, et al: Malignant thoracopulmonary small-cell ("Askin") tumor. *Am J Roentgenol* 1985; 145:517–520.
169. Firooznia H, Pudlowski R, Golimbu C, et al: Diffuse interstitial calcification of the lungs in chronic renal failure mimicking pulmonary edema. *Am J Roentgenol* 1977; 129:1103–1105.

170. Fischman RA, Marschall KE, Kislak JW, et al: Adult respiratory distress syndrome caused by *Mycoplasma pneumoniae*. *Chest* 1978; 74:471–473.
171. Fisher AMH, Kendall B, Leuven BDV: Hodgkin's disease: a radiological survey. *Clin Radiol* 1962; 13:115–127.
172. Fisher ER, Godwin JD: Extrapleural fat collections: pseudotumors and other confusing manifestations. *Am J Roentgenol* 1993; 161:47–52.
173. Fisher JK: Skin fold versus pneumothorax. *Am J Roentgenol* 1978; 130:791–792.
174. Fleischner FG: Pulmonary embolism. *Clin Radiol* 1962; 13:169–182.
175. Fleischner FG: The visible bronchial tree: a roentgen sign in pneumonic and other pulmonary consolidations. *Radiology* 1948; 50:184–189.
176. Fleischner FG, Berenberg al: Idiopathic pulmonary hemosiderosis. *Radiology* 1954; 62:522–526.
177. Flye MW, Mundinger GH, Fauci AS: Diagnostic and therapeutic aspects of the surgical approach to Wegener's granulomatosis. *J Thorac Cardiovasc Surg* 1979; 77:331–337.
178. Flynn MW, Felson B: The roentgen manifestations of thoracic actinomycosis. *Am J Roentgenol* 1970; 110:707–716.
179. Forrest JV, Shackelford GD, Bramson RT, et al: Acute mediastinal widening. *Am J Roentgenol* 1973; 117:881–885.
180. Forrest ME, Skerker LB, Nemiroff MJ: Hard metal pneumoconiosis: another cause of diffuse interstitial fibrosis. *Radiology* 1978; 128:609–612.
181. Fortier M, Mayo JR, Swenson SJ, et al: MR imaging of chest wall lesions. *Radiographics* 1994; 14:597–606.
182. Foster WL Jr, Gimenez EI, Roubidoux MA, et al: The emphysemas: radiologic-pathologic correlations. *Radiographics* 1993; 13:311–328.
183. Foy HM, Loop J, Clarke ER, et al: Radiographic study of *Mycoplasma pneumoniae* pneumonia. *Am Rev Respir Dis* 1973; 108:469–474.
184. Fraire AE, Greenberg SD, O'Neal RM, et al: Diffuse interstitial fibrosis of the lung. *Am J Clin Pathol* 1973; 59:636–647.
185. Fraser RG: The radiologist and obstructive airway disease. *Am J Roentgenol* 1974; 120:737–775.
186. Fraser RG, Paré JAP, Paré PD, et al: *Diagnosis of diseases of the chest*, ed 3. Philadelphia, WB Saunders, 1989.
187. Frederick AJ, Wiedemann HP, O'Donovan PB, et al: Computerized tomographic densitometry of the solitary pulmonary nodule using a nodule phantom. *Chest* 1989; 96:779–783.
188. Friedman AC, Fiel SB, Fisher MS, et al: Asbestos-related pleural disease and asbestosis: a comparison of CT and chest radiology. *Am J Roentgenol* 1988; 150:269–275.
189. Friedman PJ: Idiopathic and autoimmune type III–like reactions: interstitial fibrosis, vasculitis, and granulomatosis. *Semin Roentgenol* 1975; 10:43–51.
190. Friedman PJ: Lung cancer: update on staging classifications. *Am J Roentgenol* 1988; 150:261–264.
191. Fulcher AS, Proto AV, Jolles H: Cystic teratoma of the mediastinum: demonstration of fat/fluid level. *Am J Roentgenol* 1990; 154:259–260.
192. Gaensler EA, Carrington CB: Peripheral opacities in chronic eosinophilic pneumonia: the photographic negative of pulmonary edema. *Am J Roentgenol* 1977; 128:1–13.
193. Gaensler EA, Carrington CB, Contu RE: Clinical notes on respiratory diseases. *Am Thorac Soc* 1972; 10:1–16.
194. Gaensler EA, Carrington CB, Contu RE, et al: Pathological, physiological, and radiological correlations in the pneumoconioses. *Ann N Y Acad Sci* 1972; 200:574–607.
195. Gajaraj A, Johnson TH, Feist JH: Roentgen features of giant cell carcinoma of the lung. *Am J Roentgenol* 1971; 111:486–491.
196. Gallis HA: Subacute staphylococcal pneumonia in a renal transplant recipient. *Am Rev Respir Dis* 1975; 112:109–112.
197. Gamsu G, Aberle DR, Lynch D: Computed tomography in the diagnosis of asbestos-related thoracic disease. *J Thorac Imaging* 1989; 4:61–67.
198. Gamsu G, Webb WR: Computed tomography of the trachea: normal and abnormal. *Am J Roentgenol* 1982; 138:321–326.

199. Garg K, Lynch DA, Newell JD, et al: Proliferative and constrictive bronchiolitis: classification and radiologic features. *Am J Roentgenol* 1994; 162:803–808.
200. Garland LH: The rate of growth and natural duration of primary bronchial cancer. *Am J Roentgenol* 1966; 96:604–611.
201. Garland LH, Coulson W, Wollin E: The rate of growth and apparent duration of untreated primary bronchial carcinoma. *Cancer* 1963; 16:694–707.
202. de Geer G, Webb WR, Gamsu G: Normal thymus: assessment with MR and CT. *Radiology* 1986; 158:313–317.
203. Gefter WB, Conant EF: Issues and controversies in the plain-film diagnosis of asbestos-related disorders in the chest. *J Thorac Imag* 1988; 3:11–28.
204. Genereux GP: The Fleischner lecture: computed tomography of diffuse pulmonary disease. *J Thorac Imag* 1989; 4:50–87.
205. Glazer HS, Anderson DJ, Sagel SS: Bronchial impaction in lobar collapse: CT demonstration and pathologic correlation. *Am J Roentgenol* 1989; 153:485–488.
206. Glazer HS, Duncan-Meyer J, Aronberg DJ, et al: Pleural and chest wall invasion in bronchogenic carcinoma: CT evaluation. *Radiology* 1985; 157:191–194.
207. Glazer HS, Guierrez FR, Levitt RG, et al: The thoracic aorta studied by MR imaging. *Radiology* 1985; 157:149–155.
208. Glazer HS, Siegel MJ, Sagal SS: Low-attenuation mediastinal masses on CT. *Am J Roentgenol* 1989; 152:1173–1177.
209. Glazer HS, Wick MR, Anderson DJ, et al: CT of fatty thoracic masses. *Am J Roentgenol* 1992; 159:1181–1187.
210. Godwin JD: The solitary pulmonary nodule. *Radiol Clin North Am* 1983; 21:709–721.
211. Godwin JD, Merten DF, Baker ME: Paramediastinal pneumatocele: alternative explanations to gas in the pulmonary ligament. *Am J Roentgenol* 1985; 145:525–530.
212. Godwin JD, Ravin CE, Roggli VL: Fatal *Pneumocystis* pneumonia, cryptococcosis and Kaposi sarcoma in a homosexual man. *Am J Roentgenol* 1982; 138:580–581.
213. Good CA: The solitary pulmonary nodule: a problem of management. *Radiol Clin North Am* 1963; 1:429–438.
214. Good CA, Wilson TW: The solitary circumscribed pulmonary nodule. *JAMA* 1958; 166:210–215.
215. Goodman PC: Pulmonary tuberculosis in patients with acquired immunodeficiency syndrome. *J Thorac Imaging* 1990; 5:38–45.
216. Goodwin RA Jr, Snell JR Jr: The enlarging histoplasmoma. *Am Rev Respir Dis* 1969; 100:1–12.
217. Gordonson J, Birnbaum W, Jacobson G, et al: Pulmonary cryptococcosis. *Radiology* 1974; 112:557–561.
218. Gordonson J, Quinn M, Kaufman R, et al: Mediastinal lymphadenopathy and undifferentiated connective tissue disease: case report and review. *Am J Roentgenol* 1978; 131:325–328.
219. Gosink BB, Friedman PJ, Liebow AA: Bronchiolitis obliterans. *Am J Roentgenol* 1973; 117:816–832.
220. Graham JC Jr, Blanchard IT, Scatliff JH: Calcified gastric leiomyoma presenting as a mediastinal mass. *Am J Roentgenol* 1972; 114:529–531.
221. Gray JE, Taylor KW, Hobbs BB: Detection accuracy in chest radiography. *Am J Roentgenol* 1978; 131:247–253.
222. Greco FA, Oldham RK: Small-cell lung cancer. *N Engl J Med* 1979; 301:355–358.
223. Greenberg SD, Frager D, Suster B, et al: Active pulmonary tuberculosis in patients with AIDS: spectrum of radiographic findings (including a normal appearance). *Radiology* 1994; 193:115–119.
224. Greene R: Lung alterations in thoracic trauma. *J Thorac Imaging* 1987; 2:1–11.
225. Greene R: "Saber-sheath" trachea: relation to chronic obstructive pulmonary disease. *Am J Roentgenol* 1978; 130:441–445.
226. Greene R, McLoud TC, Stark P: Other malignant tumors of the lung. *Semin Roentgenol* 1977; 12:225–237.

227. Greenspan RH, Ravin CE, Polansky SM, et al: Accuracy of the chest radiograph in diagnosis of pulmonary embolism. *Invest Radiol* 1982; 17:539–543.
228. Greganti MA, Flowers WM Jr: Acute pulmonary edema after the intravenous administration of contrast media. *Radiology* 1979; 132:583–585.
229. Griscom NT, Wohl MEB, Kirkpatrick JA Jr: Lower respiratory infections: how infants differ from adults. *Radiol Clin North Am* 1978; 16:367–387.
230. Gronner AT, Ominsky SH: Plain film radiography of the chest: findings that simulate pulmonary disease. *Am J Roentgenol* 1994; 163:1343–1348.
231. Groskin SA, Panicek DM, Ewing DK, et al: Bacterial lung abscess: a review of the radiographic and clinical features of 50 cases. *J Thorac Imaging* 1991; 6(3):62–67.
232. Grossman CB, Bragg DG, Armstrong D: Roentgen manifestations of pulmonary nocardiosis. *Radiology* 1970; 96:325–330.
233. Grossman LK, Wald ER, Nair P, et al: Roentgenographic follow-up of acute pneumonia in children. *Pediatrics* 1979; 63:30–31.
234. Gruden JF, Huang L, Webb WR: AIDS-related Kaposi sarcoma of the lung: radiographic findings and staging system with bronchoscopic correlation. *Radiology* 1995; 195:545–552.
235. Gruden JF, Klein JS, Webb WR: Percutaneous transthoracic needle biopsy in AIDS: analysis in 32 patients. *Radiology* 1993; 189:567–571.
236. Guest JL Jr, Anderson JN: Osteomyelitis involving adjacent ribs. *JAMA* 1978; 239:133.
237. Gurney JW, Bates FT: Pulmonary cystic disease: comparison of *Pneumocystis carinii* pneumatoceles and bullous emphysema due to intravenous drug abuse. *Radiology* 1989; 173:27–31.
238. Gurney JW, Goodman LR: Pulmonary edema localized in the right upper lobe accompanying mitral regurgitation. *Radiology* 1989; 171:397–399.
239. Gurney JW, Schroeder BA: Upper lobe lung disease: physiologic correlates. *Radiology* 1988; 167:359–366.
240. Hadlock FP, Park SK, Awe RJ, et al: Unusual radiographic findings in adult pulmonary tuberculosis. *Am J Roentgenol* 1980; 134:1015–1018.
241. Hadlock FP, Wallace RJ Jr, Rivera M: Pulmonary septic emboli secondary to parapharyngeal abscess: postanginal sepsis. *Radiology* 1979; 130:29–33.
242. Halvorsen RA, Duncan JD, Merten DF: Pulmonary blastomycosis: radiologic manifestations. *Radiology* 1984; 150:1–5.
243. Hamman L, Rich A: Acute diffuse interstitial fibrosis of the lungs. *Johns Hopkins Med J* 1944; 74:177–212.
244. Hampton AO, Castleman B: Correlation of postmortem chest teleroentgenograms with autopsy findings: with special reference to pulmonary embolism and infarction. *Am J Roentgenol* 1940; 43:305–326.
245. Han SS, Wills JS, Allen OS: Pulmonary blastoma: case report and literature review. *Am J Roentgenol* 1976; 127:1048–1049.
246. Hanna JW, Reed JC, Choplin RH: Pleural infections: a clinical-radiologic review. *J Thorac Imaging* 1991; 6(3):68–79.
247. Haque AK: Pathology of carcinoma of lung: an update on current concepts. *J Thorac Imaging* 1991; 7(1):9–20.
248. Haramati LB, Schulman LL, Austin JHM: Lung nodules and masses after cardiac transplantation. *Radiology* 1993; 188:491–497.
249. Harnsberger HR, Armstrong JD II: Bilateral superomedial hilar displacement: a unique sign of previous mediastinal radiation. *Radiology* 1983; 147:35–36.
250. Harris VJ, Brown R: Pneumatoceles as a complication of chemical pneumonia after hydrocarbon ingestion. *Am J Roentgenol* 1975; 125:531–537.
251. Hartman TE, Müller NL, Primack SL, et al: Metastatic pulmonary calcification in patients with hypercalcemia: findings on chest radiographs and CT scans. *Am J Roentgenol* 1994; 162:799–802.
252. Hatcher CR Jr, Sehdeva J, Waters WC III, et al: Primary pulmonary cryptococcosis. *J Thorac Cardiovasc Surg* 1971; 63:39–49.

253. Heater K, Revzani L, Rubin JM: CT evaluation of empyema in the postpneumonectomy space. *Am J Roentgenol* 1985; 145:39–40.
254. Heelan RJ, Hehinger BJ, Melamed MR, et al: Non–small-cell lung cancer: results of the New York screening program. *Radiology* 1984; 151:289–293.
255. Heiberg E, Wolverson M, Sundaram M, et al: CT findings in thoracic aortic dissection. *Am J Roentgenol* 1981; 136:13–17.
256. Heithoff KB, Sane SM, Williams HJ, et al: Bronchopulmonary foregut malformations. *Am J Roentgenol* 1976; 126:46–55.
257. Heitzman ER: Bronchogenic carcinoma: radiologic-pathologic correlations. *Semin Roentgenol* 1977; 12:165–174.
258. Heitzman ER: Computed tomography of the thorax: current perspectives. *Am J Roentgenol* 1981; 136:2–12.
259. Heitzman ER: Lymphadenopathy related to anticonvulsant therapy: roentgen findings simulating lymphoma. *Radiology* 1967; 89:311–312.
260. Heitzman ER: *The lung: radiologic-pathologic correlations,* ed 2. St. Louis, Mosby, 1984.
261. Heitzman ER: *The mediastinum: radiologic correlations with anatomy and pathology,* ed 2. Berlin, Springer-Verlag, 1988.
262. Heitzman ER, Markarian B, Berger I, et al: The secondary pulmonary lobule: a practical concept for interpretation of chest radiographs. *Radiology* 1969; 93:513–519.
263. Heitzman ER, Markarian B, DeLise CT: Lymphoproliferative disorders of the thorax. *Semin Roentgenol* 1975; 10:73–81.
264. Heller RM, Janower ML, Weber AL: The radiological manifestations of malignant pleural mesothelioma. *Am J Roentgenol* 1970; 108:53–59.
265. Henry DA, Kiser PE, Scheer CE, et al: Multiple imaging evaluation of sarcoidosis. *Radiographics* 1986; 6:75–95.
266. Herman PG, Balikian JP, Seltzer SE, et al: The pulmonary-renal syndrome. *Am J Roentgenol* 1978; 130:1141–1148.
267. Hewes RC, Smith DC Lavine MH: Iatrogenic hydromediastinum simulating aortic laceration. *Am J Roentgenol* 1979; 133:817–820.
268. Hill CA: Bronchioloalveolar carcinoma: a review. *Radiology* 1984; 150:15–20.
269. Hill CA: "Tail" signs associated with pulmonary lesions: critical reappraisal. *Am J Roentgenol* 1982; 139:311–316.
270. Hillerdal G, Nou E: Large infiltrate with air bronchogram in a symptomless woman. *Chest* 1982; 82:481–482.
271. Himmelfarb E, Wells S, Rabinowitz JG: The radiologic spectrum of cardiopulmonary amyloidosis. *Chest* 1977; 72:327–332.
272. Hirakata K, Nakata H, Haratake J: Appearance of pulmonary metastases on high-resolution CT scans: comparison with histopathologic findings from autopsy specimens. *Am J Roentgenol* 1993; 161:37–43.
273. Hirsch JH, Rogers JV, Mack LA: Real-time sonography of pleural opacities. *Am J Roentgenol* 1981; 136:297–301.
274. Hoagland RJ: The clinical manifestations of infectious mononucleosis: a report of two hundred cases. *Am J Med Sci* 1960; 240:21–29.
275. Hochholzer L, Theros EG, Rosen SH: Some unusual lesions of the mediastinum: roentgenologic and pathologic features. *Semin Roentgenol* 1969; 4:74–90.
276. Hodgson CH, Good CA: Pulmonary embolism and infarction. *Med Clin North Am* 1964; 48:977–992.
277. Hoffman R, Rabens R: Evolving pulmonary nodules: multiple pulmonary arteriovenous fistulas. *Am J Roentgenol* 1974; 120:861–864.
278. Hollman AS, Adams FG: The influence of the lordotic projection on the interpretation of the chest radiograph. *Clin Radiol* 1989; 40:360–364.
279. Holt S, Ryan WF, Epstein EJ: Severe mycoplasma pneumonia. *Thorax* 1977; 32:112–115.
280. Homer MJ, Wechsler RJ, Carter BL: Mediastinal lipomatosis. CT confirmation of a normal variant. *Radiology* 1978; 128:657–661.
281. Houk VN, Moser KR: Pulmonary cryptococcosis. *Ann Intern Med* 1965; 63:583–596.

282. Hourihane JB, Owens AP: A pitfall in the diagnosis of lobar collapse. *Clin Radiol* 1989; 40:468–470.
283. Hudson AR, Halprin GM, Miller JA, et al: Pulmonary interstitial fibrosis following alveolar proteinosis. *Chest* 1974; 65:700–702.
284. Hulnick DH, Naidich DP, McCauley DJ: Pleural tuberculosis evaluated by computed tomography. *Radiology* 1983; 149:759–765.
285. Hultgren HN, Marticorena EA: High altitude pulmonary edema. *Chest* 1978; 74:372–376.
286. Hung KK Jr, Enquist RW, Bowel TE: Multiple pulmonary nodules with central cavitation. *Chest* 1976; 69:529–530.
287. Hutchinson WB, Friedenberg MJ: Intrathoracic mesothelioma. *Am J Roentgenol* 1963; 80:937–945.
288. Ikezoe J, Godwin JD, Hunt KJ, et al: Pulmonary lymphangitic carcinomatosis: chronicity of radiographic findings in long-term survivors. *Am J Roentgenol* 1995; 165:49–52.
289. Im J-G, Kong Y, Shin YM, et al: Pulmonary paragonimiasis: clinical and experimental studies. *Radiographics* 1993; 13:575–586.
290. Im J-G, Song KS, Kang HS, et al: Mediastinal tuberculous lymphadenitis: CT manifestations. *Radiology* 1987; 164:115–119.
291. Im J-G, Whang HY, Kim WS, et al: Pleuropulmonary paragonimiasis: radiologic findings in 71 patients. *Am J Roentgenol* 1992; 159:39–43.
292. Israel RH: Mycosis fungoides with rapidly progressive pulmonary infiltration. *Radiology* 1977; 125:10.
293. Itoh H, Tokunaga S, Asamoto H, et al: Radiologic-pathologic correlations of small lung nodules with special reference to peribronchiolar nodules. *Am J Roentgenol* 1978; 130:223–231.
294. Itzchak Y, Rosenthal T, Adar R, et al: Dissecting aneurysm of thoracic aorta: reappraisal of radiologic diagnosis. *Am J Roentgenol* 1975; 125:559–570.
295. Jacoby CG, Mindell HJ: Lobar consolidation in pulmonary embolism. *Radiology* 1976; 118:287–290.
296. Jagannath AS, Sos TA, Lockhart SH, et al: Aortic dissection: a statistical analysis of the usefulness of plain chest radiographic findings. *Am J Roentgenol* 1986; 147:1123–1126.
297. Janower ML, Blennerhassett JB: Lymphangitic spread of metastatic cancer to the lung. *Radiology* 1971; 101:267–273.
298. Jariwalla AG, Al-Nasiri NK: Splenosis pleurae. *Thorax* 1979; 34:123–124.
299. Jay SJ, Johanson WG Jr, Pierce AK: The radiographic resolution of *Streptococcus pneumoniae* pneumonia. *N Engl J Med* 1975; 293:798–801.
300. Joffe N: Roentgenologic findings in post-shock and postoperative pulmonary insufficiency. *Radiology* 1970; 94:369–375.
301. Joffe N: The adult respiratory distress syndrome. *Am J Roentgenol* 1974; 122:719–732.
302. Johkoh T, Ikezoe J, Tomiyama N, et al: CT findings in lymphangitic carcinomatosis of the lung: correlation with histologic findings and pulmonary function tests. *Am J Roentgenol* 1992; 15:1217–1222.
303. Jones FA, Wiedemann HP, O'Donovan PB, et al: Computerized tomographic densitometry of the solitary pulmonary nodule using a nodule phantom. *Chest* 1989; 96:779–783.
304. Jones RN, McLoud T, Rockoff SD: The radiographic pleural abnormalities in asbestos exposure: relationship to physiologic abnormalities. *J Thorac Imaging* 1988; 3:57–66.
305. Kadir S, Kalisher L, Schiller AL: Extramedullary hematopoiesis in Paget's disease of bone. *Am J Roentgenol* 1977; 129:493–495.
306. Kalifa LG, Schimmel DH, Gamsu G: Multiple chronic benign pulmonary nodules. *Radiology* 1976; 121:275–279.
307. Kangarloo H, Beachley MC, Ghahremani GG: The radiographic spectrum of pulmonary complications in burn victims. *Am J Roentgenol* 1977; 128:441–445.
308. Kantor HG: The many radiologic facies of pneumococcal pneumonia. *Am J Roentgenol* 1981; 137:1213–1220.

309. Kassner EG, Goldman HS, Elguezabal A: Cavitating lung nodules and pneumothorax in children with metastatic Wilms' tumor. *Am J Roentgenol* 1976; 126:728–733.
310. Kattan KR, Wiot JF: Cardiac rotation in left lower lobe collapse. *Radiology* 1976; 118:275–276.
311. Katz S, Stanton J, McCormick G: Miliary calcification of the lungs after treated miliary tuberculosis. *N Engl J Med* 1955; 253:135–137.
312. Kelsey CA, Moseley RD, Brogdon BG, et al: Effect of size and position on chest lesion detection. *Am J Roentgenol* 1977; 129:205–208.
313. Khan A, Herman PG, Vorwerk P, et al: Solitary pulmonary nodules: comparison of classification with standard, thin-section, and reference phantom CT. *Radiology* 1991; 179:477–481.
314. Khouri NF, Eggleston JD, Siegelman SS: Angioimmunoblastic lymphadenopathy: a cause for mediastinal nodal enlargement. *Am J Roentgenol* 1978; 130:1186–1188.
315. Khoury MB, Godwin JD, Ravin CE, et al: Thoracic cryptococcosis: immunologic competence and radiologic appearance. *Am J Roentgenol* 1984; 141:893–896.
316. Kim FM, Fennessy JJ: Pleural thickening caused by leukemic infiltration: CT findings. *Am J Roentgenol* 1994; 162:293–294.
317. Kirchner SG, Heller RM, Smith CW: Pancreatic pseudocyst of the mediastinum. *Radiology* 1977; 123:37–42.
318. Klein DL, Gamsu G, Gant TD: Intrathoracic desmoid tumor of the chest wall. *Am J Roentgenol* 1977; 129:524–525.
319. Klein J, Gamsu G: High resolution computed tomography of diffuse lung disease. *Invest Radiol* 1989; 24:805–812.
320. Klein JS, Warnock M, Webb WR, et al: Cavitating and noncavitating granulomas in AIDS patients with *Pneumocystis* pneumonitis. *Am J Roentgenol* 1989; 152:753–754.
321. Kollins SA: Computed tomography of the pulmonary parenchyma and chest wall. *Radiol Clin North Am* 1977; 15:297–308.
322. Kountz PD, Molina PL, Sagel SS: Fibrosing mediastinitis in the posterior thorax. *Am J Roentgenol* 1989; 153:489–490.
323. Kradin RL, Spirn PW, Mark EJ: Intrapulmonary lymph nodes. *Chest* 1985; 87(5):662–667.
324. Kroboth FJ, Yu VL, Reddy SC, et al: Clinicoradiographic correlation with the extent of legionnaire disease. *Am J Roentgenol* 1983; 141:263–268.
325. Krudy AG, Doppman JL, Brennan MF, et al: The detection of mediastinal parathyroid glands by computed tomography, selective arteriography and venous sampling. *Radiology* 1981; 140:739–744.
326. Kruglik GD, Reed JC, Daroca PJ: RPC from the AFIP. *Radiology* 1976; 120:583–588.
327. Kuhlman JE, Bouchardy L, Fishman EK, et al: CT and MR imaging evaluation of chest wall disorders. *Radiographics* 1994; 14:571–595.
328. Kuhlman JE, Fishman EK, Hruban RH, et al: Diseases of the chest in AIDS: CT diagnosis. *Radiographics* 1989; 9:827–857.
329. Kuhlman JE, Fishman EK, Ko-Pen Wang, et al: Esophageal duplication cyst: CT and transesophageal needle aspiration. *Am J Roentgenol* 1985; 145:531–532.
330. Kuhlman JE, Knowles MC, Fishman EK, et al: Premature bullous pulmonary damage in AIDS: CT diagnosis. *Radiology* 1989; 173:23–26.
331. Kuhlman JE, Reyes BL, Hruban RH, et al: Abnormal air-filled spaces in the lung. *Radiographics* 1993; 13:47–75.
332. Kuisk H, Sanchez JS: Desquamative interstitial pneumonia and idiopathic diffuse pulmonary fibrosis. *Am J Roentgenol* 1969; 107:258–279.
333. Kulwiec EL, Lynch DA, Aguayo SM, et al: Imaging of pulmonary histiocytosis X. *Radiographics* 1992; 12:515–526.
334. Kumpe DA, Oh KS, Wyman SM: A characteristic pulmonary finding in unilateral complete bronchial transection. *Am J Roentgenol* 1970; 110:704–706.
335. Kundel HL: Predictive value and threshold detectability of lung tumors. *Radiology* 1981; 139:25–29.
336. Kuwano K, Matsuba K, Ikeda T, et al: The diagnosis of mild emphysema. Correlation of computed tomography and pathology scores. *Am Rev Respir Dis* 1990; 141:169–178.

337. Lacronique J, Roth C, Battesti JP, et al: Chest radiological features of pulmonary histiocytosis X: a report based on 50 adult cases. *Thorax* 1982; 37:104–109.
338. Laffey KJ, Thomastow B, Jaretzki A III, et al: Systemic supply to a pulmonary arteriovenous malformation: a relative contraindication to surgery. *Am J Roentgenol* 1985; 145:720–722.
339. Landay MJ: Anterior clear space: how clear? how often? how come? *Radiology* 1994; 192:165–169.
340. Landay MJ, Christensen EE, Bynum LJ, et al: Anaerobic pleural and pulmonary infections. *Am J Roentgenol* 1980; 134:233–240.
341. Lander P, Palayew MJ: Infectious mononucleosis: a review of chest roentgenographic manifestations. *J Can Assoc Radiol* 1974; 25:303–306.
342. Landman S, Burgener F: Pulmonary manifestations in Wegener's granulomatosis. *Am J Roentgenol* 1974; 122:750–756.
343. Lane EJ, Whalen JP: A new sign of left atrial enlargement: posterior displacement of the left bronchial tree. *Radiology* 1969; 93:279–284.
344. Latour A, Shulman HS: Thoracic manifestations of renal cell carcinoma. *Radiology* 1976; 121:43–48.
345. Lau KK, Philips G, McKenzie A: Pseudotumoral paraesophageal varices. *Gastrointest Radiol* 1992; 17:193–194.
346. Lautin EM, Rosenblatt M, Friedman AC, et al: Calcification in non-Hodgkin lymphoma occuring before theray: identification on plain films and CT. *Am J Roentgenol* 1990; 155:739–740.
347. Lee KS, Kullnig P, Hartman TE, et al: Cryptogenic organizing pneumonia: CT findings in 43 patients. *Am J Roentgenol* 1994; 162:543–546.
348. Lee KS, Logan PM Primack SL, et al: Combined lobar atelectasis of the right lung: imaging findings. *Am J Roentgenol* 1994; 163:43–47.
349. Lee KS, Song KS, Lim Th, et al: Adult-onset pulmonary tuberculosis: findings on chest radiographs and CT scans. *Am J Roentgenol* 1993; 160:753–758.
350. Lee VW, Fuller JD, O'Brien MJ, et al: Pulmonary Kaposi sarcoma in patients with AIDS: scintigraphic diagnosis with sequential thallium and gallium scanning. *Radiology* 1991; 180:409–412.
351. Lees RF, Harrison RB, Williamson BRJ, et al: Radiographic findings in Rocky Mountain spotted fever. *Radiology* 1978; 129:17–20.
352. Leigh TF, Weens HS: Roentgen aspects of mediastinal lesions. *Semin Roentgenol* 1969; 4:59–67.
353. Leight GS Jr, Michaelis LL: Open lung biopsy for diagnosis of acute, diffuse pulmonary infiltrates in the immunosuppressed patient. *Chest* 1978; 73:477–482.
354. Lemire P, Trepanier A, Hubert G: Bronchocele and blocked bronchiectasis. *Am J Roentgenol* 1970; 110:687–693.
355. Lenique F, Brauner MW, Grenier P, et al: CT assessment of bronchi in sardoidosis: endoscopic and pathologic correlations. *Radiology* 1995; 194:419–423.
356. LeRoux BT: Supraphrenic herniation of perinephric fat. *Thorax* 1965; 20:376–381.
357. Lewis ER, Caskey CI, Fishman EK: Lymphoma of the lung: CT findings in 31 patients. *Am J Roentgenol* 1991; 156:711–714.
358. Lewis JE, Sheptin C: Mycoplasma pneumonia associated with abscess of the lung. *Calif Med* 1972; 117:69–72.
359. Li C, Miller WT, Jiang J: Pulmonary edema due to ingestion of organophosphate insecticide. *Am J Roentgenol* 1989; 152:265–266.
360. Libshitz HI, Atkinson GW, Israel HL: Pleural thickening as a manifestation of aspergillus superinfection. *Am J Roentgenol* 1974; 120:883–886.
361. Libshitz HI, Baber CC, Hammond CB: The pulmonary metastases of choriocarcinoma. *Obstet Gynecol* 1977; 49:412–416.
362. Libshitz HI, Southard ME: Complications of radiation therapy: the thorax. *Semin Roentgenol* 1974; 9:41–49.
363. Liebow AA: New concepts and entities in pulmonary disease. In *The Lung.* Baltimore, Williams & Wilkins, 1968.
364. Liebow AA: Pulmonary angitis and granulomatosis. *Am Rev Respir Dis* 1973; 108:1–18.

365. Liebow AA, Carrington CB: Hypersensitivity reactions involving the lung. In *Transactions and studies of the College of Physicians of Philadelphia 34*, series 4, 1966–1967:47–70.

366. Liebow AA, Carrington CB, Friedman PJ: Lymphomatoid granulomatosis. *Hum Pathol* 1972; 3:457–532.

367. Link KM, Samuels LJ, Reed JC, et al: Magnetic resonance imaging of the mediastinum. *J Thorac Imaging* 1993; 8(1):34–53.

368. Liu YC, Tomashefski JF Jr, Tomford JW, et al: Necrotizing *Pneumocystis carinii* vasculitis associated with lung necrosis and cavitation in a patient with acquired immunodeficiency syndrome. *Arch Pathol Lab Med* 1989; 113:494–497.

369. Longuet R, Phelan J, Tanous H, et al: Criteria of the silhouette sign. *Radiology* 1977; 122:581–585.

370. Louria DB: Rickettsial and parasitic infections of the lungs and embolic lung infections. In Baum GL editor, *Textbook of pulmonary diseases.* Boston, Little, Brown, 1974.

371. Lui YM, Taylor JR, Zylak CJ: Roentgenanatomical correlation of the individual human pulmonary acinus. *Radiology* 1973; 109:1–5.

372. Lundius B: Intrathoracic kidney. *Am J Roentgenol* 1975; 125:678–681.

373. Lyons HA, Calvy GL, Sammons BP: The diagnosis and classification of mediastinal masses. 1. A study of 782 cases. *Ann Intern Med* 1959; 51:897–932.

374. Madewell JE, Daroca PJ, Reed JC: RPC from the AFIP. *Radiology* 1975; 117:555–559.

375. Madewell JE, Feigin DS: Benign tumors of the lung. *Semin Roentgenol* 1977; 12:175–185.

376. Madewell JE, Stocker JT, Korsower JM: Cystic adenomatoid malformation of the lung. *Am J Roentgenol* 1975; 124:436–448.

377. Maguire R, Fauci AS, Doppman JL, et al: Unusual radiographic features of Wegener's granulomatosis. *Am J Roentgenol* 1978; 130:233–238.

378. Maher GC, Berger HW: Massive pleural effusion: malignant and nonmalignant causes in 46 patients. *Am Rev Respir Dis* 1972; 105:458–460.

379. Maile CW, Rodan BA, Godwin JD, et al: Calcification in pulmonary metastases. *Br J Radiol* 1982:55:108–113.

380. Mallens WMC, Nijhuis-Heddes JMA, Bakker W: Calcified lymph node metastases in bronchioloalveolar carcinoma. *Radiology* 1986; 161:103–104.

381. Marglin SI, Mortimer J, Castellino RA: Radiologic investigation of thoracic metastases from unknown primary sites. *J Thorac Imaging* 1987; 38–43.

382. Marglin SI, Soulen RL, Blank N, et al: Mycosis fungoides. *Radiology* 1979; 130:35–37.

383. Margolin FR, Gandy TK: Pneumonia of atypical measles. *Radiology* 1979; 131:653–655.

384. Marinelli DL, Albelda SM, Williams TM, et al: Nontuberculous mycobacterial infection in AIDS: clinical, pathologic and radiographic features. *Radiology* 1986; 160:77–82.

385. Martin W III, Choplin RH, Shertzer ME: The chest radiograph in Rocky Mountain spotted fever. *Am J Roentgenol* 1982; 139:889–893.

386. Masson RG, Tedeschi LG: Pulmonary eosinophilic granuloma with hilar adenopathy simulating sarcoidosis. *Chest* 1978; 73:682–683.

387. Masur H, Ognibene FP, Yarchoan R, et al: CD4 counts as predictors of opportunistic pneumonias in human immunodeficiency virus (HIV) infection. *Ann Intern Med* 1989; 111:223–231.

388. Matthay RA, Schwarz MI, Ellis JH Jr, et al: Pulmonary artery hypertension in chronic obstructive pulmonary disease: determination by chest radiography. *Invest Radiol* 1981; 16:95–100.

389. Mays EE: Rheumatoid pleuritis: observations in eight cases and suggestions for making the diagnosis in patients without the "typical findings." *Dis Chest* 1968; 53:202–214.

390. McAdams HP, Rosado-de-Christenson ML, Lesar M, et al: Thoracic mycoses from endemic fungi: radiologic-pathologic correlation. *Radiographics* 1995:15:255–270.

391. McAdams HP, Rosado-de-Christenson ML, Templeton PA, et al: Thoracic mycoses from opportunistic fungi: radiologic-pathologic correlation. *Radiographics* 1995; 15:271–286.

392. McGahan JP, Graves DS, Palmer PES, et al: Classic and contemporary imaging of coccidioidomycosis. *Am J Roentgenol* 1981; 136:393–404.
393. McGuinness G, Scholes JV, Jagirdar JS, et al: Unusual lymphoproliferative disorders in nine adults with HIV or AIDS: CT and pathologic findings. *Radiology* 1995; 197:59–65.
394. McHugh K, Blaquiere RM: CT features of rounded atelectasis. *Am J Roentgenol* 1989; 153:257–260.
395. McLoud, TC: Asbestos-related diseases: the role of imaging techniques. *Postgrad Radiol* 1989; 9:65–74.
396. McLoud TC, Carrington CB, Gaensler EA: Diffuse infiltrative lung disease: a new scheme for description. *Radiology* 1983; 149:353–363.
397. McLoud TC, Epler GR, Colby TV, et al: Bronchiolitis obliterans. *Radiology* 1986; 159:1–8.
398. McLoud TC, Isler RJ, Novelline RA, et al: Review: the apical cap. *Am J Roentgenol* 1981; 137:299–306.
399. McLoud TC, Kalisher L, Stark P, et al: Intrathoracic lymph node metastases from extrathoracic neoplasms. *Am J Roentgenol* 1978; 131:403–407.
400. Meighan JW: Pulmonary cryptococcosis mimicking carcinoma of the lung. *Radiology* 1972; 103:61–62.
401. Melamed M, Barker WL, Langston HT: Unusual pleural fistulas. *Am J Roentgenol* 1974; 120:876–882.
402. Meredith HC, Cogan BM, McLaulin B: Pleural aspergillosis. *Am J Roentgenol* 1978; 130:164–166.
403. Mermelstein RH, Freireich AW: Varicella pneumonia. *Ann Intern Med* 1961; 55:456–463.
404. Meszaros WT, Guzzo F, Schorsch H: Neurofibromatosis. *Am J Roentgenol* 1966; 98:557–569.
405. Meyer JE: Thoracic effects of therapeutic irradiation for breast carcinoma. *Am J Roentgenol* 1978; 130:877–885.
406. Meyer JS, Harty MP, Mahboubi S, et al: Langerhans cell histiocytosis: presentation and evolution of radiologic findings with clinical correlation. *Radiographics* 1995; 15:1135–1146.
407. Millar JK: The chest film findings in "Q" fever—a series of 35 cases. *Clin Radiol* 1978; 29:371–375.
408. Miller BH, Rosado-de-Christenson ML, McAdams HP, et al: Thoracic sarcoidosis: radiologic-pathologic correlation. *Radiographics* 1995; 15(2) 421–437.
409. Miller WT, Aronchick JM, Epstein DM, et al: The troublesome nipple shadow. *Am J Roentgenol* 1985; 145:521–523.
410. Miller WT, Cornog JL Jr, Sullivan MA: Lymphangiomyomatosis. *Am J Roentgenol* 1971; 111:565–572.
411. Miller WT, Husted J, Freiman D, et al: Bronchioloalveolar carcinoma: two clinical entities with one pathologic diagnosis. *Am J Roentgenol* 1978; 130:905–912.
412. Miller WT, MacGregor RR: Tuberculosis: frequency of unusual radiographic findings. *Am J Roentgenol* 1978; 130:867–875.
413. Miller WT Jr: Spectrum of pulmonary nontuberculous mycobacterial infection. *Radiology* 1994; 191:343–350.
414. Milne ENC, Pistolesi M, Miniati M, et al: The radiologic distinction of cardiogenic and noncardiogenic edema. *Am J Roentgenol* 1985; 144:879–894.
415. Milos M, Aberle DR, Parkinson BT, et al: Maternal pulmonary edema complicating beta-adrenergic therapy of preterm labor. *Am J Roentgenol* 1988; 151:917–918.
416. Mink JH, Bein ME, Sukov R, et al: Computed tomography of the anterior mediastinum in patients with myasthenia gravis and suspected thymoma. *Am J Roentgenol* 1978; 130:239–246.
417. Mintzer RA, Neiman HL, Reeder MM: Mucoid impaction of a bronchus. *JAMA* 1978; 240; 1397–1398.
418. Mirvis SE, Rodriguez A, Whitley NO, et al: CT evaluation of thoracic infections after major trauma. *Am J Roentgenol* 1985; 144:1183–1187.

419. Moore ADA, Godwin JD, Müller NL, et al: Pulmonary histiocytosis X: comparison of radiographic and CT findings. *Radiology* 1989; 172:249–254.
420. Morgan DE, Nath H, Sanders C, et al: Mediastinal actinomycosis. *Am J Roentgenol* 1990; 155:735–737.
421. Morgan H, Ellis K: Superior mediastinal masses: secondary to tuberculous lymphadenitis in the adult. *Am J Roentgenol* 1974; 120:893–897.
422. Moser ES Jr, Proto AV: Lung torsion: case report and literature review. *Radiology* 1987; 162:639–643.
423. Moser KM: Pulmonary embolism. *Am Rev Respir Dis* 1977; 115:829–852.
424. Mountain CF: A new international staging system for lung cancer. *Chest* 1986; 89(4 suppl):225S–233S.
425. Muhm JR, Brown LR, Crowe JK: Detection of pulmonary nodules by computed tomography. *Am J Roentgenol* 1977; 128:267–270.
426. Muhm JR, Miller WE, Fontana RS, et al: Lung cancer detected during a screening program using four-month chest radiographs. *Radiology* 1983; 148:609–615.
427. Müller NL, Guerry-Force ML, Staples CA, et al: Differential diagnosis of bronchiolitis obliterans with organizing pneumonia and usual interstitial pneumonia: clinical, functional, and radiologic findings. *Radiology* 1987; 162:151–156.
428. Müller NL, Miller RR, Webb WR, et al: Fibrosing alveolitis: CT-pathologic correlation. *Radiology* 1986; 160:585–588.
429. Müller NL, Staples CA, Miller RR: Bronchiolitis obliterans organizing pneumonia: CT features in 14 patients. *Am J Roentgenol* 1990; 154:983–987.
430. Müller NL, Webb WR, Gamsu G: Paratracheal lymphadenopathy: radiographic findings and correlation with CT. *Radiology* 1985; 156:761–765.
431. Müller NL, Webb WR, Gamsu G: Subcarinal lymph node enlargement: radiographic findings and CT correlation. *Am J Roentgenol* 1985; 145:15–19.
432. Murray HW, Masur H, Senterfit LB, et al: The protean manifestations of mycoplasma pneumoniae infection in adults. *Am J Med* 1975; 58:229–242.
433. Murray HW, Tuazon CU, Kirmani N, et al: The adult respiratory distress syndrome associated with miliary tuberculosis. *Chest* 1978; 73:37–43.
434. Naidich DP, Garay SM, Leitman BS, et al: Radiographic manifestations of pulmonary disease in the acquired immunodeficiency syndrome (AIDS). *Semin Roentgenol* 1987; 22:14–30.
435. Nakata H, Kimoto T, Nakayama T, et al: Diffuse peripheral lung disease: evaluation by high-resolution computed tomography. *Radiology* 1985; 157:181–185.
436. Nathan MH: Management of solitary pulmonary nodules. *JAMA* 1974; 227:1141–1144.
437. Nathan MH, Collins VP, Adams RA: Differentiation of benign and malignant pulmonary nodules by growth rate. *Am J Roentgenol* 1962; 79:221–232.
438. Neiman HL, Wolson AH, Berenson JE: Pulmonary and pleural manifestations of Waldenstrom's macroglobulinemia. *Radiology* 1973; 107:301–302.
439. Newman A, So SK: Bilateral neurofibroma of the intrathoracic vagus associated with Von Recklinghausen's disease. *Am J Roentgenol* 1971; 112:389–392.
440. Nordenström BEW: New trends and technique of roentgen diagnosis of bronchial carcinoma. In Simmon M, Potchen EJ, Lemay M, editors, *Frontiers of pulmonary radiology.* New York, Grune and Stratton, 1969.
441. Numan F, Islak C, Berkmen T, et al: Behcet disease: pulmonary arterial involvement in 15 cases. *Radiology* 1994; 192:465–468.
442. O'Connell RS, McLoud TC, Wilkins EW: Superior sulcus tumor: radiographic diagnosis and workup. *Am J Roentgenol* 1983; 140:25–30.
443. O'Reilly GV, Dee PM, Otteni GV: Gangrene of the lung: successful medical management of three patients. *Radiology* 1978; 126:575–579.
444. Oels HC, Harrison EG Jr, Carr DT, et al: Diffuse malignant mesothelioma of the pleura: a review of 37 cases. *Chest* 1971; 60:564–570.
445. Ogakwu M, Nwokolo C: Radiological findings in pulmonary paragonimiasis as seen in Nigeria: a review based on one hundred cases. *Br J Radiol* 1973; 46: 699–705.

446. Oldham SAA, Castillo M, Jacobson FL, et al: HIV-associated lymphocytic interstitial pneumonia: radiologic manifestations and pathologic correlation. *Radiology* 1989; 170:83–87.
447. Ominsky SH, Kricun ME: Roentgenology of sinus of Valsalva aneurysms. *Am J Roentgenol* 1975; 125:571–581.
448. Ostendorf P, Birzle H, Vogel W, et al: Pulmonary radiographic abnormalities in shock. *Radiology* 1975; 115:257–263.
449. Oswalt CE, Gates GA, Holmstrom FMG: Pulmonary edema as a complication of acute airway obstruction. *JAMA* 1977; 238:1833–1835.
450. Pagani JJ, Libshitz HI: Opportunistic fungal pneumonias in cancer patients. *Am J Roentgenol* 1981; 137:1033–1039.
451. Parra O, Ruiz J, Ojanguren I, et al: Amiodarone toxicity: recurrence of interstitial pneumonitis after withdrawal of the drug. *Eur Respir J* 1989; 2:905–907.
452. Pearlberg JL, Haggar AM, Saravolatz L: *Hemophilus influenzae* pneumonia in the adult. *Radiology* 1984; 151:23–26.
453. Pearlberg JL, Sandler MA, Beute GH, et al: TIN0M0 bronchogenic carcinoma: assessment by CT. *Radiology* 1985; 157:187–190.
454. Pendergrass EP: An evaluation of some of the radiologic patterns of small opacities in coal worker's pneumoconioses. *Am J Roentgenol* 1972; 115:457–461.
455. Phillips MJ, Knight RK, Green M: Fiberoptic bronchoscopy and diagnosis of pulmonary lesions in lymphoma and leukaemia. *Thorax* 1980; 35:19–25.
456. Pierce JW, Kerr IH: Immunologic diseases and the lung. *Radiol Clin North Am* 1978; 16:389–406.
457. Pinckney L, Parker BR: Primary coccidioidomycosis in children presenting with massive pleural effusion. *Am J Roentgenol* 1978; 130:247–249.
458. Pinsker KL: Solitary pulmonary nodule in sarcoidosis. *JAMA* 1978; 240:1379–1380.
459. Plavsic BM, Robinson AE, Freundlich IM, et al: Melanoma metastatic to the bronchus: radiologic features in two patients. *J Thorac Imaging* 1994; 9(2):67–70.
460. Podoll LN, Winkler SS: Busulfan lung. *Am J Roentgenol* 1974; 120:151–156.
461. Pope TL Jr, Armstrong P, Thompson R, et al: Pittsburgh pneumonia agent: chest film manifestations. *Am J Roentgenol* 1982; 138:237–241.
462. Potchen EJ, Bisesi MA: When is it malpractice to miss lung cancer on chest radiographs? *Radiology* 1990; 175:29–32.
463. Press GA, Glazer HS, Wassermann TH, et al: Thoracic wall involvement by Hodgkin disease and non-Hodgkin lymphoma: CT evaluation. *Radiology* 1985; 158:195–198.
464. Price JE Jr, Rigler LG: Widening of the mediastinum resulting from fat accumulation. *Radiology* 1970; 96:497–500.
465. Primack SL, Hartman TE, Hansell DM, et al: End-stage lung disease: CT findings in 61 patients. *Radiology* 1993; 189:681–686.
466. Proto AV: Conventional chest radiographs: anatomic understanding of newer observations. *Radiology* 1992; 183:593–603.
467. Proto AV, Corcoran HL, Ball JB Jr: The left paratracheal reflection. *Radiology* 1989; 171:625–628.
468. Proto AV, Lane EJ: Air in the esophagus: a frequent radiographic finding. *Am J Roentgenol* 1977; 129:433–440.
469. Proto AV, Moser ES Jr: Upper lobe volume loss: divergent and parallel patterns of vascular reorientation. *Radiographics* 1987; 7:875–887.
470. Putman CE, Loke J, Matthay RA, et al: Radiographic manifestations of acute smoke inhalation. *Am J Roentgenol* 1977; 129:865–870.
471. Putman CE, Minagi H, Blaisdell FW: The roentgen appearance of disseminated intravascular coagulation (DIC). *Radiology* 1973; 109:13–18.
472. Putman CE, Tummillo AM, Myerson DA, et al: Drowning: another plunge. *Am J Roentgenol* 1975; 125:543–548.
473. Raasch BN, Carsky EW, Lane EJ, et al: Pleural effusion: explanation of some typical appearances. *Am J Roentgenol* 1982; 139:899–904.
474. Rabinowitz JG, Busch J, Buttram WR: Pulmonary manifestations of blastomycosis. *Radiology* 1976; 120:25–32.

475. Rabinowitz JG, Cohen BA, Mendolson DS: Lymphomatoid granulomatosis. *JAMA* 1985; 254:3458–3460.

476. Raider L: Calcification in chickenpox pneumonia. *Chest* 1971; 60:504–507.

477. Ramilo J, Harris VJ, White H: Empyema as a complication of retropharyngeal and neck abscesses in children. *Radiology* 1978; 126:743–746.

478. Ramsay GC, Meyer RD: Cavitary fungus disease of the lungs. *Radiology* 1973; 109:29–32.

479. Ravin CE: Pulmonary vascularity: radiographic considerations. *J Thorac Imaging* 1988; 3:1–13.

480. Ravin CE, Smith GW, Ahern MJ, et al: Cytomegaloviral infection presenting as a solitary pulmonary nodule. *Chest* 1977; 71:220–222.

481. Reed JC: Pathologic correlations of the air-bronchogram: a reliable sign in chest radiology. *CRC Crit Rev Diagn Imaging* 1977; 10:235–255.

482. Reed JC, Choplin RH: Pulmonary and pleural complications of pneumonias. *Contemp Diagn Radiol* 1989; 12:1–5.

483. Reed JC, Hallet KK, Feigin DS: Neural tumors of the thorax: subject review from the AFIP. *Radiology* 1978; 126:9–17.

484. Reed JC, Madewell JE: The air bronchogram in interstitial disease of the lungs. *Radiology* 1975; 116:1–9.

485. Reed JC, McLelland R, Nelson P: Legionnaires' disease. *Am J Roentgenol* 1978; 131:892–894.

486. Reed JC, Reeder MM: Honeycomb lung (interstitial fibrosis). *JAMA* 1975; 231:646–647.

487. Reed JC, Sobonya RE: Morphologic analysis of foregut cysts in the thorax. *Am J Roentgenol* 1974; 120:851–860.

488. Reed JC, Sobonya RE: RPC from the AFIP. *Radiology* 1975; 117:315–319.

489. Reeder MM: Gamut: causes of pleural fluid. *Semin Roentgenol* 1977; 12:255.

490. Reeder MM: Gamut: pleural-based lesion arising from the lung, pleura, or chest wall. *Semin Roentgenol* 1977; 12:261–262.

491. Reeder MM, Felson B: *Gamuts in radiology.* Cincinnati, Audiovisual Radiology of Cincinnati, 1975.

492. Reeder MM, Hochholzer L: RPC of the month from the AFIP. *Radiology* 1969; 92:1106–1111.

493. Reeder MM, Reed JC: Solitary pulmonary nodule (< 4 cm in diameter). *JAMA* 1975; 231:1080–1082.

494. Reinke RT, Coel MN, Higgins CB: Calcified nonsyphilitic aneurysms of the sinuses of Valsalva. *Am J Roentgenol* 1974; 122:783–787.

495. Renner RR, Markarian B, Pernice NJ, et al: The apical cap. *Radiology* 1974; 110:569–573.

496. Renner RR, Pernice NJ: The apical cap. *Semin Roentgenol* 1977; 12:299–302.

497. Rice RP, Loda F: A roentgenographic analysis of respiratory syncytial virus pneumonia in infants. *Radiology* 1966; 87:1021–1027.

498. Rich S, Brundage BH: Primary pulmonary hypertension: current update. *JAMA* 1984; 251:2252–2254.

499. Rigler LG: An overview of cancer of the lung. *Semin Roentgenol* 1977; 12:161–164.

500. Rigler LG: An overview of diseases of the pleura. *Semin Roentgenol* 1977; 12:265–268.

501. Rigler LG: The natural history of untreated lung cancer. *Ann N Y Acad Sci* 1964; 114:755–766.

502. Robbins LL: The roentgenological appearance of parenchymal involvement of the lung by malignant lymphoma. *Cancer* 1953; 6:80–88.

503. Rohlfing BM: The shifting granuloma: an internal marker of atelectasis. *Radiology* 1977; 123:283–285.

504. Rohlfing BM, Webb WR, Schlobohm RM: Ventilator-related extra-alveolar air in adults. *Radiology* 1976; 121:25–31.

505. Rohlfing BM, White EA, Webb WR, et al: Hilar and mediastinal adenopathy caused by bacterial abscess of the lung. *Radiology* 1978; 128:289–293.

506. Rosado-de-Christenson ML, Frazier AA, Stocker JT, et al: Extralobar sequestration: radiologic-pathologic correlation. *Radiographics* 1993; 13:425–441.
507. Rosado-de-Christenson ML, Pugatch RD, Moran CA, et al: Thymolipoma: analysis of 27 cases. *Radiology* 1994; 193:121–126.
508. Rosai J, Levine CD: *Tumors of the thymus. Atlas of tumor pathology,* series 2. Washington, DC, Armed Forces Institute of Pathology, 1976.
509. Rosen SH, Castleman B, Liebow AA: Pulmonary alveolar proteinosis. *N Engl J Med* 1958; 258:1123–1142.
510. Rosenbloom SA, Ravin CE, Putman CE, et al: Peripheral middle lobe syndrome. *Radiology* 1983; 149:17–21.
511. Rosenow EC III: The spectrum of drug-induced pulmonary disease. *Ann Intern Med* 1972; 97:977–991.
512. Roswit B, White DC: Severe radiation injuries of the lung. *Am J Roentgenol* 1977; 129:127–136.
513. Roucos S, Tabet G, Jebara VA, et al: Thoracic splenosis. Case report and literature review. *J Thorac Cardiovasc Surg* 1990; 99:361–363.
514. Rovner AJ, Westcott JL: Pulmonary edema and respiratory insufficiency in acute pancreatitis. *Radiology* 1976; 118:513–520.
515. Rubin SA: Radiographic spectrum of pleuropulmonary tularemia. *Am J Roentgenol* 1978; 131:277–281.
516. Rubin SA: Radiology of immunologic diseases of the lung. *J Thorac Imaging* 1988; 3:21–39.
517. Ryerson GG, Lauwasssesr ME, Block AJ, et al: Legionnaires' disease: a sporadic case. *Chest* 1978; 73:113–115.
518. Saba GP II, James AE Jr, Johnson BA, et al: Pulmonary complications of narcotic abuse. *Am J Roentgenol* 1974; 122:733–739.
519. Sagel SS, Forrest JV: Multiple pulmonary nodules in an alcoholic man. *Chest* 1974; 66:571–572.
520. Sahin AA, Cöplü L, Selcuk ZT, et al: Malignant pleural mesothelioma caused by environmental exposure to asbestos or erionite in rural Turkey: CT findings in 84 patients. *Am J Roentgenol* 1993; 161:533–537.
521. Sakowitz AJ, Sakowitz BH: Disseminated cryptococcosis. *JAMA* 1976, 236:2429–2430.
522. Saltzman HA, Chick EW, Conat NF: Nocardiosis as a complication of other diseases. *Lab Invest* 1962; 11:1110–1117.
523. Saltzstein SL, Ackerman LV: Lymphadenopathy induced by anticonvulsant drugs and mimicking clinically and pathologically malignant lymphomas. *Cancer* 1959; 12:164–182.
524. Salyer WR, Salyer DC: Pleural involvement in cryptococcosis. *Chest* 1974; 66:139–140.
525. Samuel S, Kundel HL, Nodine CF, et al: Mechanism of satisfaction of search: eye position recordings in the reading of chest radiographs. *Radiology* 1995; 194:895–902.
526. Samuels ML, Howe CD, Dodd GD Jr, et al: Endobronchial malignant lymphoma. *Am J Roentgenol* 1961; 85:87–95.
527. Sandhu JS, Goodman PC: Pulmonary cysts associated with *Pneumocystis carinii* pneumonia in patients with AIDS. *Radiology* 1989; 173:33–35.
528. Sargent EN, Barnes RA, Schwinn CP: Multiple pulmonary fibroleiomyomatous hamartomas. *Am J Roentgenol* 1970; 110:694–700.
529. Sargent EN, Gordonson J, Jacobson G, et al: Bilateral pleural thickening: a manifestation of asbestosis dust exposure. *Am J Roentgenol* 1978; 131:579–585.
530. Sargent EN, Jacobson G, Gordonson JS: Pleural plaques: a signpost of asbestos dust inhalation. *Semin Roentgenol* 1977; 12:287–297.
531. Sargent EN, Jacobson G, Wilkinson EE: Diaphragmatic pleural calcification following short occupational exposure to asbestos. *Am J Roentgenol* 1972; 115:473–478.
532. Sargent EN, Wilson R, Gordonson J, et al: Granular cell myoblastoma of the trachea. *Am J Roentgenol* 1972; 114:89–92.

533. Savic B, Birtel FJ, Tholen W, et al: Lung sequestration: report of seven cases and review of 540 published cases. *Thorax* 1979; 34:96–101.
534. Savoca CJ, Austin JHM, Goldberg HI: The right paratracheal stripe. *Radiology* 1977; 122:295–301.
535. Saxon RR, Klein JS, Bar MH, et al: Pathogenesis of pulmonary edema during interleukin-2 therapy: correlation of chest radiographic and clinical findings in 54 patients. *Am J Roentgenol* 1991; 156:281–285.
536. Scatarige JC, Stitik FP: Induction of thoracic malignancy in inorganic dust pneumoconiosis. *J Thorac Imaging* 1988; 3:67–79.
537. Schachter EN, Kreisman H, Putman C: Diagnostic problems in suppurative lung disease. *Arch Intern Med* 1976; 136:167–171.
538. Schaner EG, Chang AE, Doppman JL, et al: Comparison of computed and conventional whole lung tomography in detecting pulmonary nodules: a prospective radiologic-pathologic study. *Am J Roentgenol* 1978; 131:51–54.
539. Schmitt WGH, Hübener KH, Rücker HC: Pleural calcification with persistent effusion. *Radiology* 1983; 149:633–638.
540. Schnur MJ, Austin JHM: Radiopaque hemithorax in an elderly woman. *Chest* 1979; 76:209–211.
541. Schnyder PA, Gamsu G: CT of the pretracheal retrocaval space. *Am J Roentgenol* 1981; 136:303–308.
542. Schulthess von GK, McMurdo K, Tscholakoff D, et al: Mediastinal masses: MR imaging. *Radiology* 1986; 158:289–296.
543. Schwartz EE, Holsclaw DS: Pulmonary involvement in adults with cystic fibrosis. *Am J Roentgenol* 1974; 122:708–718.
544. Schwartz EE, Teplick JG, Onesti G, et al: Pulmonary hemorrhage in renal disease: Goodpasture's syndrome and other causes. *Radiology* 1977; 122:39–46.
545. Schwartz LB, McCann RL: Traumatic false aneurysm of the common carotid artery presenting as a mediastinal mass: a case report. *J Vasc Surg* 1989; 10:281–284.
546. Schwartz MI: Pulmonary and cardiac manifestations of polymyositis-dermatomyositis. *J Thorac Imaging* 1992; 7(2):46–54.
547. Scott WW Jr, Kuhlman JE: Focal pulmonary lesions in patients with AIDS: percutaneous transthoracic needle biopsy. *Radiology* 1991; 189:419–421.
548. Seigel R, Wolson AH: The radiographic manifestations of chronic *Pneumocystis carinii* pneumonia. *Am J Roentgenol* 1977; 128:150–152.
549. Seltzer SE, Balikian JP, Birnholz JC, et al: Giant hyperplastic parathyroid gland in mediastinum—partially cystic and calcified. *Radiology* 1978; 127:43–44.
550. Septimus EJ, Awe RJ, Greenberg SD, et al: Acute tuberculous pneumonia. *Chest* 1977; 71:774–776.
551. Shackelford GD, Sacks EJ, Mullins JD, et al: Pulmonary venoocclusive disease: case report and review of the literature. *Am J Roentgenol* 1977; 128:643–648.
552. Shaffer HA Jr: Multiple leiomyomas of the esophagus. *Radiology* 1976; 118:29–34.
553. Shannon TM, Gale ME: Noncardiac manifestations of rheumatoid arthritis in the thorax. *J Thorac Imaging* 1992; 7(2):19–29.
554. Sheflin JR, Campbell JA, Thompson GP: Pulmonary blastomycosis: findings on chest radiographs in 63 patients. *Am J Roentgenol* 1990; 154:1177–1180.
555. Shin MS, Berland LL, Myers JL, et al: CT demonstration of an ossifying bronchial carcinoid simulating broncholithiasis. *Am J Roentgenol* 1989; 153:51–52.
556. Shopfner CE: Aeration disturbances secondary to pulmonary infection. *Am J Roentgenol* 1974; 120:261–273.
557. Sicuranza BJ, Tisdall LH: Amniotic fluid embolism. *N Y State J Med* 1975; 75:1517–1519.
558. Sider L, Gabriel H, Curry DR, et al: Pattern recognition of the pulmonary manifestations of AIDS on CT scans. *Radiographics* 1993; 13:771–784.
559. Sider L, Weiss AJ, Smith MD, et al: Varied appearance of AIDS-related lymphoma in the chest. *Radiology* 1989; 171:629–632.
560. Siegelman SS, Zerhouni EA, Leo FP, et al: CT of the solitary pulmonary nodule. *Am J Roentgenol* 1980; 135:1–13.

561. Siegler DIM: Lung abscess associated with mycoplasma pneumoniae infection. *Br J Dis Chest* 1973; 67:123–127.
562. Silver TM, Farber SJ, Bole GG, et al: Radiological features of mixed connective tissue disease and scleroderma-systemic lupus erythematosus overlap. *Radiology* 1976; 120:269–275.
563. Silverstein EF, Ellis K, Wolff M, et al: Pulmonary lymphangiomyomatosis. *Am J Roentgenol* 1974; 120:832–850.
564. Sinner WN, Sandstedt B: Small-cell carcinoma of the lung. *Radiology* 1976; 121:269–274.
565. Sites VR, Poland JD: Mediastinal lymphadenopathy in bubonic plague. *Am J Roentgenol* 1976; 116:567–570.
566. Sivit CJ, Schwartz AM, Rockoff SD: Kaposi's sarcoma of the lung in AIDS: radiologic-pathologic analysis. *Am J Roentgenol* 1987; 148:25–28.
567. Smathers RL, Buschi AJ, Pope TL Jr, et al: The azygous arch: normal and pathologic CT appearance. *Am J Roentgenol* 1982; 139:477–483.
568. Smith RC, Mann H, Greenspan RH, et al: Radiographic differentiation between different etiologies of pulmonary edema. *Invest Radiol* 1987; 22:859–863.
569. Smith SD, Cho CT, Brahmacupta N, et al: Pulmonary involvement with cytomegalovirus infections in children. *Arch Dis Child* 1977; 52:441–446.
570. Smith TR, Khoury PT: Aneurysm of the proximal thoracic aorta simulating neoplasm: the role of CT and angiography. *Am J Roentgenol* 1985; 144:909–910.
571. Sone S, Higashihara T, Kotake T, et al: Pulmonary manifestations in acute carbon monoxide poisoning. *Am J Roentgenol* 1974; 120:865–871.
572. Sones PJ Jr, Torres WE, Colvin RS, et al: Effectiveness of CT in evaluating intrathoracic masses. *Am J Roentgenol* 1982; 139:469–475.
573. Sostman HD, Putnam CE, Gamsu G: Review: diagnosis of chemotherapy lung. *Am J Roentgenol* 1981; 136:33–40.
574. Sostman HD, Ravin CE, Sullivan DC, et al: Use of pulmonary angiography for suspected pulmonary embolism: influence of scintigraphic diagnosis. *Am J Roentgenol* 1982; 139:673–677.
575. St. Clair EW, Rice JR, Synderman R: Pneumonitis complicating low-dose methotrexate therapy in rheumatoid arthritis. *Arch Intern Med* 1985; 145:2035–2038.
576. Stansell JD: Fungal disease in HIV-infected persons: cryptococcosis, histoplasmosis, and coccidioidomycosis. *J Thorac Imaging* 1991; 6(4):28–35.
577. Staples CA, Gamsu G, Ray CS, et al: High resolution computed tomography and lung function in asbestos-exposed workers with normal chest radiographs. *Am Rev Respir Dis* 1989; 139:1502–1508.
578. Stark DD, Federle MP, Goodman PC, et al: Differentiating lung abscess and empyema: radiography and computed tomography. *Am J Roentgenol* 1983; 141:163–167.
579. Stark P, Thordarson S, McKinney M: Manifestations of esophageal disease on plain chest radiographs. *Am J Roentgenol* 1990; 155:729–734.
580. Steele JD: The solitary pulmonary nodule. *J Thorac Cardiovasc Surg* 1963; 46:21–39.
581. Stein DS, Korvick JA, Vermund SH: CD4 + lymphocyte cell enumeration for prediction of clinical course of human immunodeficiency virus disease: a review. *J Infect Dis* 1992; 165:352–363.
582. Stein MG, Mayo J, Müller N, et al: Pulmonary lymphangitic spread of carcinoma: appearance on CT scans. *Radiology* 1987; 162:371–375.
583. Stelling CB, Woodring JH, Rehm SR: Miliary pulmonary blastomycosis. *Radiology* 1984; 150:7–13.
584. Stephan WC, Parks RD, Tempest B: Acute hypersensitivity pneumonitis associated with carbamazepine therapy. *Chest* 1978; 74:463–464.
585. Stern RC, Gamsu G, Golden JA, et al: Intrathoracic adenopathy: differential features of AIDS and diffuse lymphadenopathy syndrome. *Am J Roentgenol* 1984; 142:689–692.
586. Stitik FP, Tockman MS: Radiographic screening in the early detection of lung cancer. *Radiol Clin North Am* 1978; 16:347–366.
587. Stokes D, Sigler A, Khouri NF, et al: Unilateral hyperlucent lung (Swyer-James syn-

drome) after severe mycoplasma pneumoniae infection. *Am Rev Respir Dis* 1978; 117:145–152.

588. Stolberg HO, Patt NL, MacEwen KF, et al: Hodgkin's disease of the lung. *Am J Roentgenol* 1964; 92:96–115.

589. Stolz JL, Arger PH, Benson JM: Mushroom worker's lung disease. *Radiology* 1976; 119:61–63.

590. Streiter ML, Schneider HJ, Proto AV: Steroid-induced thoracic lipomatosis: paraspinal involvement. *Am J Roentgenol* 1982; 139:679–681.

591. Sugimoto H, Ohsawa T: Unilateral hyperlucent thorax on plain chest radiographs after neck dissection: importance of atrophy of the trapezius muscle. *Am J Roentgenol* 1994; 163:1079–1082.

592. Summer WR, Dwyer P, Hales ED, et al: Hypersensitivity pneumonitis. *Johns Hopkins Med J* 1980; 146:80–87.

593. Swensen SJ, Brown LR, Colby TV, et al: Pulmonary nodules: CT evaluation of enhancement with iodinated contrast material. *Radiology* 1995; 194:393–398.

594. Swensen SJ, Harms GF, Morin RL, et al: CT evaluation of solitary pulmonary nodules: value of 185-H reference phantom. *Am J Roentgenol* 1991; 156:925–929.

595. Swischuk LE: Bubbles in hyaline membrane disease. *Radiology* 1977; 122:417–426.

596. Talbot S, Worthington BS, Roebuck EJ: Radiographic signs of pulmonary embolism and pulmonary infarction. *Thorax* 1978; 28:198–203.

597. Talner LB, Gmelich JT, Liebow AA, et al: The syndrome of bronchial mucocele and regional hyperinflation of the lung. *Am J Roentgenol* 1970; 110:675–686.

598. Taryle DA, Potts DE, Sahn SA: The incidence and clinical correlates of parapneumonic effusions in pneumococcal pneumonia. *Chest* 1978; 74:170–173.

599. Teixidor HS, Bachman al: Multiple amyloid tumors of the lung. *Am J Roentgenol* 1971; 111:525–529.

600. Templeton AW: Malignant mediastinal teratoma with bone metastases. *Radiology* 1961; 76:245–247.

601. Teplick JG, Nedwich A, Haskin ME: Roentgenographic features of thymolipoma. *Am J Roentgenol* 1973; 117:873–877.

602. Teplick JG, Teplick SK, Haskin ME: Granular cell myoblastoma of the lung. *Am J Roentgenol* 1975; 125:890–894.

603. Theros EG: RPC of the month from the AFIP. *Radiology* 1969; 92:1557–1561.

604. Theros EG: RPC of the month from the AFIP. *Radiology* 1969; 93:677–681.

605. Theros EG: Varying manifestations of peripheral pulmonary neoplasms: a radiologic-pathologic correlative study. *Am J Roentgenol* 1977; 128:893–914.

606. Theros EG, Feigin DS: Pleural tumors and pulmonary tumors: differential diagnosis. *Semin Roentgenol* 1977; 12:239–247.

607. Theros EG, Reeder MM, Eckert JF: An exercise in radiologic-pathologic correlation. *Radiology* 1968; 90:784–791.

608. Thompson BH, Stanford W, Galvin JR, et al: Varied radiologic appearances of pulmonary aspergillosis. *Radiographics* 1995; 15:1273–1284.

609. Thompson MJ, Kubicka RA, Smith C: Evaluation of cardiopulmonary devices on chest radiographs: digital vs analog radiographs. *Am J Roentgenol* 1989; 153:1165–1168.

610. Thornhill BA, Kyunghee CC, Morehouse HT: Gastric duplication associated with pulmonary sequestration: CT manifestations. *Am J Roentgenol* 1982:138:1168–1171.

611. Thurlbeck WM, Müller NL: Emphysema: definition, imaging and quantification. *Am J Roentgenol* 1994; 163:1017–1025.

612. Thurlbeck WM, Simon G: Radiographic appearance of the chest in emphysema. *Am J Roentgenol* 1978; 130:429–440.

613. Timmons RG, Siegel JS, Metheny RS Jr: Fatal pulmonary hemorrhage complicating infectious mononucleosis. *Pa Med* 1971; 74:65–67.

614. Tocino IM, Miller MH, Fairfax WR: Distribution of pneumothorax in the supine and semirecumbent critically ill adult. *Am J Roentgenol* 1985; 144:901–905.

615. Triebwasser JH, Harris RE, Bryant RE, et al: Varicella pneumonia in adults. *Medicine* 1967; 46:409–423.

616. Tuddenham WJ: Glossary of terms for thoracic radiology: recommendations of the nomenclature committee of the Fleishner Society. *Am J Roentgenol* 1984; 143:509–517.

617. Unger JM, Schuchmann GG, Grossman JE, et al: Tears of the trachea and main bronchi caused by blunt trauma: radiologic findings. *Am J Roentgenol* 1989; 153:1175–1180.

618. Urban BA, Fishman EK, Goldman SM, et al: CT evaluation of amyloidosis: spectrum of disease. *Radiographics* 1993; 13:1295–1308.

619. Vanley GT, Huberman R, Lufkin RB: Atypical *Pneumocystis carinii* pneumonia in homosexual men with unusual immunodeficiency. *Am J Roentgenol* 1982; 138:1037–1041.

620. Vix VA: Radiographic manifestations of broncholithiasis. *Radiology* 1978; 128:295–299.

621. Vix VA: Roentgenographic manifestations of pleural disease. *Semin Roentgenol* 1977; 12:177–286.

622. Wadsworth DT, Siegel MJ, Day DL: Wegener's granulomatosis in children: chest radiographic manifestations. *Am J Roentgenol* 1994; 163:901–904.

623. Wagenvoort CA, Wagenvoort N: Primary pulmonary hypertension: a pathologic study of the lung vessels in 156 clinically diagnosed cases. *Circulation* 1970; 42:1163–1184.

624. Wagner RB, Crawford WO, Schmipf PP: Classification of parenchymal injuries of the lung. *Radiology* 1988; 167:77–82.

625. Wallace LS, Robinson AE: Unusual radiological manifestations of acquired pulmonary cysts in children. *JAMA* 1982; 248:85–87.

626. Walter JF, Rottenberg RW, Cannon WB, et al: Giant mediastinal lymph node hyperplasia (Castleman's disease):angiographic and clinical features. *Am J Roentgenol* 1978; 130:447–450.

627. Watts DM, Jones GP, Bowman GA, et al: Giant benign mesothelioma. *Ann Thorac Surg* 1989; 48:590–591.

628. Webb WR: Magnetic resonance imaging of the chest. *Curr Opin Radiol* 1989; 1:40–43.

629. Webb WR: Radiologic evaluation of the solitary pulmonary nodule. *Am J Roentgenol* 1990; 154:701–708.

630. Webb WR, Gamsu G: Cavitary pulmonary nodules with systemic lupus erythematosus: differential diagnosis. *Am J Roentgenol* 1981; 136:27–31.

631. Webb WR, Gatsonis C, Zerhouna EA, et al: CT and MR imaging in staging non–small cell bronchogenic carcinoma: report of the Radiologic Diagnostic Oncology Group. *Radiology* 1991; 178:705–713.

632. Webb WR, Müller NL, Naidich DP: Standardized terms for high-resolution computed tomography of the lung: a proposed glossary. *J Thorac Imaging* 1993; 8(3):167–175.

633. Webb WR, Sagel SS: Actinomycosis involving the chest wall: CT findings. *Am J Roentgenol* 1982; 139:1007–1009.

634. Weber WN, Margolin FE, Nielson SL: Pulmonary histiocytosis X. *Am J Roentgenol* 1969; 107:280–289.

635. Weick JK, Kiely JM, Harrison EG Jr, et al: Pleural effusion in lymphoma. *Cancer* 1973; 31:848–853.

636. Weisbrod GL, Chamberlain D, Herman SJ: Cystic change (pseudocavitation) associated with bronchioloalveolar carcinoma: a report of four patients. *J Thorac Imaging* 1995; 10(2):106–111.

637. Weisbrod GL, Todd TR: Congenital left superior vena cava with absent right superior vena cava: a cause of progressive mediastinal widening. *J Can Assoc Radiol* 1985; 36:155–157.

638. Weisbrod GL, Towers MJ, Chamberlain DW, et al. Thin-walled cystic lesions in bronchioalveolar carcinoma. *Radiology* 1992; 185:401–405.

639. Wellner LJ, Putnam CE: Imaging of occult pulmonary metastases: state of the art. *Cancer* 1986; 36:48–58.

640. Westcott JL, Volpe JP: Peripheral bronchopleural fistula: CT evaluation in 20 patients with pneumonia, empyema, or postoperative air leak. *Radiology* 1995; 196:175–181.

641. Wexler HA, Dapena MV: Congenital cystic adenomatoid malformation. *Radiology* 1978; 126:737–741.

642. Whalen JP, Lane EJ Jr: Bronchial rearrangements in pulmonary collapse as seen on the lateral radiograph. *Radiology* 1969; 93:285–288.

643. Whitcomb ME, Schwartz MI: Pleural effusion complicating intensive mediastinal radiation therapy. *Am Rev Respir Dis* 1971; 103:100–107.

644. Wiedemann HP, Matthay RA: Pulmonary manifestations of systemic lupus erythematosus. *J Thorac Imaging* 1992; 7(2):1–18.

645. Wieder S, Rabinowitz JG: Fibrous mediastinitis: a late manifestation of mediastinal histoplasmosis. *Radiology* 1977; 125:305–312.

646. Wieder S, White TJ III, Salazar J: Pulmonary artery occlusion due to histoplasmosis. *Am J Roentgenol* 1982; 138:243–251.

647. Wilen SB, Rabinowitz JG, Ulreich S, et al: Pleural involvement in sarcoidosis. *Am J Med* 1974; 57:200–209.

648. Williams JL, Moller GA: Solitary mass in the lungs of coal miners. *Am J Roentgenol* 1973; 117:765–770.

649. Williams JR, Wilcox WC: Pulmonary embolism. *Am J Roentgenol* 1963; 89:333–342.

650. Williams NS, Lewis CT: Bronchopleural fistula: a review of 86 cases. *Br J Surg* 1976; 63:520–522.

651. Wilson ES: Pleuropulmonary amebiasis. *Am J Roentgenol* 1971; 111:518–524.

652. Wimbish KJ, Agha FP, Brady TM: Bilateral pulmonary sequestration: computed tomographic appearance. *Am J Roentgenol* 1983; 140:689–690.

653. Winer-Muram HT, Rubin SA: Thoracic complications of tuberculosis. *J Thorac Imaging* 1990; 5:46–63.

654. Winterbauer RH, Belic N, Moores KD: A clinical interpretation of bilateral hilar adenopathy. *Ann Intern Med* 1973; 78:65–71.

655. Winterbauer RH, Riggins RCK, Griesman FA, et al: Pleuropulmonary manifestations of Waldenstrom's macroglobulinemia. *Chest* 1974; 66:368–375.

656. Wiot JF, Spitz HB: Atypical pulmonary tuberculosis. *Radiol Clin North Am* 1973; 11:191–196.

657. Wolson AH: Pulmonary findings in Gaucher's disease. *Am J Roentgenol* 1975; 123:712–715.

658. Wolson AH, Rohwedder JJ: Upper lobe fibrosis in ankylosing spondylitis. *Am J Roentgenol* 1975; 124:466–471.

659. Wong JSL, Weisbrod GL, Chamberlain D, et al: Bronchioloalveolar carcinoma and the air bronchogram sign: a new pathologic explanation. *J Thorac Imaging* 1994; 9(3):141–144.

660. Wood BP, Anderson VM, Mauk JE, et al: Pulmonary lymphatic air: locating "pulmonary interstitial emphysema" of the premature infant. *Am J Roentgenol* 1982; 138:809–814.

661. Woodring JH: Determining the cause of pulmonary atelectasis: a comparison of plain radiography and CT. *Am J Roentgenol* 1988; 150:757–763.

662. Woodring JH: Pitfalls in the radiologic diagnosis of lung cancer. *Am J Roentgenol* 1990; 154:1165–1175.

663. Woodring JH, Fried AM, Chuang VP: Solitary cavities of the lung: diagnostic implications of cavity wall thickness. *Am J Roentgenol* 1980; 135:1269–1271.

664. Woodring JH, Halfhill H II, Reed JC: Pulmonary strongyloidiasis: clinical and imaging features. *Am J Roentgenol* 1994; 162:537–542.

665. Woodring JH, Howard TA, Kanga JF: Congenital pulmonary venolobar syndrome revisited. *Radiographics* 1994; 14:349–369.

666. Woodring JH, King JG: Determination of normal transverse mediastinal width and mediastinal-width to chest-width (M/C) ratio in control subjects: implications for subjects with aortic or brachiocephalic arterial injury. *J Trauma* 1989; 29:1268–1272.

667. Woodring JH, Rhodes RA III: Posterosuperior mediastinal widening in aortic coarctation. *Am J Roentgenol* 1985; 144:23–25.

668. Worsley DF, Alavi A, Aronchick JM, et al: Chest radiographic findings in patients with acute pulmonary embolism: observations from the PIOPED study. *Radiology* 1993; 189:133–136.

669. Young LW, Smith DI, Glasgow LA: Pneumonia of atypical measles. *Am J Roentgenol* 1970; 110:439–448.
670. Young R, Pochaczevsky R, Pollak L, et al: Cervico-mediastinal thymic cysts. *Am J Roentgenol* 1973; 117:855–860.
671. Zagoria RJ, Choplin RH, Karstaedt N: Pulmonary gangrene as a complication of mucormycosis. *Am J Roentgenol* 1985; 114:1195–1196.
672. Zapol WM, Trelstad RL, Coffey JW, et al: Pulmonary fibrosis in severe acute respiratory failure. *Am Rev Respir Dis* 1979; 119:547–554.
673. Zeit RM, Constantin C, Lippmann M: Compression of pulmonary artery by aortic aneurysm. *JAMA* 1981; 246:1586–1587.
674. Zelefksy MN, Lutzker LG: The target sign: a new radiologic sign of septic pulmonary emboli. *Am J Roentgenol* 1977; 129:453–455.
675. Zerhouni EA, Stitik FP, Siegelman SS, et al: CT of the pulmonary nodule: a cooperative study. *Radiology* 1986; 160:319–327.
676. Ziskind MM, George RB, Weill H: Acute localized and diffuse alveolar pneumonias. *Semin Roentgenol* 1967; 2:49–60.
677. Ziter FMH Jr, Westcott JL: Supine subpulmonary pneumothorax. *Am J Roentgenol* 1981; 137:699–701.
678. Zwiebel BR, Austin JHM, Grimes MM: Bronchial carcinoid tumors: assessment with CT of location and intratumoral calcification in 31 patients. *Radiology* 1991; 179:483–486.
679. Zwirewich CV, Vedal S, Miller RR, et al: Solitary pulmonary nodule: high-resolution CT and radiologic-pathologic correlation. *Radiology* 1991; 179:469–476.
680. Zyroff J, Slovis TL, Nagler J: Pulmonary edema induced by oral methadone. *Radiology* 1974; 112:567–568.

INDEX

Italics indicate figures; *t* indicates tabular material.

A

Abdominal diseases
  and elevated diaphragm, 75
  in evaluation of pleural effusion, *44, 52–53*
Abscess
  lung, 423
  paraspinous, 168
  pulmonary, 342
  subphrenic, and elevated diaphragm, 75
Acinar opacities, 229
Acinar rosettes, 238, 282
Actinomycosis, chest wall, 9
Adenocarcinomas, 27, 29
  calcification in, 337, *349*
Adenopathy
  AIDS-related, 133, *139*
  as cause of middle mediastinal
    masses, *137*
  hilar, *148,* 153, *160, chart 298,* 301,
    302–303
    in atelectasis, 191
    bilateral, 154–155, *155*
    fine reticular opacities in, *chart 298,*
      301, 302–303
    in sarcoidosis, 131–132, 320
    and segmental and lobar
      opacities, 218
    unilateral, 153–154, *161*
  mediastinal, in usual interstitial
    pneumonia, 321
Adhesive atelectasis, *207*
  in hyaline membrane disease, 189, 194
  in pulmonary embolism, 194–195
Adult respiratory distress syndrome,
  232–233, *240*
Agammaglobulinemia, as cause of cystic
  bronchiectasis, 421
Age
  in differential diagnosis of posterior
    mediastinal masses, 168
  as parameter in diagnosing pulmonary
    nodule, 342
AIDS-related adenopathy, 133, *139*
AIDS-related diseases, 236
  and multifocal ill-defined opacities,
    263–265
Aids-related lucent lesions, 423, *429, 430, 431*
Air alveologram, 229
Air bronchograms, *227,* 229
Air trapping, as cause of hyperlucent lung,
  379–380

Airway obstruction
  as cause of atelectasis, 189
  and noncardiac pulmonary edema,
    232, *239*
Allergic alveolitis, fine nodules in, 283
Allergic bronchopulmonary
  aspergillosis, 422
Alveolar edema, 49
Alveolar proteinosis, and air-space
  consolidation, 238, *247*
Alveolitis
  allergic, fine nodules in, 283
  fibrosing, 262
Amebiasis, 259
Amiodarone, course reticular interstitial
  pattern associated with
  hypersentivity to, 318
Amyloidosis, 304–305
Amyloid tumor, biopsy in diagnosing, 190
Aneurysm
  mediastinal mass due to, 113,
    133, *140*
  and posterior mediastinal mass, *177, 178*
Angioblastic lymphadenopathy, 261
Angiography, in diagnosis of
  aneurysm, 113
Aorta
  dissection of, 95–96
  transection of, 96
Apical pleural "capping," 63
Aplastic anemia, association with
  thymomas, 110
Arteriovenous fistulas, spontaneous
  occurrence of, 342
Arteriovenous malformation (AVM), shape
  of, 342
Arthritis. *See* Rheumatoid arthritis
Asbestos exposure, 63
  association with lung cancer, 27–28
  as cause of pleural calcifications, *60,*
    64, *71*
Asbestosis, radiologic pattern of, 303
Asbestos-related plaques, 28, 63, *68*
Aspergillosis, *270*
  allergic bronchopulmonary, 422
  chest wall, 9
Aspergillus
  and diffuse air-space disease, 236
  in pulmonary gangrene, 396
Aspiration pneumonia, 235
  and segmental and lobar opacities, 216
Atelectasis, *185, 186, chart 187,* 188–189
  adhesive, *207*
    in hyaline membrane disease, 189, 194
    in pulmonary embolism, 194–195